Official Journal of the International Society of L
Official Journal of European Digestive Surgery (EDS)

Digestive Surgery

KARGER

Printed in Switzerland
on acid-free paper by
Reinhardt Druck, Basel

Appears bimonthly:
1 volume per year
(6 issues)

Guidelines for Authors

Digestive Surgery

Submission

Only original papers written in English are considered and should be sent to:

Prof. Dr. M.W. Büchler
Department of Visceral and Transplantation Surgery
University of Bern
Inselspital
CH–3010 Bern (Switzerland)

or

Prof. Dr. E.H. Farthmann
Department of Surgery
University of Freiburg
Hugstetter Strasse 55
D–79106 Freiburg (Germany)

Manuscripts should be submitted in quadruplicate (with four sets of illustrations of which one is an original), typewritten double-spaced on one side of the paper, with a wide margin.

Conditions

All manuscripts are subject to editorial review. Manuscripts are received with the explicit understanding that they are not under simultaneous consideration by any other publication. Submission of an article for publication implies the transfer of the copyright from the author to the publisher upon acceptance. Accepted papers become the permanent property of 'Digestive Surgery' and may not be reproduced by any means, in whole or in part, without the written consent of the publisher. It is the author's responsibility to obtain permission to reproduce illustrations, tables, etc. from other publications.

The journal consists of the following sections:

1. Editorials
2. Review Articles
* 3. How I Do It
4. Original Papers
5. Case Reports
6. Announcements

Special Requirements

1. Investigations Involving Human Subjects: 'Digestive Surgery' requires that investigations performed on human subjects have the prior approval of the institutional committee on human experimentation. Authors are required to submit a signed statement as to the date and details of the appropriate review. In countries where such mechanisms for approval do not exist, authors are required to submit a signed declaration that the research was carried out in accordance with the Helsinki Declaration. A similar assurance is required to document that animal experimentation was performed under appropriate circumstances.

2. Statement for Authors Submitting Original Research or Case Reports: 'The enclosed manuscript ... (Title)... has been approved by me as well as by the responsible authorities at the institute where the work has been carried out.

I certify that none of the material in this manuscript has been published previously in any form and that none of this material is currently under consideration for publication elsewhere. This includes symposia and proceedings of meetings and preliminary publications of any kind except an abstract of 400 words or less.'

(To be signed by *all* authors)

3. The undersigned also confirm that they qualify for (co-) authorship according to the 'Uniform Requirements for Manuscripts' published in the guidelines of the 'International Committee of Medical Journal Editors' in 1988 as follows: Authorship credit should be based only on substantial contributions to (a) conception and design, or analysis and interpretation of data; (b) drafting the article or revising it critically for important intellectual content; and on (c) final approval of the version to be published. Conditions (a), (b), and (c) must all be met. Participation solely in the acquisition of funding or the collection of data does not justify authorship. General supervision of the research group is also not sufficient for authorship. Any part of an article critical to its main conclusions must be the responsibility of at least one author. Persons who have contributed intellectually to the article but whose contributions do not justify authorship may be named and their particular contribution described in the section 'Acknowledgements'. Such persons must give their permission to be named.

Arrangement

Title page: The first page of each paper should indicate the title (main title underlined), the authors' names, and the institute where the work was conducted. A short title for use as running head as well as the full address of the author to whom correspondence should be sent are also required.

Full address: The exact postal address complete with postal code must be given at the bottom of the title page. Please also supply phone and fax numbers, as well as your e-mail address.

Key words: For indexing purposes, a list of 3–10 key words in English is essential.

Abstract: Each paper needs an abstract of up to 200 words. It should be organized as follows:

Background/Aims:	What is the major problem that prompted the study?
Methods:	How was the study done?
Results:	Most important findings?
Conclusion:	Most important conclusion?

Small type: Paragraphs which can or must be set in smaller type (case histories, test methods, etc.) should be indicated with a 'p' (petit) in the margin on the left-hand side.

Footnotes: Avoid footnotes. When essential, they are numbered consecutively and typed at the foot of the appropriate page.

Tables and illustrations: Tables and illustrations (both numbered in Arabic numerals) should be prepared on separate sheets. Tables require a heading and figures a legend, also prepared on a separate sheet. For the reproduction of illustrations, good drawings and original photographs are preferred; slides may also be accepted; negatives or photocopies cannot be used. Due to technical reasons, figures with a screen background should not be submitted. When possible, group several illustrations on one block for reproduction (max. size 181 × 223 mm) or provide crop marks. On the back of each illustration, indicate its number, the author's name, and 'top' with a soft pencil.

Color illustrations: Up to 6 color illustrations per page can be integrated with the text at the reduced price of CHF 660.– / USD 545.00 per page. Color illustrations are reproduced at the author's expense.

References: In the text identify references by Arabic numerals [in square brackets]. Material submitted for publication but not yet accepted should be noted as 'unpublished data' and not be included in the reference list. The list of references should include only those publications which are cited in the text. Do not alphabetize; number references in the order in which they are first mentioned in the text. The surnames of the authors followed by initials should be given. There should be no punctuation other than a comma to separate the authors. Cite all authors, 'et al' is not sufficient. Abbreviate journal names according to the Index Medicus system. (Also see International Committee of Medical Journal Editors: Uniform requirements for manuscripts submitted to biomedical journals. Br Med J 1988;296:401–405.)

Examples

(a) Papers published in periodicals: Sun J, Koto H, Chung KF: Interaction of ozone and allergen challenges on bronchial responsiveness and inflammation in sensitised guinea pigs. Int Arch Allergy Immunol 1997;112:191–195.

(b) Monographs: Matthews DE, Farewell VT: Using and Understanding Medical Statistics, ed 3, revised. Basel, Karger, 1996.

(c) Edited books: Parren PWHI, Burton DR: Antibodies against HIV-1 from phage display libraries: Mapping of an immune response and progress towards antiviral immunotherapy; in Capra JD (ed): Antibody Engineering. Chem Immunol. Basel, Karger, 1997, vol 65, pp 18–56.

Galley proofs

Unless indicated otherwise, galley proofs are sent to the first-named author and should be returned with the least possible delay. Alterations made in galley proofs, other than the correction of printer's errors, are charged to the author. No page proofs are supplied.

Reprints

Order forms and a price list are sent with the galley proofs. Orders submitted after the issue is printed are subject to considerably higher prices.

* How I Do It

Digestive Surgery is publishing articles which describe modern operative techniques in the field of Gastrointestinal Surgery.

The manuscript should be short and precise (maximum 10 typewritten double spaced pages) and should contain 1–4 figures to explain the surgical procedure.

Decisions of submitted papers within 6 weeks: A decision will be reached within 6 weeks for manuscripts submitted to the 'How I Do It' section.

KARGER

Fax +41 61 306 12 34
E-Mail karger@karger.ch
www.karger.com

The Guidelines for Authors are available at:
www.karger.com/journals/dsu/dsu_gl.htm

Digestive Surgery

General Information

Publication data: 'Digestive Surgery' is published 6 times a year. Volume 16 with 6 issues appears in 1999.

Subscription rates: Subscriptions run for a full calendar year. Prices are given per volume.

Personal subscription:
Subscription + postage and handling
CHF 259.05 + CHF 23.50 Europe
CHF 259.05 + CHF 35.50 Overseas
USD 198.00 + USD 23.50
(Must be in the name of, billed to, and paid by an individual. Order must be marked 'personal subscription'.)

Institutional subscription:
Subscription + postage and handling
CHF 925.– + CHF 29.40 Europe
CHF 925.– + CHF 44.40 Overseas
USD 707.00 + USD 29.40

Airmail postage: CHF 36.–, USD 30.00.
(Extra per volume.)

Discount subscription price:
European Digestive Surgery (EDS)
Collegium Internationale Chirurgiae Digestivae (CICD)

Microforms: Please direct all enquiries and orders to: University Microfilms Inc.
300 North Zeeb Road, P.O. Box 1346
Ann Arbor, MI 48106-1346 (USA)

Subscription orders: Orders can be placed at agencies, bookstores, directly with the Publisher
S. Karger AG, P.O. Box,
CH–4009 Basel (Switzerland)
or with any of the following distributors:
Deutschland: S. Karger GmbH, Postfach
D–79095 Freiburg
France: Librairie Luginbühl
36, bd de Latour-Maubourg, F–75007 Paris
Great Britain, Ireland: S. Karger Publishers
58 Grove Hill Road
Tunbridge Wells, Kent TN1 1SP
USA: S. Karger Publishers, Inc.
26 West Avon Road, P.O. Box 529
Farmington, CT 06085
India, Bangladesh, Sri Lanka:
S. Karger India Subscription Agency
B–5/132 Safdarjung Enclave
New Delhi-110029
Japan: Katakura Libri, Inc.
2F, Marushima Bldg, 4-6-17, Yushima,
Bunkyo-ku, Tokyo 113-0034

Change of address: Both old and new address should be sent to the subscription source.

Single issues and back volumes: Information can be obtained through the Publisher.

Advertising: Correspondence and rate requests should be addressed to the Publisher.

Bibliographic indices: This journal is regularly listed in bibliographic services, including *Current Contents®*.

Book Reviews: Books are accepted for review by special agreement.

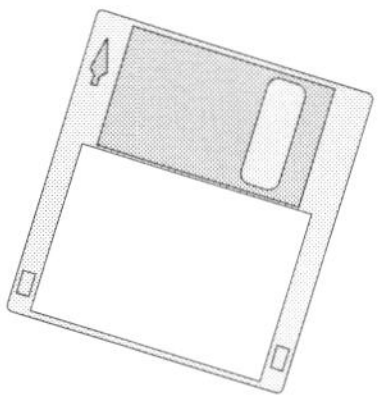

Disk Submission

A **comprehensive version** of these guidelines for the **submission of manuscripts and illustrations on disk** can be accessed online under **www.karger.com/journals/disksub.htm** or requested as a leaflet from the editorial department.

Please follow the general rules on style and arrangement in the **"Guidelines for Authors"** of the journal. Submit a **double-spaced printout** of your manuscript matching the file on disk exactly.

Technical Information

Store only data pertinent to this manuscript. Include your fonts (screen and printer fonts for Macintosh). For a **text only** manuscript, use a 3.5 inch disk. For **text and illustrations,** use 3.5 or 5.25 Magneto Optical Disc; CD-ROM (DOS or hybrid); iomage Zip/DOS (100 MB), or 44 MB, 88 MB or 200 MB SyQuest. Compress extensive data using ZIP format.

Data Description

Label your disk with the **title of the journal or book** for which it is submitted; a **short version** of the paper's title; your **name,** postal and e-mail address, fax and phone number; **hard and software** used, including the version; and the **complete list of the file names.** File names consist of eight characters before the dot identifying the file and three characters after the dot identifying the application.

Text and Format

The **preferred word-processing package is MS-Word.** Other commonly used PC text programs and ASCII formats are accepted.
Update your data when you revise subsequent to the reviewer's or editor's decision and mark revisions clearly. Manuscripts accepted for publication are subject to **copy editing:** changes and/or questions will be marked in the manuscript, which will be returned to you with your disk and the galley proofs for checking.
Enter your text continuously flush left. Do not use any layout functions. Do not split words at the end of a line. **Do not use indentations.** Use a blank line before and a hard return at the end of paragraphs.
Arrange headings flush left. Insert only **one space after punctuation marks.** Insert Greek letters, mathematical symbols etc. with your word-processing program. Use **boldface and italics** as well as sub- and superscript where appropriate.
Tables are part of the text and should be placed at the end of the text file. Separate the individual parts of a table by lines. Use the tabulator instead of spaces. Format operation data on one line in the same column. **Legends to illustrations are part of the text** and should also be listed at the end of the text file.

Illustrations

Store illustrations as separate files: do not embed them in your text. Export **line drawings/vector graphics** as TIF, EPS or WMF format. Use Photoshop for processing and retouching **scanned halftone images.** Save the original scan and the processed version. Export **black and white or color images** as TIF or EPS format in their anticipated size in print. **For detailed information** on how to submit illustration data on disk please consult the leaflet or **www.karger.com/journals/disksub.htm.**

Fax + 41 61 306 12 34
E-Mail karger@karger.ch
www.karger.com

The Journal Home Page is available at:
www.karger.com/journals/dsu

Dig Surg 1999; 16 (suppl 1): 5-7

Portal hypertension

0,01

MESOATRIAL SHUNT FOR THE TREATMENT OF BUDD-CHIARI SYNDROME

A.Emre, G.Kalaycı, O.Bilge, I.Özden, K.Acarlı, Y.Tekant, A.Ökten[1], A.Alper, O.Arıoğul
Istanbul Faculty of Medicine, Depts of General Surgery and Gastroenterology[1], Istanbul, Turkey

Shunt operations are the preferred treatment modality in acute and subacute Budd-Chiari Syndrome. However, the mesoatrial shunt using a long synthetic graft is under debate due to its risk of thrombosis. Patients undergoing this type of operation were reviewed to determine its efficacy and long term effectiveness.

Between January 1993 - 98, 12 patients with the Budd-Chiari Syndrome were treated with a mesoatrial shunt at the HPB Surgery Unit of the Istanbul Faculty of Medicine in Istanbul, Turkey. Nine patients were females and three were males with a mean age of 32 years (17-43). The median time to operation from the beginning of symptoms was three months (one month – 10 years). Ascites and hepatomegaly was found in all the patients, while pain in the right hypochondrium was present in 40% and jaundice in 25% of the patients. According to the Bismuth classification, one patient was in the acute stage of the disease, while 10 were in the subacute and one in the chronic stage. All the patients had caudate lobe hypertrophy, and three had additional thrombosis of the inferior vena cava (IVC). The remaining nine patients had severe stenosis of the IVC due to extrensic compression. The infra and suprahepatic IVC pressures were measured in all the patients as well as peroperative measurement of the superior mesenteric vein. Fourteen and/or 16 mm ringed PTFE grafts were used for the mesoatrial shunts. Mean pre-shunt pressures were 445 mmH2O (320-550), while it dropped to a mean of 200 mmH2O (110-270) after shunting. Postoperative shunt patencies were assessed by Doppler ultrasound or angiography. Two patients died in the early postoperative period. They had no thrombosis at their grafts. At a median follow-up period of three years (two months - six years), only one patient developed shunt thrombosis one year after the operation. All the remaining nine patients are well and healthy.

In conclusion, the mesoatrial shunt using a long synthetic graft is an effective option in the treatment of the Budd-Chiari Syndrome.

KARGER
Fax +41 61 306 12 34
E-Mail karger@karger.ch
www.karger.com

0,02

NATURAL VERSUS SYNTHETIC TISSUE ADHESIVES ENDOSCOPIC TREATMENT OF BLEEDING GASTRIC VARICES

El-Sefi T.[1], Saleh A.,[2] and Rashed M.Y.T.[3]

Surgical department[1], Medical department, Liver Institute, Menoufiya University[2], Medical department (HPB unit)[3]

Aims: To compare the efficacy and safety of natural (fibrin sealant) versus (N-butyl-2-cyanoacrylate) tissue adhesives in the management of bleeding gastric fundal varices.
Methods: 47 patients with bleeding large gastric fundal varices were randomly allocated to emergeny endoscopic intravariceal injections with either fibrin sealant „subsequent technique" (Gp. I, n=24) or N-butyl-2-Cyanoacrylate (GP.II, n=2). The incidence of procedure related complications and rebleeding within 4 weeks from the index bleeding were analyzed.
Results: Immediate control of bleeding was achieved in 96% in Gp. I. and 87% in Fp. II. Compications in Gp. I. included fevere of short duration in 9, post injection abdominal pain of mild severity in fifteen patients. Re-bleeding didn't occur after successful fibrin sealant therapy. Complications in Gp. II included: post-injection ulcers in all, from which re-bleeding occurred in 35 %. Distant embolisation in 2 patients (mesenteric venous occlusion in one, and left renal, I.V.C., and portal vein in the second), Malignant hyperthermia in 2, and stenosis of the cardia in one patient. In both groups, there were no complications relatd to activation of systematic coagulation fibrinolysis.
Conclusions: Fibrin sealant therapy is an efficient and safe agent for endoscopic management of bleeding gastric fundal varices.

0,03

ENDOSCOPIC EMBOLIZATION WITH FIBRIN GLUE FOR THE PREVENTION OF FIRST AND RECURRENT VARICEAL BLEEDING. SHORT AND LONG-TERM RESULTS.

Mishin I V
Department of Surgery III "N.Anestiadi",
Medical University "N.Testemitsanu", Kishinev, Republic Moldova.

Aims: The aim of this study was to evaluate the efficiency of fibrin glue (FG) as an injectate agent for endoscopic embolization (EE) of esophageal varices (EV).
Methods: From March 1995 to June 1997, twenty seven consecutive patients (18 males and 9 females; mean age, 46.1±2.4 yr) were selected for a study on EE of EV using FG, at the Department of Surgery, Hospital "St. Treime". The origin of portal hypertension was posthepatic (HBV and/or HCV) liver cirrhosis. Severity of liver disease was classified according to the Child-Pugh classification: class A/B/C-4/14/9, the mean score on admission was 8.96±0.4.
Prophylactic EE (1gr) was performed in 15 pts with high-risk EV(F2 or F3, RC sign ++ or +++) according selection criteria JRSPH(1991)and EE for prophylactic of recurrent variceal bleeding in 12 pts. An absolute criteria for exclusion was: pts who had already been treated endoscopically for EV.
FG was prepared *ex tempore*: fibrinogen(30mg/ml), thrombin (150-300units/ml), CaCl2(40mM/ml), aprotinin (3.000 KIU/ml). EE was carried out with a flexible endoscope and an original or commercial injectors by intravariceal or combined injections of FG. EE was repeated once a week until all EV has been eradicated.
Results: Characteristics of EE with FG were: total sessions in both gr.-33, total volume of sclerosant-6.6±0.5(3-11)ml, volume of FG per single varix - 3.1±0.2(2-6)ml. Only minor complications (fever, chest pains) were observed in 4(14.8%). Ulcer formation, esophageal stenosis and perforation did not occur. The therapeutic end point (Cw-Th,RC-) in both groups was achieved in all patients with a lower mean number of sessions 1.2(range 1-3). Changes in the selected hemostasis parameters were not essential, clinically there were no detectable thrombotic or hemorrhagic complications. Mean duration of follow-up was 25.6±2.4(1-44)months, during this period 9 pts died (6-hepatic failure and 3-bleeding from acute gastric and duodenal lesions).
Conclusions: This study shows that FG is an efficient and safe agent for EE of EV. However, studies in lager series and prospective randomized trials comparing FG with other sclerosant agents (inc. thrombin) are still needed before a final conclusion can be reached.

0,04

ENDOLOOP VERSUS BAND LIGATION FOR ENDOSCOPIC CONTROL OF ACUTE ESOPHAGEAL VARICEAL BLEEDING

A double blind controlled study

Rashed MYT[1], El-Sefi T[2], Boghdadi I.[3]
[1]Alexandria University HPB Unit., [2]Liver Institute, and [3]Faculty of Medicine, Menoufiya University, Egypt.

Varieceal band ligation (VBL) was developed in an attempt ot provide a treatment equivalent in efficady to schlerotherapy but with fewer local and systemic complications.

Aims: To compare emergency endoscopic band ligation versus endoscop liction.

Methods: 52 patients with acute esocpageal variceal bleeding randomized to emergency endoscopic variceal ligation using either „o" ring rubber band (GI, n=26). Incidence of various complications, failures, technical problems was analyzed.

Results: Succesful immediate control of bleeding was achieved in 69,2% in Gp I and 96% in Gp II. No major complications related to both techniques were reported. Failure in Gp. I. was due to slipping of the „O" ring. In G II. failure as due to disruption of the plastic stopper due to excessive traction on the loop. All cases of failure were converted to sclerotherapy. Average no. of rings used was 2 to 4 compared to one endoloop for each patient. Rings or endoloops were applied directly to the bleeding site. Recurrence of bleeding within 4 weeks of the index bleeding was 19% in GP I. No recurrence of bleeding in Gp. II. Postligation ulcers in both groups were comparable as regards the endoscopis appearances. Re-bleeding was more common in cases of large Varices due to partial ligation in G I. Field of vision was more clear during endoloop application. No strain was demonstrated on the endoscope during endoloop ligation. Tightening of the endoloop was an advantage in Gp. II.

Conclusions: Emergency esophasgeal ligation using endoloop technique is more effective, with less complications and technical problems.

0,05

COLOR DOPPLER SONOGRAPHY IN DETECTION OF PORTAL HYPERTENSION.

Szántová, M.
3rd Department of Medicine, Medical School of Comenius University, Bratislava, Slovakia.

Aims : The evaluation of portal hemodynamics in healthy (control group - CG) and patients with benign hyperbilirubinemia (BH), fatty liver (FL), chronic hepatitis (CHH) and cirrhosis (Ci).

Methods and Materials : The group of 262 persons (209 patients and 53 healthy controls) were examinated . Toshiba Sonolayer SSA 270 with 3.75 Mhz linear probe was used . The following ultrasonographic parameters were determinated : portal vein diameter (PVD), thickness of the gallbladder (GWT), maximal splenic diameter (SD), presence of ascites, hepatic artery diameter (HAD), maximal , minimal , peak (PFV) and mean flow velocity (MFV) in the portal vein, character and direction of the portal vein flow, presence of the spontaneous portosystemic shunts.

Results : SD enables to differentiate the healthy from the patients with FL, CHH or Ci. PVD is sensitive parameter for differentiation of patients with Ci from patients with FL, BH and healthy . Statistically significant reduction of portal vein flow was found in the course : CG – FL – Ci ($p \leq 0,05$) . GWT allows the group of Ci from all other groups to distinguish . All US parameters above mentioned allowed more sensitively degree of portal hypertension as Child-Pugh score to recognize . Patients with history of esophageal bleeding had higher degree of portal hypertension in comparision to the patients without bleeding. There was found correlation between PFV and MFV. Significant correlation of MFV with Child- Pugh score was found at a 5% level of significance. Significant coorelation of MFV and degree of esofageal varices by Paquet was found at a 9 % level of significance. Dilation of HAD in patients with Ci was found . All groups were comparible by the age and BMI with exception of group of BH and group with FL .

Conclusion : Using of CDU helps to differenciate the groups with FL from the group with CH, Ci and healthy . No differences between BH and control group were found . Using of PVD, SD, GWT, PFV, portosystemic shunts, presence of ascites allowed very sensitively degree of portal hypertension to recognize.

0,06

PORTAL HYPERTENSION CAUSED BY VENOUS MALFORMATIONS IN CHILDREN

Tasnádi G., Gorácz Gy
Heim Pál Hospital for Children, Budapest

Aims: The Early diagnosis of portal hypertension is important for possible therapy planning.

Methods: Beside of the known etiology of portal hypertension the congenital malformations of the hepatic, portal veins should be also considered. These venous malformations manifest mostly at the age of 2-3 years, causing syndrome. Cases:

1. Stenosis of the hepatic veins at their ostium in the inferior vena cava
2. Hypoplasia of the hepatic veins and inferior vena cava
3. Persisting ductus venous Arantii
4. MOVC /membranous obstruction of inferior vena cava/
5.,6.,7.: Portal ectasia, stenosis and cavernoma.

Results: The diagnosis at this age is very difficult, their treatment depends on the form of the malformation.

Conclusion: Early recognition of venous malformations besides the non invasive methods the angiographies are necessery, especially before surgical intervention. The therapy depends on the localisation /pre-, intra-, or posthepatic/ of the venous malformations.

0,07

SURGICAL TREATMENT IN CIRROTIC AND NONCIRRHOTIC PORTAL HIPERTENSION (HP)

Bancu Serban
Surgical Clinic No. III. TG-Mures, Romania

Aims: We present a personal series of 26 patients with PH, treated in the service between 1994-1998 there were 21 hepatic cirrhosis with variceal bleeding, 2 portal vein thrombosis with variceal bleeding and 3 Budd-Chiari syndromes.

Methods and results: 4 selective Warren shunts and 10 side-to-side portocaval Eck shunts were made for cirrhotic HP and 2 mesenterico-caval shunts in "H", with Goretex, for the portal vein thrombosis, with 1 postoperative death. For the Budd-Chiari syndrome we performed 1 portocaval, 1 mesenterico-caval and 1 iliaco-mesenterico-atrial shunt, with Dacron prothesis. 1 unsuccessful attempt of shunting was noted, 3 patients refused operation, undergoing to conservative treatment and schlerotherapy, 3 patients died in the intensive care unit, without operation. 17 operated patients had a good evolution.

0,08

CIRRHOSIS: ADSORPTIVE PURIFICATION AND REINFUSION OF ASCITIC FLUID

Chornomyz VD, Sarnatskaya VV, Sakhno LA, Maslenny VN, Yushko LA, Nikolaev VG.*
* - City surgery center of liver, bile duct and pancreas, Kiev, Ukraine
Institute of experimental pathology, oncology and radiobiology NAS of Ukraine, Kiev, Ukraine

Aims: The ascitic syndrome at liver cirrhosis is characterised by sequestration of blood proteins, first of all, of albumins in ascitic fluid (AF) which aggravates hypo- and disproteinemia at the background of suppresion of a synthetic liver function. The exfusion of AF large volumes increases the deficit of proteins and electrolytes, hypervolemia and other homeostasis disturbances, aggra-vates the state of patients and hemodynamic disorders.

Methods: Original method of ascitic fluid reinfusion has been used in a treatment of 12 liver cirrhosis cases, complicated by resistant to drug therapy ascitis. The concentrating and sorptional detoxification onto deliganding carbon adsorbents has been performed prior to a direct intravenous infusion.

Results: the toxicity of cirrhotic fluids before and after treatment was studied with tymocytes dye-exclusion test using cytotoxic (CTA) and cytolytic (CLA) activity parameters. After concentrating CTA of AF increased from 27,5 to 43,3 arb.units. Adsorptive purification resulted in 2,4 times reduction of CTA. CLA was absent in all cases. Purification of AF completely restored of ascitic albumin complexing abilities of all 5 main binding regions of protein globule. Activity of some binding centers after purification became even higher in comparison with the activity of healthy donors albumin appropriate centers reflecting complete removal not only hepatic toxins but also different protein-bound substances normally transporting by albumins. It means very effective restoration of functional activity of ascitic albumin after the purification of AF onto the deliganding synthetic activated carbons of the new generation.

Conclusions: Effective reinfusion of concentrated and purified AF contributed to further surgical correction of portal hypertension and ascitic syndrome. Additional clinical benefits are expected from lower hepatotoxicity of ascitic fluid after their adsorption treatment which should favour quick recovery of residual liver function.

0,09

THE RESULTS OF SURGICAL TREATMENT OF SECONDARY HYPERSPLENISM IN CIRRHOTICL PORTAL HIPERTENSION

V. Hotineanu, V. Cazacov, Z. Caragat
Medical University, Republic of Moldva, Chishinau

Aim: To analyze retrospective the patients with liver cirrhosis, operated for secondary hypersplenism, resistent to conservative treatment, during the period of 1990-1998 years. The study presents 52 patients, mean age 35,5 years. They were divided according to Child-Pugh classification into the following groups: A/B/C - 9/41/2 respectively.
Methods: The following surgical methods were applied: splenectomy (3), splenectomy, associated with: omentorenopexy (39), omentohepatofrenicopexy (2), azygo-portal transabdomenal deconnectation (4), omfalo-caval anastomosis (2) and splenorenal anastomosis (2).
Results: The early postoperativ period in 13 cases was difficult becouse of appearing the following complications: acute postplenectomical pancreatitis (4), left subdiafragmatical abcess (4), the trombosis of the stump of vena lienalis (5). The letality was 11.6% (n=6): acute hepatorenal unsufficiency (3), total pancreonecrosis (1), trombosis of pulmonary artery (1), ascite-peritonitis (1). The late postoperative period (6 months - 3 yeasrs) was studied in 29 patients. 22 of them had favorable postoperative period: asimptomatical clinico-biological station, absence of bleeding and ascites, temporary optimization of portal hemodinamics with decreasing in 15 cases of the varyxes.
Conclusion: Surgical treatment of this category of patients must be well organized and individual. The postoperative results depends from the livers functional station, presents of different kinds of complications, current patients station and adoptated surgical attitude.

0,10

Treatment of diuretic resistant ascites

Pirtskhalava T.L., Granov D.A.
Research Institute of Roentgenology & Radiation Therapy, St.Petersburg Medical Universiti, St.Petersburg, Russia

Aim: Treatment of diuretic resistant ascites is an old problem in hepatology and up to now it is unsolved. Complex use of the medicines that correct sweat and physiologic changes in patients with hepatic cirrhosis, opens new possibilities in treatment of the cirrhosis complications. Increase of the peripheral resistance due to the arteriolas of the skin surfaces and internal organs promotes the resorption of the tissues edema. Controlled hypertension increases the glomerular filtration with an increase of the diuresis amount .
Materials and methods: Six patients with a marked ascites were studied and treated. Diuretic therapy given for them did not result in regression of the ascites. They received intravenous Angiotenzinamid (a synthetic polypeptide medicine that is close by its structure to endogenic Angiotenzin II.) Considering initial low arterial blood pressure (at the average 90/65; 80-110/60-80 mm Hg) these patients intravenously received Angiotenzinamid in order to increase the arterial blood pressure up to 115-125/75-80 mm Hg. These blood pressure values were maintained at this level for long (6-8 hours).
Results: When in 30-40 minutes an optimal level of the arterial blood pressure was set up, the diuresis amount became higher and was increased by 2 - 2,5 (2 - 3,5) liters a day at the average . It is necessary simultaneously to give intravenously protein, cardiotonic, crystaloid medicines and microelements. The arterial blood pressure was back to the initial values after stopping to give Angiotenzinamid. In 2 - 3 days sensitivity to the diuretics was recovered and stayed as far as a complete regression of the ascites.
Conclusion: Thus the use of Angiotenzinamid enables to increase the peripheral resistance, to create the controlled hypertension and in this way conditions are made in order to introduce sequestrative liquid in the organism.

Abstracts

Dig Surg 1999; 16 (suppl 1): 8-10

Pancreas tumor I.

1.01

TUMOR MARKERS IN DETECTING AND STAGING OF PANCREATIC CARCINOMA

Vrettos M.E., Papavassiliou C., Mavroudis N., Métaxas T., Papameletiou V.

B' Propedeutical Surg. Clin. Aristotle University, Hippokration Hospital, Thessaloniki, Greece.

Aims: The aim of the study was to compare the sensitivity of various tumor markers (TM) in detecting pancreatic carcinoma preoperatively.

Methods: The last 6 years, in 131 patients, 78 male and 53 female, aged 34 – 80 years, operated for pancreatic Ca, the tumor markers CEA, CA 19-9 and CA 125 were estimated preoperatively. Additionally in 27 patients the tumor markers TPA, CA 15-3 and AFP were examined during the last 2 years.

Results: The obtained values were increased for CEA 40,45%, for CA 19-9 77,86%, for CA 125 47,11%, for TPA 85,18%, for CA 15-3 40,70% and for AFP 14,81%. Patients with resectable tumor showed lower values than those with no-resectable as follows: CA 19-9 68% to 83,95%, CEA 32% to 45,67%, CA 15-3 18,18% to 56,25% and CA 125 33,33% to 56,45%.

Conclusions: The higher the elevation of the tumor markers values the worst the prognosis. The comparison of the tested markers in pairs suggests that the combination of TPA with CA 19-9 gave the best results.

1.02

TURBULENT MESENTERICOPORTAL VENOUS FLOW IS A POOR PREDICTOR OF INVOLVEMENT BY PANCREATIC AND PERI-AMPULLARY TUMOURS

M J Midwinter, R M Charnley, S T Elliott*

HPB Surgery Unit and *Dept. of Radiology, Freeman Hospital, Newcastle upon Tyne.

Aim: To correlate the finding of turbulent mesentericoportal venous flow by Doppler ultrasound with the surgical assessment in patients with a suspected pancreatic or ampullary tumour.

Methods: Patients with clinically suspected pancreatic or ampullary tumours had ultrasound assessment including colour flow, pulsed and power Doppler of the superior mesenteric and portal vein (SMV/PV). The presence of morpholgical evidence of venous involvement (loss of tumour-vessel interface) and the presence of turbulent flow were recorded prospectively. Thirty patients underwent laparotomy and surgical assessment of the SMV/PV. Twenty patients had resections of their tumour and 10 had bypass procedures. For the SMV/PV to be declared free from involvement by the tumour, resection had to occur as only then can the whole of the SMV/PV can be inspected.

Results: Fourteen patients were found to have SMV/PV involvement by the tumour at laparotomy. The sensitivity and specificity of morphological evidence of involvement by ultrasound was 78.6% and 93.8% with positive and negative predictive values of 91.7% and 83.3% respectively. The sensitivity and specificity of turbulent flow in the SMV/PV alone as evidence of involvement by tumour was 71.4% and 62.5% with positive and negative predictive values of 62.5% and 71.4% respectively. Ultrasonographic evidence of morphological vascular involvement was significantly better than the presence of turbulent flow alone in determining SMV/PV involvement as assessed at surgery (McNemar's test for paired proportions, one tailed, χ^2 = 3.57, p<0.05).

Conclusion: Turbulent mesentericoportal venous flow as assessed by Doppler ultrasound is less reliable than morphological evidence of venous involvement by ultrasound in the assessment of SMV/PV involvement by pancreatic and peri-ampullary tumours.

1.03

STAGING AND RESULTS OF TREATMENT OF PANCREATIC CANCER

Jesipowicz M., Rudzki S., Jesipowicz J.

First Department of General and Transplant Surgery of Medical University of Lublin, Poland

Pancreatic cancer is known for its extremely poor prognosis, and is associated with the lowest 5-year survival rate of the cancer of lung, breast, colon, stomach and prostate. The aim of the present study is to analise survival after operative treatment for pancreatic cancer in relation to timing of preoperative history, tumor stage, kind of operation and adjuvant chemiotherapy.

In the years 1995-1998, 31 patients were operated on because of pancreatic cancer. 28 were confirmed histologically and 84,4% were adenocarcinomas. The median age of patients was 62,2 and ranged between 42 and 78 years old. 14 patients with stage I and II of cancer underwent curative operation. In 10 pancreatoduodenectomy m.Whipple with lymphadenectomy was performed, 4 patients underwent resection of the body and tail of the pancreas with lymph nodes and connective tissue. In 7 patients with III and IV stage of cancer gastro-jejuno (4 patients) and choledocho-duodeno (5 patients) anastomoses were performed. Adjuvant chemotherapy was carried out in 11 out of 21 patients with stage I, II or III. In 9 patients with stage IV of cancer we performed laparotomy. Because of fatigue and wasting of those patients chemiotherapy was not introduced.

Among patients who underwent curative operation 4 died at 7 (no chemiotherapy), 9, 10 (both underwent 6 month's chemiotherapy) and 14 months after operation. The last patient did not undergo chemiotherapy and died because of myocardial infarction. The other (10) patients of these group have survived between 6 to 30 months and are all in their observation period. 6 of them have survived more than 18 months , all the patients who underwent resection of the body and tail of the pancreas are in this group. 6 out of those 10 underwent adjuvant chemiotherapy. All patients who underwent bypass operation survival medium 9 weeks, in two of them chemiotherapy was carried out (stage III, death in 9 and 11 weeks after operation). Medium survival rate for patients who underwent laparotomy was 6 and half weeks.

On the basis of our material and a little bit short period of follow up, it seems, that the most important for survival rate is the site of the tumor (head or body and tail) and special attention to removal the lymph nodes and connective soft tissue with its regional drainage.

1.04

SURGICAL TREATMENT OF PANCREATIC CANCER AND PERIAMPULAR ZONE

A. A. Shalimov, V. M. Kopchak, A. I. Dronov, I. V. Khomyak
Institute of clinic & experimental surgery, Kyiv, Ukraine

Aims
Improvement of the results of surgical treatment in patients with pancreatic cancer.
Methods
There were examined and analysed results of medical treatment and operations performed 836 patients over the period from 1976 to 1997 years. We apply the following methods: pancreatoduodenal resection, subtotal pancreatoduodenal, local pancreatoduodenal, distal, widened and combined resections of pancreas. On localisation of tumor in the area of head of pancreas the Whipple's pancreatoduodenal resection had been performed. We reckon that the key moment of operation is the selection of optimal way of pancreatic stump treatment. We perform pancreaticoeunoanastomoses on external drainage of pancreatic duct providing by this the exception of intestinal content reflux. In summary from 1976 up to 1997 we performed 543 pancreatoduodenal resections with 9,8% of lethal outcome. On aroundpapillar cancer of pancreas and cancer Vater's papilla duodenum (T1N0M0) we perform as the most organsaving, down local resection of ventral segment of pancreas with the adjacent part of duodenum and its Vater's papilla. On defeating pancreatic body and tail of pancreas we perform widened subtotal leftsided resection on organ. We also mobilise distal segments of pancreas by the united block with paraortal, backpancreatic, pancreatosplenic lymphatic glancs and spleen. We execute and combined leftsided resection on pancreas at patients who have tumor on pancreatic body itself and pancreatic tail as well as the one which is growing inside the stomach, celiac trunk or its branches and also transverse-rimmed colon.
Results
Distant results of treatment of patients with cancer of pancreas, who were radically operated on, were as following: 63% of patients lived more than one year, 17% of patients lived more than 3 years, 3,6% - 5 years and over. Those patients who had cancer of periampular zone respectively: 74% of patients lived 1 year, 42% lived 3 years, and 32% lived 5 years and over.

1.05

SURGICAL TREATMENT OF PANCREATIC CANCER (Pca) – OUR TEN YEARS EXPERIENCE

R. Dobrila- Dintinjana, M. Uravić, A. Depolo, M. Rubinić, D. Kovač, N. Ivaniš, Z. Tomše
Digestive Surgery Clinic, Internal Clinic, Pathology Dept. University Hospital Rijeka, CROATIA

Aims: to obtain 10 years experience of surgical treatment for pancreatic cancer (Pca).
Methods: from 1. 01. 1988- 31. 12. 1997. 146 patients underwent operation in our Clinic because of pancreatic adenocarcinoma. The tumors were confirmed histologically. Patients with duodenal, bile duct, islet cell or ampullary carcinoma were excluded. Only 16(11%) patients underwent curative operation, exploration was done in 20(14%) patients, and paliative operations in 110(75%) patients.
Results: It was 88(60%) men and 58(40%)women, age from 26- 90 years (average 62, 5 y). Cancerous proces was localised in head of pancreas in 88(60%)of patients, in body 16(11%), head+ body 21(14%), in tail at 1(0, 7%) and in whole pancreas at 20(13, 7%) patients. Early postoperative mortality rate was 13, 7%(20 patients). No gender or age had implications on early mortality. But men had higher early mortality rate (p> 0, 01). 15 patients (10, 27%) survived over 12 months, and 6 patients (4, 11%) survived over 24 months. Significantly more men (p> 0, 01) were longer survivors, but mean surviving time is same between genders.
Conclusions: The male and female ratio of Pca was 1, 51: 1.Only 16(11%) patients received curative operation. The average time for 50% survival of patients who received operation was longer than supportive treatment. There was not significant diference between the survival time of the patients with Pca of head, body, tail and whole gland. One year surviving rate was 10, 27%(15 patients), and 6 patients(4, 11%) are long survivcrs (over 24 months). The most longer surviving has man, now 72 years old, who had tumor of pancreatic body, and after hemipancreatectomy and splenectomy is still living (65 months).

1.06

RESULTS OF DIFFERENT SURGICAL METHODS OF PANCREATIC HEAD AND PERIAMPULLARY TUMORS

Kovács I., Tóth P., Árkossy P., Veres L., Sápy P.
2nd Department of Surgery, University Medical School of Debrecen, Hungary

Aims: The surgical treatment of the tumors of the head of pancreas and the periampullary tumors are the same, nevertheless the pathological behaviour of the two groups of tumors are different. The aim of this study was the comparison of operative outcome, nutritional recovery and survival of patients who underwent standard Whipple pancreatoduodenectomy(WP), pylorus-preserving pancreatoduodenectomy(PPPD) and palliative therapy of these tumors.
Methods: In the period from Jan. 1992 to 1998 we observed 76 patients with tumor located in the head of pancreas and 26 patients with periampullary tumors. These included 19 tumors originated from the ampulla of Vater and 7 from the distal common bile duct. Symptomatic pancreas tumors were generally diagnosed by transabdominal ultrasonography, computer tomography and ERCP. Facultative angiography, video-laparoscopy in combination with sonography and peritoneal lavage are providing important information about the spread of the tumor to archive satisfactory palliation endoscopically or surgically. Tumor markers such as CEA, CA 19-9 and CA 125 were also studied.
Results: The operability rate was 20(26%) in pancreatic head tumors and 16(69%) in periampullary tumors. Considering the 36 resections: 11 WP, 20 PPPD and 5 cases of local excision for tumor of ampulla. The mortality rate was 2(7%). We found that elevated serum level of CA 19-9 is the most sensitive marker among the tumor markers of the malignant pancreatic tumors. After non resectional treatment, in 4 cases(6%) patients died in the postoperative period. After resection postoperative complications were in 8(22%) patients. Delayed gastric emptying was more common in the PPPD group resulting in longer hospitalisation. In the PPPD group there was a better nutritional recovery and also the increase of both body weight and serum albumin level.There was no other significant difference between the survival of WP and PPPD group, but we found much better survival in patients with periampullary tumor.
Conclusions: Improved surgical techniques and improved perioperative management together decrease the surgical risk. Our data provided many evidences about the advantage of PPPD in patients with malignant periampullary and pancreas head tumors. There is no any difference between the survival rates of WP and PPPD but the long term results and quality of life are much better after PPPD.

1.07

D. Henne-Bruns, I. Vogel, J. Lüttges*, G. Klöppel *, B. Kremer.
Department of Surgery, Christian-Albrecht-University Kiel, Germany, *)
Department of Pathology, Christian-Albrecht-University Kiel, Germany

Results after Regional and Extended Lymphadenectomy in Patients with Ductal Adenocarcinoma of the Pancreas Head.

Aim: The value of extended lymphadenectomy (LA) in patients with pancreatic cancer is still discussed controversely. Therefore it was the aim of the study to evaluate the influence of regional versus extended LA on survival in patients with pancreatic adenocarcinomas.
Patients and Methods: Between 10/88 and 3/98 72 patients with ductal adenocarcinoma of the pancreas underwent partial duodeno-pancreatectomy with either regional (n = 26) or extended (n = 46) LA.
The outcome of the two groups was compared by constructing survival curves and evaluating demographic, intraoperative and histopathologic data from all patients with R0-resections (n =58).
Results: Mortality was 3.8% after regional and 6.5% after extended LA. A comparison of R0 resected patients showed no significant differences in long-term survival between the two groups. Only tumor stage (5-year-survival in stage I/II was 63% compared to 15% in stage III/ IV, p = 0.0087), tumor grade (p = 0.0022) and portal vein involvement (p = 0.0063) had a significant influence on survival, regardless of the type of operation.
For patients with nodal involvement (5-year survival of patients in N0 Stage 46,9% compared to 15% for N1 stage patients) a trend (p =0.081) was observed regarding the prognosis indepent from the type of operation.
Conclusion: Our data suggest that no further improvement of the survival rate can be achieved by extended LA compared to regional lymphadenectomy in patients with ductal adenocarcinomas of the head of the pancreas.

1,08

COMPLEMENT RESISTANCE FACTORS CD 55 AND CD 59 FREQUENTLY OCCUR IN PANCREATIC AND IN GASTROINTESTINAL CANCER BUT RARELY IN THE CORRESPONDING NORMAL TISSUE

Del Bello F., Juhl, H

Dept. of General and Thoracic Surgery, University of Kiel, Germany

Aims: Complement resistance factors CD 55 and CD 59 have been found in various malignancies. Their occurrence interfere with an effective antibody therapy by the inhibition of the classical pathway of complement. Furthermore the expression of CD 55 and CD 59 might be an immunological escape mechanism of malignant cells. So far, no comprehensive study has investigated the expression of CD 55 and CD 59 in pancreatic and other gastrointestinal cancers.
Methods: The expression of CD 55 and CD 59 in pancreatic and gastrointestinal cancer was studied in comparison to the corresponding normal tissue and clinical data, e.g. tumor stage and grading. 63 pancreatic and gastrointestinal tumor samples and their corresponding normal tissue have been immunostained for CD 55 and CD 59..Additionally, tumor tissue was stained for the expression of 17-1A antigen which has been shown to be a promising target for adjuvant antibody therapy of colon cancer..
Results: Expression of CD 55 was seen in 47% of the pancreatic, 63% of the gastric and 77% of the colorectal cancer tissue (normal tissue: 25%,0% and 11%). CD 59 was positive in 71%, 50% and 68% (normal tissue: 50%, 20% and 11%)Coexpression of CD 55 and CD 59 was seen in 29% of pancreatic, 38% of gastric and 41 % of colon cancer samples. In contrast normal pancreatic tissue showed both resistance factors only in 12%, and none of the normal gastric and colon samples expressed CD 55 and CD 59 in parallel. The expression of CD 55 and CD 59 was independent of tumor stage and grading. 17-1A antigen was present in 83% of the pancreatic, 26% of the gastric and 73% of the colon cancer samples. A coexpression of 17-1A with CD 55 and CD 59 was found in 60%, 20% and 46% of the tumor tissue.
Conclusion: This study suggests CD 55 and CD 59 as protective immune escape factors in carcinogenetic process of pancreatic-, gastric- and colorectal cancer which might also limit the effect of an antibody therapy in patients with gastrointestinal malignancies.

Dig Surg 1999; 16 (suppl 1): 11-13

HPB research I.

2,01

THE SIGNIFICANCE OF NM-23 H1 PROTEIN EXPRESSION IN PRIMARY LIVER CARCINOMA

Trotovsek B, Gadzijev EM, Marolt V .
Dep. of abdominal surgery, University medical centre, Ljubljana, Slovenia.

Aims: The purpose of this study was to investigate prognostic factors and significance of nm-23 H1 protein expression in tumour and surrounding liver tissue in patients treated with liver resection for primary liver carcinoma (PLC) by immunohistochemical staining with anti nm-23 H1 antibody. The main goal was to evaluate whether the expression of antimetastatic nm-23 H1 protein is associated with tumour stage, clinicopathologic findings and patient survival.
Methods : A retrospective analysis of medical records was performed for 56 patients identified through the Registry of Cancer, Slovenia as having been treated with liver resection for PLC in University medical centre, Ljubljana. Clinical characteristics were noted including age, sex, history of alcohol abuse, hepatitis B and/or C positivity, TNM staging, serum alpha-feto protein (AFP), macroscopic and microscopic tumour characteristics, patency of portal vasculature, treatment received and ultimate survival from the beginning of treatment. The presence of nm-23 H1 protein was studied using mouse monoclonal antibody directed against the internal domain of nm-23 H1 protein in a 1:50 dilution (Novocastra Lab UK). As avidin-biotin-complex technique was employed, the secondary antibody was a biotinylated rabbit anti-mouse immunoglobulin (DAKO, Denmark). Negative controls were performed in the absence of primary antibodies against nm-23 H1 protein. The intensity of tumour staining was classified into two grades: negative, when staining of tumour was less intense then in surrounding nontumorous liver tissue and positive, when staining of tumour was more intensive.
Results : Positive expression of nm-23 H1 protein in tumorous tissue was associated with tumours of TNM stage 1 and 2 ($p<0.05$). There was no statistically significant correlation between presence of satellite nodes, macroscopic type of growth, vascular invasion and number of tumours and expression of nm-23 H1 protein in tumorous tissue. By univariate analysis the nm-23 expression in tumorous tissue was not associated with improved overall survival. The mean survival time in the group of patients with stronger expression of nm-23 H1 protein in tumourous tissue was 42 months comparing to 33 months in nm-23 H1 negative group. The difference was not statistically significant.
Conclusion : Although the correlation between expression of nm-23 H1 protein and some favourable prognostic factors as absence of cirrhosis, low TNM stage was observed, the beneficial effect of nonreduced expression of nm-23 H1 protein in tumourous tissue on survival of the patients was not confirmed.

2,02

HEPATIC PATHOLOGIC CHANGES AFTER LIVER ISCHEMIC DAMAGE IN JAUNDICED RATS

Karavias D, Tsamandas AC*, Tepetes K, Mirra L, Agriantoni M, Androulakis J
Departments of Surgery and *Pathology University of Patras, Greece

Aims: Cholestatic liver is known to be more susceptible to ischemia than the normal one. In this study we assessed the histopathologic features of hepatic ischemic damage and liver regeneration, in rats with experimental obstructive jaundice.

Methods: The study comprised 80 male Wistar rats assigned randomly in 3 categories: I (n=10) sham operation, II (n=40) ligation of hepatic artery and portal vein (total liver ischemia-TLI), and III (n=30) common bile duct ligation (BDL). Rats from category II sacrificed 15 (IIA), 30 (IIB) and 60 min (IIC) after TLI was done. Ten days after BDL, 10 rats of category III underwent euthanasia, whereas the remaining 30, underwent TLI and sacrificed after 15 min (IIIB), 30 min (IIIC), and 60 min (IIID). Liver wedge biopsies (left anterior lobe) were obtained and histologic examination included H&E, and immunohistochemical stains for cytokeratin AE3, α1-antitrypsin (α1AT), and antigen Ki67. Immunohistochemical results for Ki67 were expressed as the percentage of nuclear stained positive cells/500 cells.

Results: Livers sections from group IIIA (BDL) showed large duct obstruction features, and these from category II (TLI), ischemic changes including centrilobular hepatocellular swelling and necrosis, hepatocanalicular cholestasis, and mild portal mononuclear/mixed inflammation. Sections from groups IIIB, IIIC, IIID (all BDL+TLI) displayed together changes of large duct obstruction and ischemia, and in groups IIIC (BDL+30 min TLI), and IIID (BDL+60 min TLI) necrosis of the large bile ducts was present. The total liver parenchymal area affected (% necrosis) was higher in groups IIID, and IIIC compared to groups IIIB ($p< 0.05$), and IIC, IIB, IIA ($p<0.01$). All 60 TLI-liver biopsies, developed features of liver regeneration originated from zone 2, extended to zone 1 and occasionally to zone 3. Immunohistochemical stains revealed cells positive to AE1 and cells positive to á1AT. Proliferation rate (% Ki67+ cells) was higher in group IIA compared to groups IIB , IIC, IIIA, ($p<0.05$), and groups IIIC, and IIID ($p<0.0$).

Conclusions: Liver ischemia induces more severe hepatocyte damage in livers with obstructive cholangiopathy than in normal ones. Liver reparative process is mediated mainly by proliferation of non-necrotic cells that express hepatocellular or ductular epithelial features. The proliferation rate of hepatocytes (degree of regeneration) is lower when liver ischemia and obstructive jaundice co-exist.

2,03

SIGNIFICANCE OF nm23 mRNA EXPRESSION IN HUMAN HEPATOCELLULAR CARCINOMA

Fan Chun,Zhang Yangde, Wan Xiaoping, Linianfeng, Lu Huanyuan
National Hepatobilitary and Enteric Surgery Research Center, Ministry of Health
Changsha, Hunan, China

It has sbeen proposed than nm23-H1, a candidate suppressor gene for metastasis, plays an important role in the metqastasis of human tumors. In order to investigate its role in the human hepatocellular carcinoma (HCC), 12 matched pairs of tumorous and adjacent nontumorous lifer tissues of hepatectomy from patients with HCC were studied by quantitative reverse transcription-PCR. The results of these molecular studies were correlated with the clinicopathologic features of the patients. Nm23-H1 transcript was expressed in all neoplastic and adjacent nontumorous liver tissue. The level of expression, however, did not correlate well with the extension or metastatic potential of the tumors. Instead, in 9 (75%) of 12 HCC, nm23-H1 expression was higher in the tumorous tissues, compared with the adjacent nontumorous tissues, and significantly higher levels of nm23-H1 mRNA expression was detected in HCC with poor differentiation (Edmonson classification, III and IV) than those with moderate differentiation (I and II). Southern blot analysis of nm23-Hl gene revealed neither amplification nor loss. of heterozygosity of all HCC tissues examined. Direct sequencing of the nm23-H1 gene in all HCC tissues detected no mutations. These findings suggested that increased nm23-1 mRNA expression is correlated with HCCtumor progression.

KARGER
Fax +41 61 306 12 34
E-Mail karger@karger.ch
www.karger.com

2,04

DISSEMINATED TUMOR CELLS IN PATIENTS WITH HEPATOBILIARY CARCINOMA

Deleré Y, Vogel I, Juhl H, Henne-Bruns D, Kremer B

Dept. for General and Thoracic Surgery, University of Kiel, Germany

Aims: Previously we could demonstrate that detection of disseminated tumor cells in the bone marrow and the peritoneal cavity of patients with colorectal and gastric cancer can be performed by immunocytological methods with a high sensitivity. In this study we wanted to analyse if disseminated tumor cells can also be detected also in patients with hepatobiliary carcinoma (hepatocellular carcinoma (HCC), carcinoma of the papilla vateri, gall bladder carcinoma) and if their detection seems to correlate with patients survival prognosis either.
Methods: Prior to operation we aspirated bone marrow (BM) from the iliac crest and performed a lavage of the peritoneal cavity (PC). 13 peritoneal samples (PC) and 11 bone marrow samples (BM) of 14 patients with hepatocellular carcinoma, 13 PC and 15 BM of 18 patients with carcinoma of the papilla vateri and 8 PC and 8 BM of 9 patients with gall bladder carcinoma were analysed with a pannel of monoclonal antibodies. Indirect immunperoxydase staining using the mab KI-1 (Cytokeratin), C1P83 (CEA), Ca 19-9, 17-1A, Ra 96 (Mucin), C 54 (epithelial membran antigene) and AFP were performed.
Results: For patients with HCC the detection rate in both compartments was 35.75% (5/14) with 14.3% (2/14) in the bone marrow (BM) and 35.75% (5/14) in the peritoneal cavity (PC) samples. In patients with carcinoma of the papilla vateri the overall detection rate was 27.7% (5/18), in BM 16.6% (3/18) and 16.6% (3/18) in the PC. 77.7% of patients with gall bladder carcinoma were positive in BM or PC, 44.4% (4/9) in BM and 66.6% (6/9) in the PC. Analyses of postoperative survival showed that patients who tested negative in any sample seems to have a better survival prognosis than patients who tested positive.
Conclusions: For for the first time we could show that parallel to our previous studies in patients with gastrointestinal carcinoma disseminated tumor cells can be detected in patients with hepatobiliary carcinoma. Even in hepatobiliary carcinoma the detection of tumor cells in bone marrow and/or peritoneal cavity seems to correlate to patients survival prognosis.

2,05

CD 34 EXPRESSION IN CHRONIC LIVER DISEASE AND HEPATOCELLULAR CARCINOMA (HCC).

Puleo S, Fraggetta F °, Di Carlo I, Lombardo R, Azzarello G, Vasquez E °.

First Surgical Clinic, ° Department of Pathology, University of Catania, Catania, Italy

Capillarisation of hepatic sinusoids is a well recognized phenomen occurring in long standing liver disease, in hepatic cirrhosis as well as in hepatocellular carcinoma.
Aim.
To study immunohistochemically the expression and distribution of CD 34 in chronic liver diesease and hepatocellular carcinoma in order to evaluate the possible diagnostic implication of this marker.

Materials and methods.
Sixty-five samples of liver tissue, showing different degrees of chronic inflammation and fibrosis and histological features of hepatocellular carcinoma were included in the study. The specimens were fixed in formalin and embedded in paraffin and a immunohistochemical investigation was performed by the standard avidin-biotin-peroxidase complex method with CD 34.

Results.
The sinusoids of liver affected by different degrees of chronic active hepatitis showed no or focal immunostaining for CD 34; an increased immunoreactivity was observed in the periportal sinusoids of the cirrhotic nodules whereas a diffuse and strong staining was observed in the overall HCC as well as in the hepatocellular adenoma tested.

Conclusion. In HCC, immunoreactivity for CD 34 represents an effective method to evaluate angiogenesis and to distinguish well-differentiated HCC from non-neoplastic liver. Its role in clinical stage and prognostic evaluation

2,06

DNA-IMAGE-CYTOMETRY AND P53/KI-67 STATUS OF RESECTED COLORECTAL LIVER METASTASES - ARE THERE THERAPEUTICAL CONSEQUENCES?

Riesener KP, Kasperk R, König M, Biesterfeld S, Jacob C**, Füzesi L**, Schumpelick V*
Department of Surgery, *Institute of Pathology, University Hospital, RWTH Aachen, **Institute of Pathology, University of Göttingen, Germany

Aims
Resection of colorectal hepatic metastases provides the only chance of cure in this stage of disease. Nevertheless, in spite of presumed R0-resections the overall recurrence rate reaches 60-80%. The role of an adjuvant regional chemotherapy remains controversial, as several studies were not able to prove a survival benefit. The aim of our study was to define risk groups of recurrence by cytometry or immunhistochemistry and the possible influence of an adjuvant chemotherapy in these groups.
Methods
Between 1986 and 1995 R0-resection of colorectal hepatic metastases was performed in 104 patients. 49 patients were additionally treated by an adjuvant hepatic arterial chemotherapy (HAI). DNA-Image-Cytometry of the resected metastases was performed in 55 patients, p53 and Ki-67 immunhistochemistry in 67 and 51 patients, respectively.
Results
Expression of Ki-67 did not markedly influence survival following hepatic resection, while p53 was slightly correlated with the prognosis. A maximum single cell ploidy of more than 9c was followed by a significant decrease in survival time. Postoperative HAI showed an improvement of survival only in the group of patients with 9c Exceeding events, while the other groups were unaffected.
Conclusions
Our study demonstrates an improvement of survival time after adjuvant HAI only in patients with an expected poor prognosis as evidenced by the results of DNA-Image-Cytometry. Thus the results of cytometry might be valuable in defining risk groups before HAI.

2,07

COLORECTAL TUMOUR CELL EXPRESSION OF E-CADHERIN AND IMMUNE EVASION. THE PATHWAY TO METASTASIS.

Mr K Seymour, Dr B K Shenton, Mr R M Charnley, Dr J A Kirby. Department of Surgical and Reproductive Science, Medical school, University of Newcastle upon Tyne, Framlington Place, NE2 4HH, UK

Background. E-cadherin is a cell adhesion molecule, expressed by all epithelial cells, with tumour suppresser functions. Reduction of E-cadherin is common amongst the common epithelial malignancies and positively associated with invasion and liver metastasis and worse prognosis, features currently ascribed to its role in homotypic adhesion. CD103 is a receptor ligand for E-cadherin expressed by the large subset of lymphocytes associated with immune surveillance of the mucosal surfaces. We have examined the effect of up-regulation of E-cadherin on the ability of lymphocytes to bind and kill colorectal tumour cells.

Method. The inflammatory cytokines, TNF-α and IL_2 alone and in combination, Tamoxifen, and Paclitaxel were screened for their ability to up-regulate E-cadherin on HT-29 cells. Quantitative expression of E-cadherin was assessed by flow cytometry. Fluorescent standards were generated using a mixture of standardised fluorochrome conjugated fluorospheres. Adhesion between E-cadherin up regulated HT-29 cells and a lymphocyte line expressing CD103 (MOLT-16) was examined by flow cytometry. Cells were distinguished from one another by labelling HT-29 with anti-epithelial antigen (FITC) and lymphocytes with anti CD45 (PerCP). Incorporation of Flow-Count fluorospheres allowed accurate estimations of rosetting ratios. The susceptibility of HT-29 to killing was assayed by colourimetric transformation of MTT in 96 well plates.

Results. Tamoxifen has no effect on HT-29 expression of E-cadherin. E-cadherin is down regulated by both TNF-α and IL_2 ($p<0.01$), there is no synergy. Paclitaxel significantly up regulates E-cadherin expression on HT-29 cells at a dose of $4x10^{-9}M$ ($p<0.01$). The up regulation of E-cadherin resulted in increased binding of lymphocytes to the HT29-cells, rosetting ratios were reduced from 3 HT-29 per lymphocyte for un-treated cells to 2 HT-29 per lymphocyte bound for cells treated with paclitaxel ($p=0.028$). Co-incubation of lymphocytes with E-cadherin up-regulated HT-29 resulted in increased cell death ($p<0.01$).

Conclusions. E-cadherin is up regulated by paclitaxel but not by tamoxifen or inflamatory cytokines on HT-29 cells. $CD103^+$ lymphocytes bind more avidly to HT-29 with up regulated E-cadherin and result in more tumour cell death in vitro. These results suggest a role for E-cadherin in tumour immunology and its reduction may facilitate liver metastasis from epithelial malignancies in a way independent from reduced homotypic adhesion.

2.08

CORRELATION BETWEEN CHEMOTHERAPEUTIC MEDICINES' SENSITIVITY OF COLORECTAL CARCINOMA AND MUTATIONS OF P53 GENE

Fan Chun, Zhang Yangde, Shen Hong, Wan Xiaoping, Li Lianfeng
Xiangya Hospital, Hunan Medical University,
Changsha, Hunan 410008, P.R.China

Utilizing MTT colorimetrics for chemotherapeutic medicines' sensitivity of colorectal carcinoma and PCR-SSCP technique for analyzing mutations of P53 gene, we observed 20 patients with colorectal carcinoma. The result shows that colorectal carcinoma cells are the most sensitive to 5-Fu (IR=54.7%?14.1%), less sensitive to MMC (IR=43.9% VS 10.8%, p<0.05) and ADM (IR=43.9% VS 9.4%, p<0.05), and resistant to DDP (IR=25.9% VS 12.8%, p<0.01). The mutation percentage of P53 gene is 45% (9/20). A positive correlation was found between sensitivities of MMC and ADM and mutations of P53 gene (rmmc = 0.589, radm = 0 624, p<0.05). This correlation proved that the effects in colorectal carcinoma induced by chemotherapeutic medicines such as MMC and ADM+ depended on p53 gene. However, no correlation was demonstrated between sensitivities of 5-Fu and DDP and mutations of p53 gene. This will suggest us some other possible genes such as c-myc, c-fos, Bcl-2 and ras gene take a important controlling role in the process of 5-Fu and DDP killing colorectal carcinoma cells.

2.09

CONTRIBUTORY ROLE OF MICROPEROXIDASE DERIVED FROM MITOCHONDRIAL CYTOCHROME C IN DEVELOPMENT OF ACUTE NECROTIZING PANCREATITIS.

Sledzinski Z.', Wozniak M.2, Ostrowski M.M.2, Kossowska E.2, Jankowski K.2
1 lst Department of Surgery, Medical University of Gdansk, Poland
2 Department of Biochemistry, Medical University of Gdansk, Poland

Detailed mechanisms of fulminant pancreatic cell death during acute pancreatitis (AP) is still a matter of intensive debate although harmful role of autodigestion of pancreatic tissue seems to be evident hallmark of the disease. Inverse relationship of acinar cell necrosis versus apoptosis in relation to severity of AP has been well docutnented. Oizr previous study demonstrated time dependence in changes of level of lipid hydroperoxides (LOOI~ peaked at 3h after cerulein infusion but returned to almost control level after subsequent 3h. Interestingly despite disappearance of LOOH, evident progression of morphological alteration of pancreatic tissue was clearly visible. Our study aimed to clarify these discrepancies. Taking into account possible secondary pathway of free radical production in pancreatic LOOH decomposition we hypothesised that intracellular proteolytic degradation of hemoproteins like cytochrome c can provide efficient trigger of free radicals from LOOH. Eighteen rats were divided into two equal groups: group 1 acted as control, rats were injected with 0.9% NaCI; group 2 rats had five hourly injections of cerulein 40 wg/mg. Rat pancreatae were removed, trimmed of connective tissue and homogenised in 0.15M KCI + IOmM Tris HCl pH 7.4. Pancreatic acinar cell cytosol obtained after 1 h centrifugation of postmitochondrial supernatant incubated with native cytochrome c (1 Omg/ml) has been found to generate nücroperoxidase from cytochrome c ouy if respective rats were treated with cerutein. Microperoxidase lias been found to generate free radicals from synthetic hydroperoxidase ButOOH 40 times more efficiently tlien parent molecule cytochrome c. Since cytochrome c has been recognised as essential molecule for controlled cell death i.e. apoptosis, our results point on "switch on" mechanism of pancreatic cell death. Intracellular proteolysis of cytochrome c can exacerbatE oxidative stress being responsible of switching over the mode of cell death from apoptosis to necrosis.

Dig Surg 1999; 16 (suppl 1): 14-16

HPB imaging

3.01

THE ROLE OF ULTRASOUND MEASUREMENT OF LIVER ATTENUATION IN PATIENTS WITH CHRONIC DIFFUSE LIVER DISEASES

Szebeni Á., Satrapa J., Tolvaj Gy., Dávid K.
MI Central Hospital, Hungary; Deutsche Krebsforschungszentrum, Germany

Aims: In vivo measurement of liver attenuation by ultrasound (US) in healthy subjects and in patients with chronic diffuse liver diseases (CDLD) and to correlate the results with body mass index (BMI) and subcutaneous fat thickness of the skin.

Methods: 46 normal subjects and 83 patients with CDLD were examined. Two basic groups of „bright livers" were formed according to attenuation, the low attenuation type (DI.) of 52 and the high attenuation type (DII.) of 31 patients. Attenuation of the liver was determined by US scanning of the liver and a reference phantom in the same set up and evaluating their digitized image by a special software. Subcutaneous fat thickness and BMI (body weight[kg]/body height^2[m^2]) was measured simultaneously with US scanning of the liver.

Results: Attenuation of the liver in the three patient groups (normal, DI. and DII.) was correlated with BMI and subcutaneous fat thickness of the patients. It was found that in cases of normal liver and in type DI. bright liver the examined parameters showed no significant differences. On the contrary, in type DII. bright livers, relevant parameters showed higher values than in the other two patient groups.

Conclusions: It was concluded that type DII. bright liver pattern in patients with CDLD may be in connection with obesity.

3.02

ULTRASONIC CHANGES OF RADICAL SURGICAL SEGMENTED INTESTINE'S TREATMENT RESULTS

Chizhikov N.V., Oparina O.N.
The Region Hospital of War-Veterans, Penza, Russia

Aim: to demonstrate the opportunities of ultrasonic examination in the context of clinic-labour forecast and the necessity of medical reablement of the patients after radical surgical treatment of the segmented intestine cancer.

Methods: 118 patients having gone through radical surgical treatment of the segmented intestine cancer were examined on their liver, cholecystis and pancreas by ultrasonics within 4 to 19 years after the operation. There were 64 men and 54 women within the age of 26 and 63 years among them. There were 39 right-side hemicolectomies, 4 transverse segmented intestine resections, 15 left-side hemicolectomies and 60 sigmoid resections fulfilled.

Results: 67 (56,7%) patients showed no pathological echostructural changes. There was liver metastasis found in 4 (3,4%) patients. 47 (29,8%) patients showed the next changes: 18 chronic cholecystitis, 10 chronic persistent hepatitis, 7 fatty liver degeneration, 3 chronic cholecysto-pancreatitis, 2 chronic pancreatitis, 2 chronic calculous cholecystitis. 5 patients showed the damages of several body-organs: 3 - chronic cholecystitis and hepatis, 1 - chronic pancreatitis and fatty liver degeneration, 1 chronic cholecysto-pancreatitis and hepatitis. The most frequent ultrasonic changes were discovered in 30 (25,4%) patients after the right-side hemicolectomy.

Conclusions: The ultrasonic examination makes it possible to discover metastatic and chronic inflammatory changes in liver, cholecystis and pancreas of the patients which can influence the clinic-labour forecast and the arrangements of medical reablement.

3.03

COLOR DOPPLER ULTRASONOGRAPHY IN DETECTING VASCULAR INVOLVEMENT BY PANCREATIC CANCER

Pirski M.L., Nowakowski M. Lukianski M., Kostro J.
I Department of Surgery Medical Universitz of Gdansk, Poland

Aims: The aim of this study was to asses the accuracy of color Doppler imaging in diagnosis vessels involvement by pancreatic cancer.
Methods: Since May 1996 color Doppler USG was routinely performed in all patients treated for pancreatic cancer. All 51 patients (30M, 21F) were submitted to the study. Age of them was 37-76 yr, (mean 58). Cancer staging according to the AJCC/TNM classification was as follows: I-16 (31%), II-14 (28%), III-20 (39%), IV-1 (2%). USG tests were performed with Ultramark - machine with convex probe operating at 2-4 Mhz. The morphological lesions of the vessels were evaluated according to the criteria proposed by Angeli: grade O-no contact with the tumor, 1-contact continuity less then 2 cm, 2-contact more 2 cm or vascular compressions, 3-encasement or thrombosis, Sonographic diagnosis was compared with surgical findings.
Results: Out of 51 patients tested sonographically 50 (98%) were submitted tu surgery, in remaining 1 (2%) there was clear evidence of cancer dissemination. In 50 (98%) out of 51 patients the tumor was identified in USG. At exploration 28 (56%) of 50 patients had pancreatic resection (grade 0-14, grade 1-14 patients). In 16 of them had Whipple procedure and 6 Traverso-Longmire operation. Four had subtotal and 2 distal pancreatectomy. In 4 cases of this group USG indicated vascular involvement (false positive results in 4 patients). In 1 patient Doppler test did not reveal vascular involvement (false negative-1). In the remaining 22 patients (44%) only palliative procedures were performed (9 laparotomies, 13 bilioenteric anastomosis). Vascular involvement in Dopler test was foung in 3 cases (false negative), 14 were grade 2 and 5 were grade 3. The sensitive, specifity and overall accuracy of color Doppler imaging were 87%, 86% and 86% respectively.
Conclusions: Color Doppler is a sensitive and specific imaging test technique in detecting vascular involvement by pancreatic cancer. Resectability of the pancreatic cancer can be assessed by this method.

KARGER
Fax +41 61 306 12 34
E-Mail karger@karger.ch
www.karger.com

3.04

THE CONTRIBUTION OF INTRAOPERATIVE ULTRASONOGRAPHY IN THE SURGICAL TREATMENT OF HEPATIC CYSTS

G. Skroubis (*), K. Tepetes (*), D. Karnabatidis (**) and C. Vagianos (*)
From the Department of Surgery (*), and the Department of Radiology (**), University Hospital of Patras, Rion Patras, Greece

Aim: In this study, we attempted to evaluate the possible usefulness of intraoperative ultrasonography in the surgery of hepatic cysts.

Methods: Eleven cases of hepatic hydatid cysts and one case of complicated polycystic liver disease are presented. In all the above mentioned cases intraoperative ultrasonography was used, in order to facilitate the surgical technique.
Results: Intraoperative ultrasonography (I.O.U.) proved to be very useful during surgery for hepatic hydatid disease for two reasons. Firstly was able to reveal deep sited cysts and therefore guide the access, and secondly proved precious to show small "satellite" cysts. In the case of the complicated polycystic liver disease I.O.U. was used not only to guide the access and the fenestration of deep-sited cysts, but was very useful as well, to preserve normal liver parenchyma between the cysts. In addition, I.O.U. was helpful to locate the major hepatic vessels, in the distorted anatomy of the disease, avoiding this way any inadvertent injury.
Conclusion: In conclusion, we think that I.O.U. is a valuable intraoperative guiding technique, improving the safety and perhaps the efficacy in surgery for hepatic cysts.

3.05

RESECTABILITY AND STRATEGY IN LIVER SURGERY: ASSESSMENT BY INTRAOPERATIVE ULTRASONOGRAPHY

Tranberg K-G, Ohlsson B, Lindell G, Möller PH, Pålsson B, Willner J
Departments of Surgery and Radiology, University of Lund, Sweden

Aim: To determine the value of preoperative computed tomography (CT) and ultrasonography (US), intraoperative ultrasonography (IOUS) and surgical assessment (SA) with respect to resectability and strategy in liver surgery.

Method: This is a prospective study of 87 patients, undergoing laparotomy for anticipated hepatic resection at 90 occasions. Nineteen patients had primary liver cancer, 55 had liver metastases, 10 had benign tumours and 6 patients had no liver tumour.

Results: A correct description of the number and location of all tumours was given by CT, US, IOUS and SA in 40, 41, 70 and 73 % of the examinations, respectively. Tumour number was underestimated in 33-38 % of the preoperative investigations (US and CT) and in 19-22 % of the intraoperative assessments (SA and IOUS). Incorrect location of the tumour(s) occurred in 14-20 % of the preoperative investigations and in 4 % at IOUS and SA. A correct assessment of resectability was given by CT, US, IOUS and SA in 80, 85, 99 and 97 % of the examinations, respectively. For tumours detected by only one intraoperative modality, IOUS detected deeply located tumours whereas SA detected superficially located tumours. IOUS provided new information at 29 (32 %) occasions and changed the surgical strategy during 11 (12 %) of the operations: resection was abandoned in 8, and a lesser or more extensive resection was performed in one and two patients, respectively.

Conclusion: IOUS is a valuable method for detection of liver tumours and is helpful in the assessment of resectability in liver resection.

3.06

LAPAROSCOPIC ULTRASOUND IN THE MANAGEMENT OF LIVER TUMORS

V. Sorin, G. Gvirz*, I. Avni**, A. Czerniac
Deps. of Surgery, Ultrasond* and Gastroenterology**
E. Wolfson Medical Center, Holom, Israel

Aim: To assess the role of laparoscopic ultrasound (LAPUS) in the management of liver mass.

Methods: Patient with hepatic mass diagnosed previously by US and CT-scan underwent LAPUS (Sharplan Usight laparoscopic US system, Israel; 8MHZ laparoscopic US probe). TNM staging was evaluated together with interrelation with vascular and biliary structures and presence of additional masses. US guided biopsy was performed in equivocal cases.

Results: 72 patients (32 male, 40 female, age range 25-80) with suspicious liver mass underwent LAPUS. There were 34 patients with suspected primary hepatic tumor and 38 with metastatic lesions. Additional information was obtained in 53 cases (74%) of which LAPUS biopsy was performed in 37 cases. This resulted in changes of therapeutic approach in 43 patients (60%). Unnecessary laparotomy was prevented in 18 patients (25%). The LAPUS study gave false results in 6 patients (8,3%).

Conclusions: Laparoscopic US is a highly effective modality for evaluation of liver mass, which improves selection of patients for surgical treatment.

3.07

C. Pasquali, C. Sperti, * F. Chierichetti, A. Canton, A. Ferronato, * G. Ferlin , S. Pedrazzoli.
Dept. of Medical and Surgical Sciences, Surgery - University of Padova, and * Nuclear Medicine - Castelfranco V. Hospital, Italy.

18 FDG-PET IMAGING IN THE DIFFERENTIAL DIAGNOSIS OF PANCREATIC CYSTIC LESIONS.

Differential diagnosis among cystic lesions of the pancreas, that include cystic neoplasms, is still difficult. The main problem is to distinguish malignant cysts from benign lesions (expecially pseudocysts and serous cystadenomas). Encouraging results inthe diagnosis of pancreatic cancer have been reported by using positron emission tomography (PET) with fluorine 18-labelled fluorodeoxyglucose (FDG).
Aim of the study was to evaluate the usefulness of PET in detecting malignant cystic lesions of the pancreas.
From June 1995 to December 1998, 31 patients with suspected pancreatic cystic tumor (24 cases) or suspected intraductal mucin hypersecreting neoplasm (IMHN; 7 cases) were prospectively investigated with 18-FDG-PET after abdominal ultrasound, helical CT scan and/or MRI. PET imaging was performed 60 min after iv. injection of 18-FDG (12 mCi). A focal tracer uptake in the pancreatic region was considered positive when the stadardized uptake value (SUV) was > 2.5. Diagnosis was confirmed by surgery in all patients.
Pathological examination showed: cystadenocarcinoma (n = 5), mucinous cystadenoma (n = 4), serous cystadenoma (n = 3), solitary true cyst (n = 3), benign IMHN (n = 4), malignant IMHN (n = 1), endocrine cystic tumor (n =2), pseudocyst (n = 5), papillary-cystic tumor (n =1), cystic lymphangioma (n = 1), adenocarcinoma with cystic necrosis (n =1), enterogenous cyst of the duodenum (n = 1). PET showed abnormal focal uptake with high SUV (range 2.6 - 7.8) in 4/5 cystadenocarcinomas, 1/1 malignant IMHN, 1/1 papillary cystic tumors, 2/2 endocrine tumors, 1/4 mucinous cystadenomas and in the case of adenocarcinoma with cystic degeneration. All serous adenomas and other benign lesions were negative. Sensitivity and specificity of PET and CT scan in predicting malignant lesions were 90, 96 % for PET and 80 and 86 % for CT respectively.
PET seems to be helpful in detecting malignancy and border-line neoplasms witin pancreatic cystic lesions.

3.08

CLINICAL VALUE OF WHOLE-BODY POSITRON EMISSION TOMOGRAPHY IN RESECTABLE COLORECTAL LIVER METASTASES

B. Topal, R. Aerts, F. Pennickx, L. Filez, L. Mortelmans, UZ Gasthuisberg, Catholic University of Leuven, Belgium

Aim: Liver resection for colorectal metastasis can be carried out with a mortality less than 5% and is associated with a 35% 5-year survival. The aim of this prospective study is to be evaluate whether patient selection can be improved with properative whole-body PET scan.

Methods: Between July 1990 and June 1998, 77 patients were considered to be eligible for liver resection after conventional investigation for colorectal liver metastases. 23 patients presented with synchronous and 54 with metachronous metastases. In all of these patients a whole body PET scan with [^{18}F]fluorodeoxyglucose (FDG) was performed.

Results: In 4 patients PET provided supplementary information to conventional investigation: detection of pervic recurrence (2), oesophageal cancer (1), and cerebral metastasis (1). PET confirmed liver metastasis in all patients, except in 2 with a small lesion (15 mm), and was partially false negative in 4 patients with small hepatic lesions. PET could not detect small perioteneal metastases in 2 patients. Among these 8 patients 4 were proven to be inoperable at the time of surgery. PET was false positive in 8 patients, suspected pelvic rrecurrencd (2), suspicion of pulmonary metastases (4) and ceervical lymphadenopathies (2).

Conclusions: PET seems to have a small benefit (5%) in improving patient selection for liver resection with a curative intent. Small metastatic lesions in the liver and periotneum are not dfetected with PET (10 % false negatives). Suspicion of pulmonary metastases, peripheral lymphadenopathies, and pe.vic recurrence have to be further infvestigated before surgery (10% false positives). Further study is needed with regard to the detection of small hepatic and peritoneal metastases, and the interpretation of spots with increased activity in the lungs and peripheral lymphnodes.

3.09

HEPATOLITHIASIS: PRE-OPERATIVE ASSESSMENT WITH MRCP VS ERCP

Jan YY, Yeh TS, Chen MF, Tseng JH*
Division of First General Surgery and Radiology*, Chang Gung University, Chang Gung Memorial Hospital, Linkou Center, Taoyuan, Taiwan

Purpose: Magnetic resorance cholangio-pancreatography (MRCP) in a new, non-invasive imaging technique for the visualization of the bile ducts and pancreatic duct. No contrast medium injection is used. The aim of this study was to assess the feasibility of MRCP versus ERCP for the pre-operative evaluation in patient with hepatolithiasis.

Materials and methods: During the period between July 1997 and Sept. 1998, prospective study of MRCP vs ERCP for pre-operative evaluation in patients with hepatolithiasis was performed. There are 11 male and 23 females, age ranged from 32 to 71 years old. Pre-operative diagnosis of stone location and bile duct stricture in hepatolithiasis by MRCP and ERCP were compared. The final diagnosis of the stone location and bile duct strictures were confirmed by the operative finding, choledochoscopic examination and T-tube cholangiography.

Results: Correct diagnosis of stone location with filling defects in hepatolithiasis by the MRCP vs ERCP study were 97% vs 55% ($p < 0.05$). Correct diagnosis of bile duct strictures in hepatolithiasis by the MRCP vs ERCP study were 100% vs 55% ($p < 0.05$).

Conclusions: MRCP is a safe, non-invasive and effective procedure than ERCP for the pre-operative evaluation the stone location and bile duct stricture in patients with hepatolithiasis.

Dig Surg 1999; 16 (suppl 1): 17-19

Pancreas tumor II.

4,01

NEOADJUVANT CHEMORADIOTHERAPY FOR SURGICAL TREATMENT IN PANCREATIC CANCER: PRELIMINARY RESULTS.

Doglietto G.B., Alfieri S., Cellini N.*, Morganti A.*, Pacelli F., Papa V.
Department of Digestive Surgery and Radiotherapy* - Catholic University – Rome – Italy

AIMS
Prognosis of pancreatic cancer is poor even when the tumor is completely resected. In attempt to improve resectability and disease control, we used neoadjuvant chemoradiation in a combined modality therapy protocol for patients with cefalopancreatic cancer. The aim of this study is to report preliminary results in terms of morbidity, mortality, acute toxicity and response.
METHODS
During the period October 1995-May 1998 20 patients (11 males, 9 females; mean age:60.1 years; median follow-up:28 months) with resectable (8 cases) or unresectable (12 cases) tumor of head of the pancreas received external beam radiation (39.6 Gy) plus 5-FU (continuous i.v. infusion at 1000 mg/m²/day for the first fuor days). After 1 month, patients were restaged for possible surgical resection. After tumor resection, electron-beam intraoperative radiation therapy (10 Gy) was given before recontruction. Thereafter, in resected patients, adjuvant chemotherapy was infused (6 courses: 5-FU, Mit C, Adriamicin).
RESULTS
During neoadjuvant chemoradiation, no patients developed 3-4 acute toxicity. Twentyfive per cent (3/12) patients with unresectable tumors had tumor downstaging. None showed complete responses. Twenty per cent (4/20) had minimal tumor response. Three cases showed disease progression after neoadjuvant chemoradiation. Nine patients underwent surgical resection plus IORT. The morbidity rate was 22%. One patient died in the post-operative period. The overall median survival time was 9.4 months (18.5 and 8.3 in resected and unresected patients respectively).
CONCLUSIONS
Our preliminary results suggest that pre-operative 5-FU chemoradiation was well tolerated and may result in tumor downstaging, but the response-rate is still low. The combined radiosurgical treatment may control better recurrence and prolong survival.

4,02

NEOPLASMS OF THE PANCREAS

G, Karatzas Gr. Kouraklis, A. Karayiannakis, A. Papachristodoulou, M. Safioleas, J. Gogas.
Second Propedeutic Department of Surgery, University of Athens School of Medicine. Athens, Greece.

The authors report the results obtained of 125 patients with pancreatic neoplasms in our surgical department, the last decade.
There were 107 carcinomas, 10 cystadenomas or cystadenocarcinomas and 8 endocrine tumours. The operations performed as far as the carcinoma is concerned were palliative in 75% and resective in 25%. All the endocrine tumours were excised either with enucleation or with a pancreatectomy.
The last decade we abandoned the nillistic theory about the surgical teatment of carcinoma of the pancreas and because of the improvement of pre-operative evaluation, we have done 32 pancreatectomies without operative mortality.
The results we had were satisfactory and the survival time was improved drastically with adjuvant chemotherapy.
It is worthwhile to notify that the 5 year survival remains zero.

4,03

PANCREATIC CANCER - DIAGNOSIS, METHODS OF TREATMENT AND RESULTS

Pirski, M.I., Kostro J., Lukianski M., Witkowski P., Raczyńska S., Eledsinski Z.
I. Department ofSurgery Medical University of Gdansk, Poland

Aim: The aim of this study was to estimate diagnosis, methods and results in the treatment of pancreatic cancer.

Methods: In 1994 - 1998. 135 patients (63 F, 72 M) were treated for pancreatic cancer. Age ranged 38-91 years (mean 58). Staging of the lesions by CT (AJCC/TNM scale) qualified: I stage - 55 (41%), II - 20 (15%), III - 52 (38 %), IV - 8 (6%).

Results: Surgery was undertaken in 130 patients (96%) and 5 had conservative treatment. In 61 cases out of 130 resectable procedures (45%) were done: 26 - Whipple resection, 8 - Traverso - Longmire, 20 - total pancreeatectomy, and on 7 distal pancreatoectomy. The final diagnosis was established on the basis of needle biopsy or wedge biopsy samples (93%), while lymph nodes were negative. In the remaining 4 cases (7%) cancer cells were found only during the examination of the whole resected specimen. Bypass anastomoses were performed in 53 cases (41%) and laparotomy in 26 (20%). Postoperative complications leading to death occurred in 7 patients (5,4%): infection of mesenteric prothesis in 1, intracranial hemorrhage in 1, tumor dissemination in 3, pulmonary edema in 1.The follow up in the resected group was 1 - 49 months. One year survival rate was 64% (n=39), 4-years - 31%. After bypass anastomoses survival was 2-14 months (mean 5,7 months) and after laparotomy 1-13 (mean 4 mts). All patients treated conservatively died within 1 month.
Conclusions: The most useful among imaging techniques are CT and ERCP.

KARGER
Fax +41 61 306 12 34
E-Mail karger@karger.ch
www.karger.com

4,04

PANCREATODUODENECTOMY WITH PANCREATODUCTUS-JEJUNOSTOMY

R. Bracco, J. Grondona, A. Michetti and S. Bugosen. Clínica Pueyrredón of Mar del Plata and Centro Médico Martín y Omar of San Isidro, Buenos Aires, Argentina.

Resections offer the only chance of cure for pancreatic cancer, however, concern remains regarding the morbidity and mortality of pancreatoduodenectomy. A variety of techniques have been reported for dealing with the pancreatic remnant. In this video, the operation of a 61 years old male patient with a mucinoid cysto-adenocarcinoma of the head of the pancreas is presented. Asymptomatic and silent jaundice had appeared three weeks before admission. Ultrasonography showed only intra and extrahepatic bile ducts dilatation without a tumor imaging. Magnetic resonance cholangio-pancreatography showed a stop in the intra-pancreatic portion of the bile duct with an hypointense imaging of 0.5 cm. in diameter. Surgical approach with bilateral subcostal incision was performed. After cholecystectomy, the resection of the choledochus, gastric antrum, head of the pancreas and the four portions of the duodenum were performed. With the ultrasound dissector the uncinate process of the head of the pancreas was easily freed from the portal vein where the smallest vessels were coagulated and the larger closed with metal clips or ligated with sutures. The end-to-side pancreatojejunostomy was performed as follows: anterior and posterior layers between the pancreatic capsule and the serosa of the jejunum and, anterior and posterior layers between the Wirsung duct and a small enterotomy with accurate mucosa-to-mucosa approximation. In spite of the fine diameter of the Wirsung duct -approximately 2 mm- the use of magnification and fine monofilament sutures allowed a safe anastomosis. End-to-side hepatojejunostomy and end-to-side gastrojejunostomy in the same loop of the jejunum were carried out. No operative complications were observed and the hospital-stay was of 8 days.
The pancreatoductus-jejunostomy dimished the incidence of the operative anastomotic leaks and ensures the long-term permeability of the Wirsung duct flow.

4,05

A RETROSPRECTIVE TRIAL OF PANCREATICO-GASTROSTOMY 8PG9 VERSUS PANCREATICO-JEJUNOSTOMY (PJ) AFTER PANCREATICO-DUODENECTOMY (PD)

Csók V., Keleti G., Molnár P., De Negri N., Bálint G., Gergely Sz.
St. László Hosp. Budapest, Hungary

Aims: The leading postoperative complication after PD is the pancreatic fistula resulting from a pancreatic anastomosis leak. The authors investigate, whether there is a difference between the incidence rate of pancreatic anastomosis leak after PG and PJ on the basis of a retrospective single instituion trial.
Methods: Between January 1988 and December 1997 95 patients underwent PD due to malignant disease, 75 tumor of the head of pancreas and 20 tumor of the Vater-papilla. 80 patients (84.2%) had an obstructive jaundice at the time of the laparotomy. Pancreaticoduodenal resection was performed as a partial pancreatectomy (classic resection or pylorus preseving modification) with PG in 44 and PJ in 51 cases. The majority of the PJ included an end to side, duct to mucosa anastomosis.
Results: The overall mortality rate was 5.2% (5/95) and the morbidity rate 53.7% (51/95). The overall incidence of pancreatic anastomosis leak was 12,35% (13/95). The incidence of pancreatic fistula was higher after PG than PJ, 9% versus 17.6% but the bleeding, required reoperation was higher in the PG group - 13.6% versus 3.9%. There was no significant difference among the two group for the length of hospital stay.
Conclusions: This retrospective single institution study demonstrates that pancreatic fistula is a common complication after PD. These data support the hypothesis, that after PG less the pancreatic anastomosis leak than in the cases with PJ, but the number of the postoperativ bleeding and delayed gastric empty are higher.

4,06

PANCREATIC DUCT OCCLUSION (PDO) WITH FIBRIN SEALANT (FS) FOR THE PROTECTION OF THE PANCREATIC-DIGESTIVE ANASTOMOSIS.

Waclawiczek HW.
Ist Surgical Dept. and Ludwig-Boltzmann-Institute for Experimental and Gastroenterol. Surg., Landeskliniken Salzburg, A-5020 Salzburg, Austria

The pancreatic-digestive anastomosis is then highly endangered when a normal lienal pancreatic tissue after pancreatic head resection has to be anastomosed with the jejunum. In the literature many procedures for the permanent as well as the temporary elimination of the exocrine pancreatic secretion are known which in most cases is responsible for the anastomosis-related complications. In animal experiments we could show the efficiency of PDO with FS for the protection of this anastomosis; in the meantime we could gain great experience with this method in clinical trials.
Methods:
Since 1987 we subjected 101 patients to partial duodenopancreatectomies (Whipple's procedure) due to pancreatic head or peri-ampullary carcinomas. After typical pancreatic head resection the duct of the remaining lienal pancreas was intubated with a thin catheter and then occluded with an average of 2 (± 0.4) ml FS. A high concentration of aprotinin (antifibrinolytic substance) of 20.000 I.U./ml added to the sealant is required to prevent a premature dissolution prior to the 5th postoperative day. Then the remaining pancreas was anastomosed in single-layer fashion.
Results:
The postoperative lethality rate amounted to 1.9 % (n = 2) and was not method-related. In 3 cases bile fistulas occurred, in one a partial liver necrosis and in another one a colonic necrosis, which required relaparotomies. No postoperative pancreatic fistulas occurred. A remarkable fact is that postoperatively only 5 of the patients suffered from exocrine and only 3 from endocrine, insulin-dependent insufficiencies.
Conclusion:
The PDO with FS represents a safe and effective method for the protection of the pancreatic-digestive anastomosis and can therefore be recommended for Whipple's procedure.

4,07

PYLORUS-PRESERVING (P.P) PANCREATODUODENECTOMY (PD) WITH PANCREATIC STUMP OCCLUSION.

L.Papastamatiou, L.Lapidakis, G.Papoutsis.
Dep.of Surgery, Apostle Paul Hosp.-KAT Athens HELLAS.

Resection of malignancies causing obstructive jaundice still present high mortality and morbidity rates. To the standard Whipple procedure a lot of modifications are proposed, aiming mainly to reduce early postoperative mortality. From those modifications p.p.P.D. seems to be popular among surgeons.The crucial point is the management of the pancreatic remnant, as complications of pancreatic anastomoses increase mortality rates. The suture of the pancreatic stump, although described over than 20 years ago did not win wide surgeons confidence.

The extension of Whipple procedure seems as an excessive operation, when its results are compared with those of more conservative resections. The combination of p.p.P.D. with simple occlusion of the pancreatic stump and elective suture of the main pancreatic duct has been the procedure of choice in the treatment of resectable carcinomas of the pancreatic head and the periampullary region. Thus, 17 patients (7 pancr.cancers, 3 duodenal tumors, 3 lower bile duct cancers, 4 ampulla tumors) were subjected to this operative procedure. The operative tactic comprised subtotal P.D. occlusion of the pancreatic remnant with a TA 55 stapler, after elective ligation of the main pancreatic duct, when possible and fixation of the bile duct stump to the jejunal loop, before its end to end to the duodenal remnant anastomosis, lately by the use of a BAR (Valtrac) ring. The mean operative time was 105 min and the mean blood units needed 2.4. No mortality occured, but morbidity rate was high, comprising in 8 patients pancreatic external fistula (47%). All 8 cases were treated conservatively and fistulae healed spontaneously in a mean time of 2.8 months (15d-6m).
Later on 2 of the above cases a pancreatic pseudocyst developped-one spontaneously absorbed, one still (8m) under observation.
It is concluded that p.p.P.D. with pancreatic stump occlusion is a quiq and safe procedure, which deserves a wider use in the treatment of malignant obstructive jaundice.

4,08

ADENOCARCINOMA OF PAPILLA VATERI-APPLIED TREATMENT

Saric P., Djurovic D-. Vukmirovic B.
Department of General Surgery
Health centre „dr. R. Simonovic"-Vojvodjanska,
Zombor, Yugoslavia

Adenomatous changes on the Papila Vateri are evident with c.3% of the patients operated on the biliary tract. Three forms of adenocarcinoma may lend themselves to macroscopic examination: a tiny, firm, calculus-like change, a pseudopolipous formation and an ulcerous laesion of duodenum wall. Cholangiographic differentiation of the changes with sclerotized papillitis is insuitable. due to the regularly resulting.
Presentation of applied principle of oncologic surgery in the treatment adenocarcinoma of papilla Vateri.
Patient, S.J. in his 60s, showed signs of fluctuating icterus 4 months ago after which cholecystectomy with biopsy of the 1st gland of the choledochus was performed ex tempore-benign. Choledochotomy is applied to explore the distal choledochus while puspose of duodenotomy is to incspect the area of the papilla Vateri, where firm infiltrate may be found which then is sampled for PH analysis. The final stage of the operation is papilloplasty. PH finding: the glands of the papilla protrude into the cosiderably proliferated surrounding fibrous tissue. After 3 month, with CT and ERCP, an operation as per Wipple is performed. Transduodenal excision is indicated with pseudo-polypous carcinomatous laesions on condition that the gland of the choledochus is not affected by a carcinoma. Polypous formation displays relatively low biological activity. With remaining two cases cephalic duodenopancreatectomy is indicated, which is radical solution applied most often. Carcinoma of papilla slowly spreads to neighbouring strictures enabling thus relatively easy operative intervention. Operative mortality rate ranges between 6% and 35% of the patients.

4,09

NEW RECONSTRUCTIONAL METHOD IN THE SURGICAL TREATMENT OF CARCINOMA OF PAPILLA OF VATER

P.Árkossy, P.Tóth, I.Kovács, P.Sápy
2nd Department of Surgery of University Medical School of Debrecen, Hungary

Aims: The radical operation of the papilla of Vater is the pancreatoduodenectomy. The mortality rate of the surgical treatment of the carcinoma of the Vater's papilla decreased in the last decade, but there is a high risk of the reconstructional procedures of the remnant pancreas regarding the complications of the anastomoses. The authors introduced a new type of reconstructional procedure to decrease the complications.
Methods: Between 1991 and 1997, 87 pancreatoduodenectomy procedures were performed for chronic pancreatitis, carcinoma of the pancreas and papilla of Vater. 28 patients were operated on for carcinoma of the papilla of Vater. In 18 of these cases pancreatoduodenectomy was performed. Of the 18 cases using the pylorus-preserving pancreatoduodenectomy, 12 cases involved pancreatogastrostomy using a single layer suture, while in 6 cases the new reconstructional method was used: after the removal of the pancreatic head and body an end to side, duct to mucosa type anastomosis was executed between the pancreatic duct and a Roux-en jejunal loop. The second anastomosis of the procedure was an end to side choledochojejunostomy, the third was an end to side duodenojejunostomy. The duodenojejunostomy was performed about 40 cm far from the pancreatic anastomosis, keeping food far from the pancreas against peristaltic waves.
Results: Two patients had reoperations for partial suture insuffitiency of the pancreatogastrostomic anastomosis. In these patients the pancreas was softer and more glandular. In these cases the tissue held sutures less well, requiring knotting to be done more carefully to avoid rupture. I such situations we used new type of reconstructional procedure.
Conclusion: This method of reconstruction allows for spontaneous closure and safe drainage of potential insufficient pancreaticojejunostomy. The recovered patients suppord future favourable usage of this new reconstructional surgical procedure.

Dig Surg 1999; 16 (suppl 1): 20-22

HPB research II.

5.01

ENDOTHELIN AND ENDOTHELIN ANTAGONISTS DO NOT INFLUENCE ICG-KINETICS AFTER HEPATIC ISCHEMIA IN RATS.

Riesener KP, Matziolis G, Kasperk R, Schmid-Schönbein G*, Hektor J*, Schumpelick V
Dept. of Surgery, Institute of Physiology*, RWTH Aachen, 52057 Aachen, Germany

Aims: The vasoactive peptid endothelin is considered responsible for ischemia-reperfusion injuries following hepatic warm ischemia. Indocyanine green (ICG) clearance serves as a valuable liver function test in men and is used in our animal experiments for evaluation of the postischemic liver function influenced by endothelin and the receptor antagonists BQ 123 and LU 302872.
Methods: Experiments were performed in 112 male Sprague-Dawley rats. Following a midline laparotomy hepatic warm ischemia was induced by selective occlusion of the left and median lobe for 15 and 30 minutes, respectively. Portal entrapment was not observed, as the blood was able to pass the right and caudate hepatic lobe during ischemia. Following reperfusion the latter segments were resected, thus only postischemic tissue was left in situ. After 15 minutes 0,5 mg/kg body weight ICG were injected as a bolus. The distribution of ICG was followed using in-vivo fluorescence photometry of the caval vein, liver, kidney, and duodenum.
Results: Hepatic vasoconstriction was observed in animals pretreated with endothelin. Postischemic ICG-kinetics were not markedly influenced by endothelin or BQ 123. Endothelin enhanced the postischemic transaminase levels compared to BQ 123 or controls without treatment. In contrast, the combined ETA- and ETB-antagonist LU 302872 led to a decrease in venous ICG-clearance and biliary ICG-excretion. This was paralleled by an increase of the bilirubin level against controls.
Conclusions: In-vivo-ICG-fluorescence-photometry allows the intraoperative measurement of the ICG-kinetics in small animals. While endothelin and BQ 123 did not markedly influence hepatic anion transport function following warm ischemia, LU 302872 deteriorated venous ICG clearance and biliary ICG-excretion with and without the influence of ischemia. The endothelin-derived disturbance of hepatic microcirculation following warm ischemia does not markedly influence hepatic function parameters in rats.

5.02

EFFECTS OF SUPEROXIDE ANIONS AND HYPOXIA INACTIVATE ENDOTHELIUM-DERIVED RELAXING ISCHEMIC-REPERFUSION IN RATS

Fan Chun, Wan Xiaoping, et al
National Hepatobiliary and Enteric Surgery Research Center, Ministry ofHealth, Changsha, Hunan, 410008 P.R.China

The animal model of intestinal ischemic-reperfusion was set up by 1 hour of total occlusion of superior mesenteric artery followed by 1 hour of reperfusion. The endothelin-1 (ET-1) of the plasma and intestinal tissue were investigated in all 23 rats which were divided into three group:
Sham group (n=8), intestinal ischemic-reperfusion model group (n-7),
Superoxidase (SOD) (15000u/kg) -treated group (n=8). The results show that ET-1 of the plasma and intestinal tissue was significantly increased in intestinal ischemic-reperfusion group and was significantly decreased in SOD-treated group than intestinal ischemic-reperfusion group.

This study suggests that SOD suppressed effectually elevation of ET-1 in plasma and tissue during intestinal ischemic-reperfusion in rats.

5.03

INDUCTION OF ADHESION MOLECULE EXPRESSION IN LIVER ISCHAEMIA/REPERFUSION INJURY IS ASSOCIATED WITH IMPAIRED PARENCHYMAL PERFUSION

El-Wahsh M., Seifalian AM, Fuller BF, Rolles K, Davidson BR
University Department of Surgery, Royal Free and University College Medical School, The Royal Free Hospital, London, U.K.

Aims: During liver transplantation Ischaemia reperfusion (I/R) injury initiates a cascade of events leading to intensified interactions between circulating host cells and graft endothelium. The endothelium adhesion molecules are a main component of this process. The relationship between intracellular adhesion molecule-1 (ICAM-1) expression and the hepatic parenchymal microcirculation (HPM) of I/R injury has not been established.

Methods: Sprague-Dawley rats (n=24) underwent laparotomy for liver exposure. Control group (n=6) were compared with those undergoing partial liver ischaemia for 30 (group1), 45 (group2) and 60 min (group3) respectively, followed by 60 min reperfusion (all groups n=6). HPM was measured by laser Doppler flowmetry (flux unit) on the left lobe of the liver. Liver biopsies were taken at the end of reperfusion period. ICAM-1 expression was demonstrated by immunohistochemistry graded 0-3.

Results: Data expressed as mean±SE.

	Control	Gp1	Gp2	Gp3
HPM (flux unit)	230±18	140±21*	54±3*	40±7*
ICAM-1 (score)	0.5±0.2	1.3±0.2#	2.3±0.3#	2.8±0.2#

*p<0.0001 and #p<0.0001 vs control (two way ANOVA analysis)

Conclusions: Ischaemia/Reperfusion injury of the liver produces significant induction of ICAM-1 expression, which corresponds with the progressive reduction in parenchymal perfusion.

KARGER
Fax +41 61 306 12 34
E-Mail karger@karger.ch
www.karger.com

5.04

ENCHANCING PORTAL BLOOD FLOW WITH AN IMPLANTED PORTAL PUMP IMPROVED LIVER FUNCTION AND HEPATIC HAEMODYNAMICS IN A CIRRHOTIC PORCINE MODEL

Jiao L.R.[1], Havlik R.[1], Seifalian A.M.[2], Li Y.[1], Marseille O.[3], Kerkhoffs W[3], Davidson BR[2]
[1]Liver Surgery Section, Imperial Collegr School of Medicine, Hammersmith Hospital and [2]Hepatic Haemodynamic Laboratory, University Department of Surgery, Royal Free Hospital and School of Medicine, London, United Kingdom, [3]Institute of Helmholtz, University of Technology, Aachen, Germany

Aims: To asses the sort term effect of mechanically pumping the portal blood flow on hepatic haemodynamics and liver function in a cirrhotic animal model.
Methods: Large white pigs underwent laparotomy and exposure of the liver: group 1 (n-6) were normal controls, group 2 (n-6) cirrhotic. Cirrhosis was established by ligaton of common bile duct. Total hepatic blood flow (THBF) was measured by a Transonic Medical Flowmeter system. At baseline, the hepatic haemodynamics and liver function were compared between normal and cirrhotic pigs. Portal blood flow as then enhanced in the cirrhotic group using a miniature portal pump designed for human implantation. The portal blod flow was increased by 50% of the baseline value over one hour. During this period, the haemodynamic parameters were monitored continuously. Liver function was assessed pre and post portal pumping with liver function test, hepatic gluconeogenesis, alkalisation and indocyanine green clearance.
Results: Cirrhotic animals showed a significant increase in portal pressure (14±3 vs 8±2mmHg, p=0.002, mean ± sd vs controls), increased total hepatic blood flow (37±10 vs 25±4 ml/min/kg, p=0.01) and raised portal vascular resistance (p=0.03). There was a grossly abnormal liver function test, a reduced intrahepatic glucogenesis and intrahapatic and systemic metabolic acidosis.
Following one hour enhanced portal inflow in cirrhotic livers, the portal pressure in the mesentery reduced (14±3 to 6±3 mmHg, p=0.001 as did the intrahepatic portal resistance (p=0.04). Liver function was shown to have improved dramatically characterised by hepatic alkalisation (7.26±0.02 vs 7.19±0.06, pre vs post pumping p=0.02), an increased production of glucose (8±1 vs 4±1 mmol/L, p<0.001) and an increased intrahepatic ICG clearance (0.121±0.017 vs 0.027±0.003 min^{-1}, p=0.01). However, the liver function test was not changedf after one hour portal pumping.
Conclusion: A short term enhanced portal pumping in a cirrhotic animal improves hepatic haemodynamics and liver function.

5.05

PIG LIVING LIVER TRANSPLANTATION USING A VASCULAR PROSTHESIS TO REPLACE THE INTRAHEPATIC VENA CAVA

*B. Nardo, F. Catena, P. Turi, G. Cavallari, F. De Vincentis, M. Simoncini *, A. Faenza, R. Bellusci, G. Fuga, A. Principe, A. Mazziotti, A. Cavallari.*
Clinica Chirugica II, Sem. Medica*, University of Bologna, Bologna ITALY

Aims: This study aimed to determine whether the porcine model could be adapted to accomodate living donor liver transplantation (LLT). Because the pig hepatic anatomy precludes a standard approach, a study was designed to evaluate the results using a segment of vascular prosthesis to replace the intrahepatic portion of the IVC with establishment of hepatic venous drainage into the graft.
Methods: A total of 10 LLT were performed using 20 pigs. After the left hepatectomy, the intrahepatic IVC was replaced with a modified aorto-iliac prosthesis, anastomosing the proximal (aortic limb) to the infradiaphragmatic IVC, one distal iliac limb to infra hepatic IVC and the other (after shortening) to establish hepatic venous drainage after transplant. Conventional venous bypass was used, and no immunosuppressive therapy was administered. The mean body weight ratio of the donors to the recipients was 82.0 % ± 7.4 %. The relative weight of the left graft to the recipient's own liver was 65.5 % ± 13.3 %. The mean anhepatic time was 43.4 ± 4.6 min. The mean total cold ischemic time of the graft was 186 min ± 32 min.
Results: All donors survived the 10 day post hepatectomy observation period. Eight of the 10 transplanted pigs survived at least 2 days (mean, 7.6 day; range 3-13 days). No evidence of caval graft thrombosis was observed.
Conclusions: At the best of our knowledge this study shows for the first time that the replacement of the recipient intrahepatic IVC by a vascular prosthesis allows to overcome the major technical obstacle which have limited the use of pigs in LLT experimental models.

5.06

EFFECT OF REDUCED GLUTATHIONE ON INTERCELLULAR ADHESION MOLECULE-1 EXPRESSION IN REPERFUSED LIVER GRAFT.

El-Wahsh M., Fuller BJ, Seifalian AM, Davidson BR, Rolles K
University Department of Surgery and Liver Transplant Unit, Royal Free and University College Medical School, The Royal Free Hospital, London, UK.

Aim: To investigate the effect of adding glutathione (GSH) to the liver perfusate on Intercellular Adhesion Molecule-1 (ICAM-1) expression of a cold preserved plus reperfused liver graft.

Methods: Livers of Sprague-Dawley rats (n=24) were flushed with UW solution and preserved for 4 h (group 1, n=6) or 18 h (group 2, n=6). In additional group (n=6), GSH was added to the UW solution and preserved for 4 h. Livers were biopsied at the end of reperfusion. Control group (n=6) underwent laparotomy for liver exposure and biopsy alone. ICAM-1 expression was assessed by immunohistochemistry and graded 0-3.

Results: Data are expressed as mean±SE. Table shows the effect of GSH addition to the perfusion solution.

	control	Gp1	Gp2	GSH Gp
ICAM-1 (score)	0.50±0.22	2.33±0.21*&	2.50±0.22*&	1.33±0.21

*P < 0.0004 vs control (Two way ANOVA analysis), &P<0.0182 vs GSH group.

Conclusion: The addition of GSH, as oxygen free radical scavenger to the cold storage solution can reduced ICAM-1induction.

5.07

DIFFERENTIAL UPREGULATION OF CELLULAR ADHESION MOLECULES AT THE SITES OF OXIDATIVE STRESS DURING THE EARLY COURSE OF EXPERIMENTAL ACUTE PANCREATITIS.

G. Telek°, R. Ducroc° J.Y. Scoazec, J. Chariot°, G. Feldmann*, C. Rozé°.*
INSERM U410°, U327*, Faculté de Médecine Xavier Bichat, Paris, France.

Aims: Acinar injury in acute necrotizing pancreatitis (ANP) results in upregulation of cellular adhesion molecules (CAMs) on periacinar endothelial cells and cytokine release. The adherent polymorphonuclear leukocytes (PMNs) become activated to release oxygen free radicals (OFRs) and harmful enzymes. An uncontrolled inflammatory cascade may be locally, systemically deleterious. We have developed a novel technique based on the cerium capture method to detect histologically the formation of OFRs in vivo. Reaction of OFR-s with $CeCl_3$ results in cerium-perhydroxide precipitations, which can be detected by their laser reflecting properties using reflectance confocal laser scanning microscopy (CLSM). In parallel the fluorescence channels can be used to demonstrate immunolabeled CAMs. We show CAM protein expression in relation to oxidative stress in ANP. CAM gene activation was measured by semiquantive RT-PCR (MIMIC). **Methods:** Classic Taurocholate ANP was induced in Wistar rats. After 1, 2, 8, 24h the animals were perfused with $CeCl_3$ solution (20 mM) through the abdominal aorta, then sacrificed. Control rats received the same $CeCl_3$ perfusion. Indirect immunofluorescence (IF) was performed on serial frozen sections of pancreata to label E-selectin, P-selectin, ICAM-1, VCAM-1 molecules. Observation of CAM-IF, cerium reflectance and cell types was performed by CLSM. From non-perfused animals total pancreatic mRNA was reverse transcribed into cDNA, which was amplified using specific primers for the above CAM-s together with MIMIC Internal Standards of the respective CAM primers. Competition between known amounts of MIMIC and unknown quantities of pancreatic CAM cDNA allows quantification. **Results:** The capillaries in normal pancreata showed sparse P-selectin and ICAM-1 positivity. Reflectance signals were negligible. At 1, 2h of ANP increased endothelial P-selectin, and ICAM-1 immunoreactivity was observed. Strong, OFR-derived cerium reflectance signals were detected in the acinar cells near CAM positive pancreatic capillaries, frequently with adherent PMN-s. PMN-s presented weak, mostly intracellular reflectance signals. At 8, 24h intense PMN infiltration, strong, mostly perinecrotic P-selectin, and ICAM-1, but moderately increased E-selectin, and VCAM-1 expression was observed. Acinar OFR signals were weakened, in contrast, PMN-s showed intense OFR production. **CONCLUSION:** CAM-s are upregulated early in experimental ANP at the sites of acinar OFR production in a specific, time dependent pattern, with rapid and strikingly high P-selectin and increased ICAM, but modestly elevated E-selectin and VCAM expression. Adherence to CAMs may play a role in the activation of leukocytes. At the earliest time points the major source of OFRs seems to be the acinus (Xanthine-oxidase), later the activated PMN-s, thereby contributing to the organ damage.

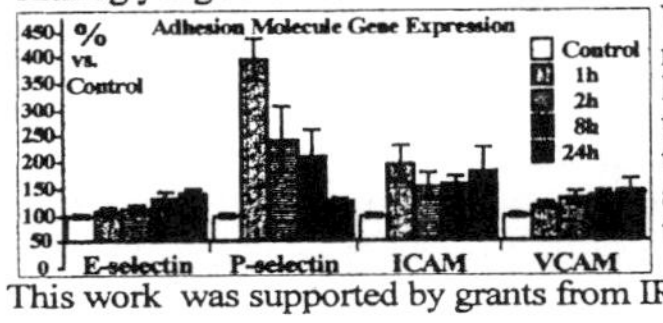

This work was supported by grants from IRMAD Foundation and Solvay Pharma.

5.08

COMBINATION THERAPY IN FULMINANT ACUTE PANCREATITIS

Andersson R., Sun ZW, Haraldsen P, Lasson Å, Wang XD
Department of Surgery, Lund University Hospital, Sweden

Aims: The majority of deaths related to acute pancreatitis (AP) is related to multiple organ dysfunction (MODS), where an increase in endothelial barrier permeability probably plays a central role, as does alterations in cytokine response and protease inhibitor levels. Previous experimental studies have implied beneficial effects of pretreatment and early treatment of platelet activating factor (PAF) inhibitors and antibodies against adhesion molecules. The aim of the present study was to evaluate single and combination therapies in fulminant AP.
Methods: AP was induced by intraductal infusion of taurodeoxycholate in the rat. Microvascular endothelial permeability was evaluated by leakage of radiolabelled human serum albumin. Plasma protease inhibitor levels were determined as were serum levels of interleukines (1 (and 6) and morfology (light and electron microscopy). Treatment was performed one or three hours after induction of AP with the PAF inhibitor lexipafant, monoclonal antibodies (MAb) against PECAM-1, the antioxidant NAC, lexipafant + PECAM-1 MAb, NAC + lexipafant, NAC + PECAM-1 Mab or lexipafant + PECAM-1 MAb + NAC. Determinations were performed 6 hours after induction of AP.
Results: AP resulted in a significant increase ($p < 0.01$) in endothelial barrier permeability in all organs stud and consumption on protease inhibitors. In general, the antioxidant NAC was sufficient in normalizing the changes though less effective in the lungs. Treatment with lexipafant or PECAM-1 MAb only resulted in partial restoration of the alterations, not reaching normal levels
($p < 0.05$ vs sham). The combination of lexipafant and NAC or even more efficiantly, especially in the lungs, of PECAM-1 MAb and NAC, restored integrity of the endothelial barrier to at least levels seen in sham operated animals.
Conclusions: Treatment with a PAF inhibitor (lexipafant) or monoclonal antibodies against PECAM-1 were only partly effective in restoring endothelial barrier dysfunction in fulminant acute pancreatitis. The antioxidant NAC and especially combinations of NAC and lexipafant or PECAM-1 antibodies were efficient, speaking in favour of multimodal therapy in the treatment of endothelial barrier dysfunction and the prevention of organ failure.

5.09

FUSIDINE AND THE CYTOKINE RESPONSE IN AN EXPERIMENTAL MODEL OF ACUTE PANCREATITIS

[1]Osman M. O., [2]El-Sefi T., [1]Lausten S.B., [3]Jacobsen N.O., [4]Larsen C.G., [1]Jensen S.L.
Depts. of [1]Surgery, [3]Pathology and [4]Dermatology, Aarhus University, Denmark and Department of Surgery, [2]Liver Institute, Menoufiya University, Egypt.

Aims : To test the potential effects of sodium fusidate (Fusidine) on the course of severe AP in rabbits.

Methods : AP was induced in 20 rabbits by retrograde injection of 5% chenodeoxycholic acid in the pancreatic duct. The rabbits were allocated to pretreatment with intravenous physiological saline or sodium fusidate (80 mg/kg) 30 min. beforethe induction of AP. Serum amylase, lipase,TNF-α, IL-8, glucose, calcium and leucocytic count were measured every three hours for a total of 12 hours. By the end of the experiment, ascitic fluid was collected and the pancreatic, lung, and kidney tissues were obtained for histology.

Results : Pretreatment with sodium fusidate reduced the mortality rate from 60% to 30% ($p< 0.05$) and the output of ascitic fluid ($p< 0.001$). Serum TNF-α and IL-8 were significantly reduced in the treated group from 5 min. up to 9 hours. The leucopenia observed after 3 hours in the untreated group was significantly improved ($p<0.001$). By contrast, both treated and untreated rabbits had similar biochemical changes including amylase, lipase, glucose and calcium as well as histologic changes in the pancreas and lungs.

Conclusions: Pretreatment with sodium fusidate resulted in a considerable reduction in mortality and ascitic fluid output in rabbits with bile-induced AP, probably by lowering the TNF-α and IL-8 blood levels. However, pretreatment with sodium fusidate did not alter the local or systemic manifestations of AP. Thus, other cytokines than TNF-α and IL-8 are likely to mediate the local and systemic manifestations of AP.

5.10

INTERSTITIAL LASER-INDUCED THERMOTHERAPY OF A RAT LIVER TUMOUR: EFFECT OF TEMPERATURE AND HEPATIC INFLOW OCCLUSION

Tranberg K-G, Sturesson C, Ivarsson K, Stenram U, Andersson-Engels S
Departments of Surgery, Physics and Pathology, University of Lund, Sweden

Aim: Interstitial laser-induced thermotherapy (ILT) was used to treat rat liver tumours at suboptimal temperatures. The aim was to investigate the influence of temperature and temporary hepatic inflow occlusion (HIO) on tumour growth and blood perfusion.

Method: A dimethylhydrazine-induced adenocarcinoma was implanted into the left lateral lobe of the rat liver. Thermotherapy was performed utilising a Nd:YAG laser with a plane-cut fibre placed in the tumour. Liver tumours were treated with ILT, giving 44°C at the tumour border for 30 min, HIO only, or a combination of these methods. Interstitial laser Doppler flowmetry was used to measure hepatic perfusion at the tumour border during and after heat treatment, for a total time of 60 min. Tumour growth was assessed 6 days after treatment.

Results: Six days after treatment a significant reduction in tumour growth was found in both laser-treated groups as compared to control. Tumours subjected to the combined treatment of HIO and ILT displayed lower perfusion 30 min after treatment and reduced growth as compared to tumours treated with either method alone.

Conclusion: A combination of hepatic inflow occlusion and interstitial laser heating lowered tumour growth, as compared to either method alone. The increased efficiency was associated with an immediate effect on tumour blood perfusion.

Dig Surg 1999; 16 (suppl 1): 23-25

Chronic pancreatitis

T.L. Hwang	*H.M. Chen*	*6,01*
M.F. Chen		
M. Santoro	*M. De Luca*	*6,02*
C. Chiacchio	*V. Forestieri*	
P. Forestieri		
Á. Pap		*6,03*
I. Kovács	*P. Tóth*	*6,04*
P. Árkosy	*L. Veres*	
Zs. Szentkereszty	*P. Sápy*	
L. Kotsis	*Sz. Kostic*	*6,05*
Z. Salló	*B. Erdélyi*	*6,06*
T. Horváth	*E. Orosz*	
Gy. Farkas	*E. Nagy*	*6,07*
Z. Morvay	*L. Leindler*	
A.K. Zacharof	*C. Ptrogiannopoulos*	*6,08*
H. Zacharof		
A. Magyar	*L. Flautner*	*6,09*
T.F. Tihanyi	*I. Pulay*	
V. Usatoff	*A. Isla*	*6,10*
A. Hadi	*T. Worthington*	
R.C.N. Williamson		

6,01

SURGICAL TREATMENT OF CHRONIC OBSTRUCTIVE PANCREATITIS

Hwang TL, Chen HM, Chen MF
Department of Surgery, Chang Gung Memorial Hospital, Chang Gung University, Taipei, TAIWAN

Aim: Chronic obstructive pancreatitis usually manifests with intractable pain and recurrent episodes of chronic pancreatic inflammation. The side-to-side pancreaticojejunostomy is used for these patients with a large pancreatic duct. But for the patients with small pancreatic duct, the optimal surgical procedure needs to be evaluated.

Methods: For the patients with small pancreatic duct, we used end to side pancreaticojejunostomy instead of pancreaticoduodenectomy in recent two years. The results were compared between two groups. Fourteen patients, all were male, with chronic obstructive pancreatitis were included. The sufferred from intractable abdominal pain with or without steatorrhea. Preoperative MR-CP or ERCP confirmed the diagnosis. Seven patients (Group A) underwent distal pancreatectomy plus end-to-side pancreatico-jejunostomy, and the other seven patients (Group B) underwent pancreaticoduodenectomy were compared.

Results: The operative time was significantly shorter in the group A. There were no operative morbidity in the patients of group A. The postoperative follow up of patients in group A had better outcome with body weight gain and no stertorrhea, all of them were complete pain relief. The patients in group B had less better outcome and body weight gain, but high incidence of postoperative DM.

Conclusions: We concluded that distal pancreatectomy with end-to-side pancreaticojejunostomy provided a better surgical treatment for the patients with chronic obstructive pancreatitis and small pancreatic duct.

6,02

LONG-TERM RESULTS AFTER SURGICAL DERIVATIVE TREATMENT FOR CHRONIC PANCREATITIS.

Santoro M, De Luca M., Chiacchio C., Forestieri V. and Forestieri P.
Chair of Oncological Surgery, "Federico II" University of Naples, Italy.

Background: the purpose of this short report has been the evaluation of results after surgical derivative treatment in patients affected by chronic pancreatitis observed in the last twenty years.
Material and Methods: from September1977 to September 1997, 228 patients (180 males, 48 females with a mean age of 41.6 years) suffering form chronic pancreatitis have been valued. Main aetiologic factors were: alcoholic (41%); obstructive (54%); other causes (5%). 103 patients (45%) suffered from diabetes (49 type 1 and 54 type 2); pseudocysts were detected in 154 patients (68%); main pancreatic duct was larger than 7 mm in 218 patients (96%) while calcifications were found in 164 (72%). Principal symptoms were: severe pain (71%), moderate pain (24%), jaundice (38%), digestive disorders (84%); palpable mass (24%).
Results and Conclusions: mortality rate was 1.7% (2 patients died after surgical treatment for massive hemorrhage and 2 for MOF); 19 patients (8.3%) developed important abdominal complications (17 pancreatic fistulas) treated with medical care in a mean lenght of time of 43 days (range 23-52). After a median follow-up of 10 years (range 1-18), the following results have been obtained: 29 patients (13%) died most frequently of cancer (19 cases), 12 of them developed a pancreatic carcinoma; 43 pts (19%) suffered from type 2 diabetes after surgery (mean interval 4 years, range 1-8); moreover, 34 out of the 54 type 2 preoperative diabetics needed insulin after a mean interval of 4.5 years; 198 patients (87%) referred significant pain reduction while 65% of them were painless at 5 years. Preoperative body-weight loss was statistically significant and surgery resulted in a significant and progressive gain with a peak after 3-4 years (mean 67.7 Kg). These data confirmed that surgery seems to affect positively pain and weight gain; besides, it was safely performed with a short number of important complications. In conclusion, according to our experience, derivative procedures should be the surgical treatment of choice, whenever possible, in patients suffering from chronic pancreatitis.

References:

1. A. Bonora, M. Falconi, C. Bassi et al. Long-term results in 364 patients submitted to surgical derivative procedures for chronic pancreatitis. Ital J Gastroenterol 1994; 26 (5):255.

6,02

MULTIPLE STENTS FOR BILIARY STENOSIS CAUSED BY CHRONIC PANCREATITIS

Á. Pap
Gastroenterology, MAV Hospital, Budapest, Hungary

Common bile duct (CBD) stenosis due to fibrosis and/or inflammation is a prevalent complication of chronic calcifying pancreatitis (CCP). Endoscopic stenting is the method of choice for CBD obstruction because recovery from relapses regularly results in resolution of stenosis. However, clogging of endoprosthesis with suppurative cholangitis is a frequent complication during the long period necessary for resolution of stenosis. 62 pts with biliary stenosis due to CCP were admitted to our institution from 1/93 to 12/96 (46 males and 16 females, mean age 45 yrs, range 30-75 yrs), 20 pts (32%) had previous pancreatic surgery. 44 pts received a simple 10F drain because of a recent attack of CCP. In other 16 pts with more stable CCP 2 large stents, in 2 similar cases 3x10F stents were placed into the common bile duct during a 3-6 month accommodation period. In 10 pts (16%) a temporary naso-biliary drainage was necessary to prevent suppurative cholangitis and early clogging of the stents. Pts were controlled by US and laboratory tests at 3 mos and ERCP at 6 mos. Stent obstruction occurred in 33% of the pts with one drain only (mean time 12 mos). The others recovered from the biliary stenosis or they were supplied with a 2nd stent. Biliary drainage remained satisfactory for about 22 mos in the pts with multiple stents and occlusion occurred only in 3/18 cases (17%). In 5 pts the stents were extracted because free movements of drains were evident at the 3rd endoscopy. In one pt. the stents spontaneously disappeared from the common bile duct. The remaining pts are doing well with stents. Conclusion: endoscopic stenting can replace surgical bypass for biliary stenosis caused by CCP. Multiple stents may dilate the strictures progressively and remain patent for the long recovery period.

KARGER
Fax +41 61 306 12 34
E-Mail karger@karger.ch
www.karger.com

6.04

STRATEGIES IN THE MANAGEMENT OF MEDIASTINAL PANCREATIC PSEUDOCYST. CASE REPORT AND REVIEW OF LITERATURE

Kovács L., Tóth P., Árkossy P., Veres L., Szentkereszty Zs., Sápy P
2nd Department of Surgery, University Medical School of Debrecen, Hungary

Aims: Pancreatic pseudocysts remain a challenging problem in pancreatitis. Pancreatic mediastinal pseudocyst is a rare condition. Sixty-five cases have been reported in the English language literature over the past 25 years. Extrapancreatic fluid collections occur most commonly in the lesser sac,but are also frequently seen in the anterior and posterior pararenal spaces. Less common sites include the mediastinum, liver, retroperitoneum, spleen or pelvis. Currently, there is some debate concerning the appropriate management of large pancreatic pseudocysts. We present the clinical and praeoperative findings of such cases, the results of operative treatment and review of literature to chose the conservative treatment or CT guided percutaneous drainage as an alternative to surgical teratment.

Methods: The last five years 103 patients were treated with pancreatic pseudocysts. 12 patients underwent CT guided percutaneous drainage. 89 patients had enteric drainage. Cystectomy were performed in two cases. Cysto-gastrostomy in 33, Juras intervention in 12, cysto-duodenostomy in 20, Wirsungo-cysto-jejunostomy in 7, Wirsungo-cysto-gastrostomy in 13 and splenectomy with pancreatic tail resection in 1 case were performed. Three patients had mediastinal pseudocyst. The pseudocyst size was greater than 10cm in diameter in 14 patients. The most common primary causes were chronic alcoholics, gallstones inducated secondary pancreatitis and trauma. The indications of interventions were fever, sepsis, pain, biliary obstructions and gastric outlet obstruction, in cases with mediastinal pseudocyst were chest or back pain, dysphagia, dyspnoe, nausea vomiting and weight loss.

Results: The mediastinal pseudocysts entered the mediastinum through the esophageal or aortic hiatus in two cases, in one case through the foramen Morgagni. Several reports described direct penetration through the diapragm. After adequate internal drainage the mediastinal mass and components are rapidly disappear, included clinical manifestations and compliences. There was no perioperative death.

Conclusions: The operative management of pancreatic pseudocysts aims to evacuate the cyst contents and prevent the serious complications of cyst rupture, haemorrhage, infections, intestinal obstruction, external compression of heart and lung. Although our experience treating mediastinal pancreatic pseudocysts is limited, it would seem the most expedient method is an internal drainage procedure, preferably cysto-gastrostomy.

6.05

TRANSDIAPHRAGMATIC CYST-JEJUNOSTOMY WITH ROUX EN-Y LOOP FOR AN EXCLUSIVELY MEDIASTINAL PANCREATIC PSEUDOCYST

Kotsis L,Kostic Sz.
Thoracic Surgical Clinic Budapes,Hungary

Diagnostical and surgical aspects of an exclusively pancreatic pseudocyst is presented. On admission the patient had an softtissue density in the retrocardiac area with left pleural effusion on chest x-ray.Based on the displacement of the distal esophagus,suspicion of a pseudocyst in the posterior mediastinum has been confirmed by echocardiography. Etanol abuse in history and abnormal high amylase level of the pleural effusion suggested pancreatic origin of the pseudocyst.At left thoraco-laparotomy the large (9oo ml) mediastinal pseudocyst surrounded the aorta and was adherent to the diaphragm,having a high concentration of amylase.Decompression was established with a retrocolic and gatric Roux-en-Y loop by transdiaphragmatic cyst-jejunostomy. The patient recovered uneventfully.During follow up (1o years) there was no sign of recurrence.Internal drainage with cyst-jejunostomy on the lower portion of an exclusively mediastinal pseudocyst may be considered as the method of choice for definitive treatment.

6.06

SURGICAL MANAGEMENT OF PANCREATIC PSEUDOANEURYSM

Salló Z. Erdélyi B., Horváth T., Orosz E.

Markhot Ferenc County Hospital, Eger, Hungary
Department of General and Vascular Surgery

Aim of this study was to determine the value of the surgical management of pancreatic pseudoaneurysm.
Methods. In the last 9 years 12 patients were treated at the authors department with pancreatic pseudoaneurysm. The authors analyze retrospective the data of these patients. They also analyze the diagnostic and therapeutical methods.
Results. Radiological procedures such as ultrasound (US), computed tomography (CT) and angiography are essential in precise morphological localization and extent of these complications. All the patients were treated succesfully by operation. The operation has to goals: to manage the pseudoaneurysm feeding artery and to treat the synchronous pancreatic disease. In 10 cases the selective feeding artery ligation was performed simultaneously with additional operations (pancreatic resection, splenectomy, drainage). In two cases the feeding artery was ligated from the interior of the pseeudoaneurysm. Two reoparations for septic complication occured and in two cases the external pancreatic fistula closed on the effect of conservative therapy.
Conclusion. Surgical management is usefull in the treatment of pancreatic pseudoanerysm and remains the base therapy by the side of the interventional radiological procedures. Authors stress the importance of accurate preoparative diagnosis and they call attention to the advantage of selective feeding artery ligation.

6.07

Surgical and radiological management of vascular complications following necrotizing pancreatitis

Farkas Gy., Nagy E., Morvay Z.*, Leindler L.*
Department of Surgery and Institute of Radiology*, A. Szent-Györgyi Medical University, Szeged, Hungary

Aims: Major arterial hemorrhage associated with pancreatic pseudocysts or abscess following necrotizing pancreatitis presents a life-threatening complication. This study was undertaken to analyze the role of the radiological and surgical management in the diagnosis and treatment of this complication.
Methods: In the past 10 years, 12 patients with arterial hemorrhage were identified. Nine patients presented with intracystic bleeding, and 3 with intrapancreatic abscess. Evidence of pseudocyst or abscess bleeding was revealed in 9 patients by a contrast-enhanced CT scan, and the site of the bleeding was identified by means of selective visceral angiography in 6 patients. The rupture of a major artery was identified perioperatively in 3 patients. Seven patients had splenic artery bleeding, 4 gastroduodenal artery bleeding, and 1 superior mesenteric artery bleeding.
Results: Angiographic embolization for control of the hemorrhage was applied in 6 patients before operation. All 12 patients underwent surgical therapy: transcystic arterial ligation and internal pancreatic pseudocyst drainage in 5 cases, distal pancreatectomy in 4 cases, and Beger's pancreatic head resection in 3 cases. No rebleeding or mortality occurred in the postoperative period.
Conclusions: Accurate diagnosis through a dynamic CT scan and angiography and control of the bleeding with angiographic embolization improved the outcome of the surgical therapy, which is recommended to be pancreatic resection or internal drainage with transcystic arterial ligation.

6.08

CHRONIC PANCREATITIS AND PRIMARY HYPERPARATHYROIDISM.

Antonis.K.Zacharof,C.Petrogiannopoulos,H.Zacharof.
2nd Department of Internal Medicine,Hellenic Red Cross Hospital,Athens,Hellas.

Objective: The frequency of chronic pancreatitis in primary hyperparathyroidism has decreased substantiality due to earlier diagnosis and operative treatment.
Patients and Methods: We investigated from the year 1983 to 1997,two hundred and forty five hospitalized patients with chronic pancreatitis in a prospective long term study to verify this topic.
Results: Over the last fifteen years,245 hospitalized patients with chronic pancreatitis have been studied. One hundred and ninety nine patients suffered from alcohol-induced (88% with calcifications) and 46 from non-alcohol-induced chronic pancreatitis (77% with calcifications).Primary hyperparathyroidism was found in 4 patients (3 males, 1 female), i.e 8.7% of non-alcohol-induced chronic pancreatitis. In 3 patients with primary painless chronic calcific pancreatitis the condition was diagnosed twice incidentally and once because of diabetes mellitus. Chronic pancreatitis was diagnosed in 3 patients before the onset of primary hyperparathyroidism and once simultaneously. In all patients the chronic pancreatitis was initially misinterpreted as alcohol-induced. Severe exocrine pancreatic insufficiency was present in 2 of 4 patients and diabetes mellitus in 3 of 4 patients. At the time of diagnosis of primary hyperparathyroidism, mean serum calcium was 12,32±1,72 mg/dl (3.08 ± 0.43 mmol/l).
Conclusions: The primary hyperparathyroidism continues to be a considerable cause for non alcoholic chronic pancreatitis.

6.09

SURGERY OF CHRONIC PANCREATIC PSEUDOCYSTS. RESULTS OF TEN YEAR'S.

A. Magyar, L. Flautner, T.F. Tihanyi, I. Pulay

1st Department of Surgery, Semmelweis University Medical School, Hungary

Authors analysed retrospectively data of 1060 patients underwent 1305 operations for pancreatic pseudocysts complicating chronic pancreatitis (CP) in between 1987-1996. The surgical procedures of choice were drainage (D) procedures in 84.4%, resection in 15.6%. The majority (87%) of D procedures were internal. The traditional Juras operation (4%) was mainly replaced by posterior cysto-gastrostomy (8%). We preferred blunt forced cysto-duodenostomy (70%) and only 1.7% cysto-jejunostomy were performed. Efforts have been made to resolve the morphological alterations of the duct of Wirsung caused by CP. This has been achieved by pancreatic duct decompression procedures such as cysto-Wirsungo-gastrostomy (14.4%), and sphincteroplasty of the papilla of Vater. These decompressive procedures with the internal D of the pseudocyst represent the combined operation group (54.2%). The morbidity was 12.9%. The early postoperative mortality was 1.51%, and was significantly more frequent in cases of complications requiring reoperations (3%). Conclusions: The best operations for CP pseudocysts have been the internal D procedures. The treatment of CP may require combined surgical procedure. The cystogastric and cystoduodenal anastomosis are just as effective, but with shorter operation time, as the Roux-en-Y cysto-jejunostomies recommended by others in the literature. The overall mortality rate has not been significantly affected by the combined surgical procedures.

6.10

THORACOSCOPIC SPLANCHINECTOMY FOR THE RELIEF OF PAIN IN CHRONIC

Usatoff, V., Isla A., Hadi A., Worthington T., Williamson RCN
Imperial College of Medicine
Hammersmith Hospital, London

Aims: The aim of this study was to assess the efficacy and feasability of performing video assisted thoracoscopic splanchnicectomy (TS) for the relief of pain associated with chronic pancreatitis in patients who had failed conventional treatment.

Methods: Thirteen patients with end stage chronic pancreatitis were offered a TS on the basis of its apparent efficacy in previously published series*. Most of these patients had undergone definitive pancreatic surgery and several attempts at percutaneous coeliac plexus block. The majority were long-term opiate users. The procedure was carried out in the later at thoracotomy position with the aid of double lumen endotracheal intubation and selective lung collapse. A total of 17 procedures were performed, initially the left side and then the right side of pain relief was not achieved. All patients were asked to complete a ten day diary accounting their analgesia requirements and a visual analog record of their daily pain before and after the procedure.

Results: We found that the operation could be performed with no mortality and low morbidity. The response in terms of post operative pain scores and analgesia requirements was not significantly different to preoperative levels.

Conclusions: TS for the relief of pain in patients with end-stage pain associated with chronic pancreatitis in this small series, does not seem to be effective. The procedure was however safe and easy to perform and in light of other more encouraging reports, it may need to be offered to patients before opiate use becomes a long-term problem.

*Maher JW., Johlin FC., Pearson D. Thoracoscopic splanchnicectomy for chronic pancreatitis pain. Surgery 1996. 120:603-10.

Dig Surg 1999; 16 (suppl 1): 26-28

Acute pancreatitis I.

7.01

AMINOPROCALCITONIN ASSAY ON ADMISSION IMPROVES THE PREDICTION OF SEVERITY OF ACUTE PANCREATITIS

Ammori BJ, Becker KL**, Kite P*, Barclay GR***, Snider RH**, Nylén ES**, White JC**, Martin IG, Larvin M, McMahon MJ
Academic Surgical Unit and *Department of Microbiology, The General Infirmary, Leeds, UK. **George Washington University, Washington, DC, USA. *** Blood Transfusion Services, The Royal Infirmary, Edinburgh.

AIMS: The early prediction of disease severity in patients with acute pancreatitis is important for optimal clinical management. Several components of procalcitonin (precalcitonin peptides; PCPs) are sensitive markers of inflammation and infection, and might be of value to predict severe pancreatitis. The aims of this study were to investigate the role of plasma levels of PCPs as an early indicator of severity in patients with acute pancreatitis, and to relate plasma PCPs changes to APACHE II, endotoxaemia, and the subsequent development of sepsis and death. **METHODS:** Plasma PCPs, endotoxin and antiendotoxin core antibodies were determined on admission. Admission and 24 hours APACHE II scores were calculated. C-reactive protein (CRP) was measured daily and a peak was identified. The concentration of PCPs was determined by radioimmunoassay. Attacks were classified as mild or severe according to the Atlanta criteria. **RESULTS:** There were 69 patients: 55 mild and 14 severe attacks. Patients with severe attacks had significantly greater APACHE II scores at 24 hours (median 11 vs 8, p=0.02) and peak CRP concentrations (median 202 *vs* 98 mg/l, p<0.001) compared with mild attacks. Admission PCPs concentrations were significantly greater in patients with severe attacks compared with mild (median 126 *vs* 25 fmol/ml, p=0.016), and in those who developed septic complications, fatal or not, compared to other attacks (median 247 *vs* 26.5 fmol/ml, p=0.025). By receiver operating characteristic analysis, the best cutoff level of PCPs for prediction of severe attacks was 32 fmol/ml, with higher sensitivity and specificity compared with admission APACHE II of >7 (75% *vs* 69% and 75% *vs* 45% respectively). A positive correlation was observed between admission plasma levels of PCPs and endotoxin (r=0.5, p<0.001). **CONCLUSION:** The assay of plasma PCPs during the first day of admission to hospital in patients with acute pancreatitis provided an improved prediction of severity compared to the APACHE II scoring system.

7.02

THE ROLE OF GASTROINTESTINAL ANASTOMOSIS IN THE GALLSTONE ILEUS

Michail P., Pikoulis E., Delis S., Kalahanis N., Papalambros E., Bastounis E.
First Department of Surgery, University of Athens, Medical School, Athens, Greece

Aim: The purpose of this study is to describe our experience in this rare entity and to point out the role of gastrointestinal anastomosis in the surgical treatment of gallstone ileus.
Methods: The last 5 years in the A' surgical clinic of Laiko Hospital, University of Athens 6 cases of obstructive gallstone ileus were treated surgically. The patients presented with obstructive small bowel ileus. The diagnostic approach included the x-rays of the abdomen. Gallstone was documented radiologically in one case and air in the biliary tree in 3patients. The surgical treatment included the excision of the stone with enterostomy, cholecystectomy and closure of the fistula at the same operation. In two cases with a more then 3cm in diameter duodenal defect we proceed to perform a truncal vagotomy with drainage.
Results: Morbidity included atelectasis (1 patient) and wound infection (2 patients). In one case of postoperative duodenal obstruction a truncal vagotomy and drainage was performed in the immediate post-operative period. No post-op deaths were noted.
Conclusion: Truncal vagotomy and gastrointestinal anastomosis must be performed in gallstone ileus if the closure of the duodenal defect unsafe (increase possibility of postoperative leakage or duodenal stenosis).

7.03

EARLY EBDOSCOPIC SPHINCTEROTOMY IN GALLSTONE-ASSOCIATED PANCREATITIS

Dobosz M., Babicki A., Dobrowolski S., Osęka T., Gruca Z., Wajda Z.
II Dept.of General, Gastroenterological, Endocrinological Surgery Medical University of Gdańsk, Poland

Several studies indicate that early ERCP and endoscopic sphincterotomy improve the outcome in gallstone-associated pancreatitis. The aim of the present study was to evaluate the velue of early (within the first 12 hours after the onset of the disease) endoscopic papillotomy in patients with biliary acute pancreatitis. Twenty four patients were qualified into the study. All the patients underwent emergency ERCP. The criteria for ERCP examination included: elevated serum and urine alpha-amylase activity, serum bilirubin level > 2 mg%, gallstones or widened common bile duct, and signs of pancreatitis in USG examination. In 14 patients ERCP revealed impacted stone in the ampulla of Vater, in 6 patients the ampulla was swollen, without impacted stone, in 4 patients the ampulla was macroscopically unchanged. In all the patients endoscopic papillotomy was performed. A rapid improvement of the abdominal complaints among all the patients was observed. The alpha amylase activity in serum and urine decreased from 1492 u/l and 20848 u/l to 304 u/l and 1762 u/l within two days respectively. The mean APACHE score calculated on the admission diminished from 5.2 pts. to 1.4 pts. within the 48 hours. One patients died due to acute cardiac insufficiency on the four day after the endoscopy. No complications related to endoscopic treatment were observed. Fifteen patients underwent elective cholecystectomy within 7-16 days after the onset of pancreatitis. In all the patients computed tomography revealed the oedematous form of the disease and no pancreatic necrosis was observed. The authors conclude that early ERCP with endoscopic papillotomy is beneficial in patients with gallstone-acute pancreatitis, results rapid improvement in their clinical status, and prevent from pancreatic necrosis development.

KARGER
Fax +41 61 306 12 34
E-Mail karger@karger.ch
www.karger.com

7.04

THE ROLE OF SOMATOSTATIN AND ITS ANALOGUE OCTREOTICE IN PATIENTS WITH ACUTE PANCREATITIS

Konstadoulakis M.M., Gomatos I.P., Milonaki D-. Latsaragalos S., Manouras S., Androulakis G.
1st Department of Propaedeutic Surgery, Hippocration Hospital, Athens Medical School

Aims: In this study we evaluated the effect of somatostatin (somastin) and octreotide (sandostatin) in the outcome of patients with acute pancreatitis.

Methods: We examined 60 patients with acute pancreatits. The diagnosis was based on abdominal CT scan findings. Twenty patients (group A) received somatostatin, while 40 patients received octreotide (group B).

Results: The mean hospital stay for the two groups of patients was 15.2 days (median 14, SD=4,4) and 17 days (median 13 SD=12) respectively. The mortality rate was 10% for group A (1.2-31.7%, 95% confidence intervals) and 17.5% for group B 7.3-32.7%, 95% confidence intervals).

Conclusions: The administration of inhibitors of the exocrine secretion of the pancreas is followed by a shorter hospital stay as well as a lower mortality rate in patients with acute pancreatitis. It seems that the sooner these patients start receiving this treatment, the better they respond to it.

7.05

INTENSIVE CARE OF MULTIPLE ORGAN FAILURE FOLLOWING ACUTE NECROTISING PANCREATITIS

Tarjányi M., Pulay I, Tihanyi T, Darvas K, *Kiss K., ** Vámos Z, Flautner L. Semmelweis Medical University, 1st Department of Surgery, *Department of Radiology, **Haemobil Kft., Budapest, Hungary

Aims: Multiple organ failure is a very serious complication of acute infected necrotising pancreatitis. The mortality rate of sterile (10 %) and infected (15-40%) pancreatic necrosis is different. The aim of the study was to establish the cause and frequency of respiratory complicationts and the frequency of kidney failure.

Methods: A group of 79 patients with multiple organ failure (MOF) syndrome were studied induced by acute necrotising pancreatitis. MOF was diagnosed, if the patient had 5 or more score points after Goris. Statistical analysis was done using Student test. All patients were on respirator therapy and the cause of respiratory complications were analysed retrospectively during one year. The rate of renal failure was 68 %, among them 27 required hemodialysis (HD) or hemofiltration (HF) and one of them got plasmaferesis treatment as well..

Results: The survival rate of patients suffering of MOF and acute necrotising pancreatitis was 28 %. The origin of MOF was mostly sepsis and septic shock, but sometimes the origin of SIRS (systematic inflammatory response system) is possible. MOF points of survivors were 7 (5-9) and non-survivors 10 (7-14), the difference is significant ($p<0,001$). Ranson scores of survivors were 3 and non survivors 5. There were no difference between the number of operations: Survivors underwent an average of 3,5 (1-9) and non-survivors 3 (1-8) operations. Surgical intervention was mostly necrectomy of pancreas and lavage. The most frequent pulmonary complications were pleural effusion and atelectasie. The renal replacement therapy was mainly intermittent treatment: 6/27 patients survived. The micro-organisms found in septic complications were most frequently: *Enterobacteriacae spp., Staphylococcus, Pseudomonas aer.* and *Candida albicans.*

Conclusions: The prognosis of patient suffering of MOF is poor.Early prevention of each organ dysfunction, especially pulmonary and renal failure is mandatory. We have to apply targeted adequate antibiotic treatment. This may complement the surgical intervention and the complex intensive therapy. Team work is necessary, anaesthesist, surgeons, nephrologist, microbiologist and other disciplines.

7.06

IMPORTANCE OF EARLY JEJUNAL FEEDING IN NECROTISING PANCREATITIS AND AFTER ESOPHAGECTOMY

Hallay J.[1], Bakó A.[1], Szappanos M.[1], Sápy P.[1], Sz. Kiss S.[1], Sipka S.[2]
[1] 2nd Department of Surgery Debrecen H4004
[2] 3rd Department of Internal Medicine Debrecen H4004

Does jejunally administered glutamin rich oligopeptid food protect against multi organ failure and shorten the hospital stay of patients who have been operated for esophagus cancer or pancreatic necrosis?
In 1998 there were 10 patients with esophagus cancer and 3 with necrotising pancreatitis who were investigated in our clinic. Their immunological status, body composition and antropometric data were mesured pre- and postoperatively. Early glutamin rich jejunal feeding was started with Stresson feed and slowly increased from 500 to 2000 ml through a 3 days period.
Nitrogen balance, body composition, protein, albumin, immunglobulin level, complement factors and acute phase plasma protein level were followed up.
The investigated parameters mentioned above proved the efficency of early glutamin rich jejunal feeding.

S. Bengmark, Fracs, FRCPS
Nutrition 1998, 14:563-572
S. Cunningham-Rundles, D. Holin
Nutrition 1998, 14:573-579
D.W. Wilmore, J.K. Shabert
Nutrition 1998, 14:618-626

7.07

TREATMENT OF PANCREANECROSIS OPERATIONS COMPLICATIONS

Glabai V., Danilov M., Temirsultanov R., Makarova V.
Department of Surgery,
Moscow Medical Academy, Moscow Russia

During the period from 1991 until 1998, 166 patients were operated for infected necrotising pancreatitis, 63 of them developed different complications in early and late periods. There were 6 mortalities.

Immediately after the operations for infected necrotising pancreatitis, the only serious complication was blood vessel erosion and bleeding (4 patients). Timely operations of 3 patients proved to be successful. The other complication during the early periods was the development of external fistula of colon (3 pts), of duodenum (1 pt), and stomach (3 pt); only one patient with external fistula of colon was operated. 3 patients developed internal fistulae, cystoduodenum (1 pt), stomach cyst fistula (3 pt), plevracyst fistula (3 pts), colon-pancreatic fistula (2 pts). The last two types required surgical treatment.

During the late periods the most common complication was the pancreatic cyst (16 pts), in 3 cases - with the development of pancreatic ascites; 19 patients, after open packing, developed ventral hernias, and 16 - external pancreatic fistla.

In 3 cyst patients the US-puncture method was used. The other 13 required surgical treatment. 5 patients had distal resection of pancreas, 8 had different types of internal drainage. Internal drainage was also performed for external pancreatic fistula patients. Also, 19 patients were operated for ventral hernias.

In conclusion, early complications seldom occur as a result of "open packing" and, we also, believe that the treatment of different types of infected pancreatic necrosis operation complications demands early diagnosis, and its type should selected on a case-by-case basis.

7.08

SPLEEN RUPTURE DURING ACUTE PANCREATITIS.

TWO CASES REPORT. LITERATURE REVIEW.

Habib E., Elhadad A.

R. Ballanger Hospital, Aulnay Sous Bois, France

Introduction: Spleen rupture is an infrequent complication during acute pancreatitis. The diagnosis is often made during operation.
Cases Report: A 31 years old male was admitted because of an acute pancreatitis with hypovolemic shock and acute respiratory failure which needed assisted ventilation. CT scan showed an heterogeneous pancreas and extra-pancreatic fat necrosis. On D+3, bleeding shock appeared. During laparotomy, 3 litres of clotted blood were drained. Clots were more important near to a ruptured spleen. A splenectomy has been undertaken. Histology analysis showed a normal splenic parenchyma with haemorragic dissociation and sub-capsular haematoma. A 45 years old women was admitted because of an acute pancreatitis developed on chronic pancreatitis. CT Scan showed an enlargement of the head of the pancreas. At D+11, she developed a hypovolemic shock with acute anaemia. During laparotomy, 3 litres of clotted blood were drained. Clots were more important near to a decapsulated spleen. Splenectomy was undertaken.
Discussion: On literature review (1900-1998), we found 41 cases of splenic complications during acute pancreatitis (39%) or during chronic pancreatitis complicated by an acute pancreatitis (61%). Patients suffered from pain in the epigastrium (44%) or in the left upper quadrant (71%) during 5 days before admission. They had guardness (46%) and a mass in left upper quadrant (22%). Spleen rupture symptoms occurred 3 days after admission and surgery has been undertaken 10 days after admission. The preoperative diagnosis was spleen rupture in 17% of the cases. During surgery, there was a spleen rupture (51%) a spleen decapsulation (11%) and an intrasplenic haematoma (44%). There was an acute pancreatitis (46%) or a chronic pancreatitis (29%). Patients underwent a splenectomy (53%) or a splenopancreatectomy (32%). Post-operative complications (20%) and reoperations (15%) were frequent as for postoperative death (13%).
Conclusion: Splenic complications during pancreatitis causes rapid aggravation of clinical status of the patient. If splenic complication is not diagnosed, patient prognosis is worsened and death may occur.

Dig Surg 1999; 16 (suppl 1): 29-30

HPB pathology

8,01

Body composition of patients with obstructive jaundice.
Effect of hydration and relieve of obstruction.

L. Lupo, A. Gallerani, A. Veglia, V. Porcelli, O. Pannarale, P. Ricci, V. Memeo - Dept Emergenza e Trapianti d'Organo, Sez. Chirurgia Gen. e Trapianto di fegato, Universitŕ di Bari, Italy

Background: A negative water balance has been reported as a potential factor for acute renal failure in patients with obstructive jaundice (OJ).

Aim: To evaluate the effect of hydration and resolution of obstruction on body composition and water distribution.

Patients & Methods: Total body water (TBW), Extra- (ECW) and Intra-cellular water (ICW) and Body cell mass (BCM) were assessed by Bio-Impedance Analysis (BIA), by measuring Resistance (R) and Reactance (Xc) in 23 patients with bilirubin >10 mg. Measurements were taken before and after i.v. aministration of 40 ml/kg/die of Ringer's solution for 3 days and after jaundice was resolved. Weight, Hct, Bilirubin, Albumin, osmolarity, fluid balance and creatinine were also monitored. Statistics: Median values; Mann-Withney test.

Results: After hydration TBW and ECW increased: 37.5 vs 36.2 and 17.5 vs 15.6 ($p < 0.05$), and HCT and Osmolarity decreased: 32 vs 35 ($p < 0.01$) and 283 vs 290. No change of Creatinine was observed. After resolution of jaundice Weight, TBW, and BCM were reduced: -3 Kg , 34.9 vs 36.2, 20.6 vs 23, but ECW increased: 17 vs 15.6; $p < 0.05$.

Conclusions: In patients with OJ administration of a large volume of cristalloids preserves renal function. Changes observed after resolution of jaundice may reflect the effect of catabolism.

8,02

PHOTODYNAMIC THERAPY FOR CHOLANGIOCARCINOMA;
an in vitro study with the photosensitizers mTHPC and PEG-mTHPC.

Bordui M*, Schuitmaker JJ**, Terpstra OT*
*Department of Surgery, **Department of Ophthalmology,
LUMC, Leiden, The Netherlands

AIMS: Photodynamic therapy (PDT) combines the use of a light sensitive drug and light to destruct tumors. In this study the possibility of using PDT for cholangiocarcinoma treatment with the second generation photosensitizers, mTHPC and PEG-mTHPC, a water-soluble derivative of mTHPC, was investigated in vitro to determine the uptake, effectiveness, toxicity and the localisation of the photosensitizers.
METHODS: Two cell lines were used. A human cholangiocarcinoma cell line and as a control a non-cancer BHK cell line, cultured in DMEM with supplements. After incubation with the photosensitizers the cells were illuminated with light of the appropriate wavelength (652 nm).
The cellular uptake was determined by extraction, the PDT effects were assessed with the MTT assay. Localisation of the photosensitizers was determined with the use of a confocal laser scanning microscope.
RESULTS: The results showed that mTHPC is located in the cytoplasm and not in the nucleus, mitochondria or lysosomes. Both cell lines showed a similar uptake maximum of mTHPC within 12 hours. PEG-mTHPC uptake was very minimal, probably due to high hydrophilicity. The effectiveness of mTHPC in both cell lines is very high, all cells are killed with low levels of light energy (<30 J/cm^2) and low photosensitizer concentrations (<2μg/ml), resulting in short treatment times. PEG-mTHPC proved to be not effective in these cell lines.
CONCLUSIONS: In a human cholangiocarcinoma cell line PDT with mTHPC as photosensitizer, in low concentrations, induces 100% cell death.

8,03

DISTRIBUTION OF METALLOTHIONEIN IN THE LIVER AFTER 70% PARTIAL HEPATECTOMY IN RATS.

Theocharis SE, Skaltsas S, Spiliopoulou C, Margeli AP, Koutselinis A. Department of Forensic Medicine and Toxicology, University of Athens, Medical School, Athens, Greece.

Aims: Metallothioneins (MTs), a set of ubiquitous low molecular weight proteins, mainly implicated in metal ion detoxification . In the present study, we investigated the expression of hepatic MT during hepatocyte regeneration induced after 70 % partial hepatectomy (PH) in rats.
Methods: Male Wistar rats (180-220 g) were subjected to 70% PH and sacrificed at 0, 4, 8, 12, 16, 20, 24, 28, 36, 48, 60 and 72 h after PH. The rate of tritiated thymidine incorporation into hepatic DNA, the enzymatic activity of thymidine kinase in liver tissue and the assessment of mitotic index in hepatocytes, were used as indices of regeneration. The serum and liver tissue Zinc (Zn) concentration were also estimated using Atomic Absorption Spectrophotometry. MT expression in the liver tissue was detected immunohistochemically.
Results: Tritiate thymidine incorporation into hepatic DNA, hepatic thymidine kinase activity and mitotic index pexcibited marked oscillations after 70% PH with peaks at 24 and 28 h post-hepatectomy. MT expression became prominent as early as 12 h after PH in the nuclei of hepatocytes. At the time intervals of 20-28 h post-hepatectomy intense cytoplasmic and nuclear MT expression was noted in all hepatocytes. A positive correlation was found among liver MT expression and liver tissue Zn content while an inverse one was noted among liver MT expression and serum Zn concentration.
Conclusions: Induction of MT expression was observed in the liver after 70% PH in rats, presenting peak at the time of maximum hepatocellular proliferation. Our data suggest that MT expression correlated to high liver tissue Zn content, partitipating in the accumulation of this metal involved to DNA replication, in the liver.

KARGER
Fax +41 61 306 12 34
E-Mail karger@karger.ch
www.karger.com

8.04

INVESTIGATION OF HEPATIC MICROVASCULATURE IN FATTY LIVER BY INTRAVITAL MICROSCOPY

Agarwal AK., Piasecki C, Seifalian AM, Davidson BR
University Department of Surgery and Liver Transplantation Unit, Royal Free and University College Medical School, London NW3 2QG, U.K.

Aims: Steatosis is a major cause of graft dysfunction following transplantation. The vascular change associated with fatty change have not been established. The aim of this study was to assess the hepatic microvasculature in fatty and normal rat livers using *in vivo* microscopy.
Methods: Two groups of SD rats were studied. Group I comprised of 6 rats fed on a normal rat diet. In group II steatosis was induced by feeding 2% cholesterol diet for 20 weeks. The hepatic microvasculature was assessed using *in-vivo* fluorescence microscopy. Plasma was labelled with FITC-dextran (Fluorescein isothiocyanate-dextran). Changes in sinusoidal blood perfusion and microvascular structure were observed and quantified using computerised image analysis of video microscopy images.
Results: Acinar perfusion was markedly impaired in the fatty livers and was accompanied by a lower percentage of perfused sinusoids compared to the normal control rats (P<0.01). Fatty livers were found to have narrow and irregular sinusoids with blood cell adhesions to the endothelium. Hepatic cord widths in fatty rats were significantly greater than in controls indicating swelling of the parenchymal and sinusoidal lining cells.
Conclusions: Steatosis results in extensive abnormalities in hepatic microvasculature resulting in impaired hemodynamics. These microvascular changes may make the fatty livers more prone to ischaemia-reperfusion injury.

8.05

Treatment of hepatic colorectal micrometastases with human angiostatin

Drixler TA[1], Gebbink MF[2], Ritchie ED[1], Aarsman CJ[2], Reyerkerk A[2], Voest EE[2] Borel Rinkes IH.
Departments of Surgery[1] and Medical Oncology[2], University Medical Centre, Utrecht, The Netherlands

Aims: (1) To optimize the antiangiogenic and antitumoral effects of angiostatin (AS) by comparing bi-daily bolus injections with continuous administration of human AS; (2) To test the antitumoral effect of AS in a murine model of hepatic colorectal micrometastases.
Methods: Balb/c mice were used. AS was generated by proteolysis of human plasminogen with pancreatic elastase. Antiangiogenic effect was measured by the corneal neovascularisation assay (model 1) in which bFGF-induced corneal angiogenesis is used to test putative angiostatic peptides. Antitumoral effects were quantified using two tumor models: (model 2) a subcutaneous primary tumor was obtained by sc injection of 10^6 C-26 cells (murine colorectal carcinoma). Tumor volume was measured daily; (model 3) a colorectal liver metastases model following intrasplenic injection of 10^5 C-26 cells. Wet liver weight (WLW) and tumor surface area in liver slides (ratio tumor/non-tumoral tissue) were measured on days 7 and 14. Mice were treated either by daily bolus injections (sc) or by continuous (Alzet® pump; sc) administration of angiostatin for up to 14 days to reach a daily dose of 100 mg/kg. Control mice received PBS.
Results: Antiangiogenic effect (model 1): continuous administration was significantly better than bi-daily bolus injection resulting in 93% and 71% inhibition, respectively (p<0.01). Antitumoral effect (model 2): growth inhibition of sc tumors was significantly greater in mice receiving continuous AS, than in mice treated with bolus injections (tumor volume in mm^3±SD: control=1848±38; AS bolus=919±94; AS continuous=105±16; p<0.005). Antitumoral effect (model 3): growth inhibition of liver metastases was significantly better in mice treated continuously with AS (tumor surface area in %±SD: control=97±2; AS bolus=81±10; AS continuous=43±6; p<0.005). Similar results were obtained using WLW (grams±SD): control=3.78±0.15; AS bolus=2.97±0.06; AS continuous=2.23±0.13; control=1.35±0.06; p<0.005).
Conclusion: At the dose level of 100 mg/kg/day continuous administration of AS dramatically improves its antiangiogenic and antitumoral actions. AS is capable of inhibiting of colorectal liver metastasis. This may present an interesting new therapeutic approach in the treatment of hepatic colorectal micrometastases.

8.06

ISLETS OF LANGERHANS ENCAPSULATED WITH A TISSUE ENGINEERED CARTILAGE LAYER FOR IMMUNOISOLATION MAINTAIN LONG-TERM INSULIN SECRETION

Pollok JM, Begemann JF, Török É, Kaufmann PM, Kluth D, Broelsch CE, Izbicki JR, Rogiers X
Departments of Hepatobiliary and Transplantation, Paediatric, and General Surgery, University of Hamburg, Germany

Aims: We demonstrate maintained in vitro secretory function of islets of Langerhans within a tissue engineered capsule of chondrocytes and cartilage matrix, which may serve as an immunoisolation barrier utilizing the immunoprivileged properties of the cartilage matrix. This immunoisolation approach might offer a therapeutic strategy for patients with type I diabetes mellitus.

Methods: Islets of Langerhans were isolated from Lewis rats. 50 islets were seeded on a 0.5x1x0.06 cm biodegradable, highly porous polyglycolic acid (PGA) polymer scaffold (density 52 mg/cc). After an attachment period of 12 hours the islets on polymer were encapsulated with a monolayer of bovine chondrocytes, previously isolated and grown in culture (n=44). Encapsulated constructs and controls were kept under standard culture conditions using a supplemented M-199 medium for one month (30 days). Culture medium was exchanged every 24 hours. The insulin content of the culture medium was measured using a radio-immuno-assay (RIA). Histological and insulin immunohistochemical studies were performed on the specimens after one month in culture.

Results: Histology demonstrated viability of the islets, completely encapsulated with a thin chondrocyte layer after one month in culture. Immunohistochemistry showed positive staining for insulin after one month in culture. The insulin content of the culture medium of encapsulated constructs demonstrated a maintained insulin secretion, only slowly decreasing from 115 iE/ml on day one to 53 iE/ml/construct on day 30.

Conclusions: We demonstrated maintained insulin secretion of islets of Langerhans encapsulated with a tissue engineered chondrocyte capsule for one month in vitro. We demonstrated viability and preservation of specific islet cell function.

8.07

Adhesion formation following laparoscopic cholecystectomy: experimental animal study

Gamal EM., Metzger P., Mikó I., Ender F., Kiss J., Furka I.
Department of Surgery, H.I. Univ. For Health Sciences, Budapest & Institute of Experimental Surgery, Debrecen Univ. of Medicine, Debrecen, Hungary

Aim of the study: to detect adhesion formation following laparoscopic cholecystectomy in large experimental animals in comparison with a control group of conventional cholecystectomy.
Methods: from the period 1993-1997. sixty hands-on laparoscopic cholesystectomies had been performed in animal models by 40 surgeons during courses arranged for teaching laparoscopic cholecytectomy. Re-laparoscopy was then performed three and six months following the operations to detect adhesions and late postoperative complications. In 40% of the animals (24), where no the intraoperative complicatons complications – such as bleeding or perforation of the gallbladder – occured, and the removal of the gallbladder took place in the fibroaerolar layer, no adhesion formation was observed. Adhesions to the liver bed were discovered in 30% of the animals (18%) where only minimal intraoperative bleeding occured. In those cases, where severe intraoperative bleeding had been accompained by the perforation of the gallbladder formation of adhesionto the liver bed and the abdominal wall was significantly high. these adhesions were only found in the right upper quadrant of the abdomen. In a control group of 5 similar animal conventional cholecystectomy had been performed. without any complications. In all cases in the control group adhesion formation to the liver bed and the abdominal wall was significantly high.
Conclusion: it seems that adhesion formation during laparoscopic cholecystectomy is highly related to the frequency of intraoperative complications.

Dig Surg 1999; 16 (suppl 1): 31-33

HPB Laparoscopy I.

9,01

ANTIMICROBIAL PROPHYLAXIS IN EFFECTIVE LAPAROSCOPIC CHOLECYSTECTOMY: A RETROSPECTIVE STUDY OF 2,400 CONSECUTIVE CASES. WAYS, RESULTS, COST-EFFECTIVENESS.

Darom A., Stamou K.M., Mylonaki D., Manouras A-. Lateryannakis J., Androulakis F.A.
A' Propaedeutic Surgical Clinic, Medical School, University of Athens

Aims: We report a retrospective study of 2400 consecutive cases of Laparoscopic Cholecystectomy controlled in four groups. The aim is to define the effects of timing and length of intravenous antimicrobial prophylaxis on a) septic complications, b) the duration of hospitalization and c) the overall cost of the procedure.

Methods: We devoded our patients in four groups:
Group A: No prophylaxis, or postoperativ antimicrobial therapy (n=837).
Group B: Intraoperativ single dose of 2nd generation cephalosporine (n=312).
Group C: Intraoperative plus three doses (24hrs) of 2nd generation cephalosporine (n=843).
Group D: Intraoperative and six doses (48hrs) of 2nd generation cephalosporine (n=408).
For all groups, the general assumptions were: absence of Acute Cholecystitis, absence of active inflammatory process, and no preoperative antibiotic induction for other causes.

Results: Patients receiving prophylaxis had statistically significantly less (p>0,005) postoperative septic complicaions then patients who did not receive prophylaxis. Among patients that did receive prophylaxis, Group C appeared to have the best overall results and also proved to be the most cost-effective.

Conclusions: Patients undergoing Elective Laparoscopic Cholestectomy should receive antimicrobial prophylaxis in order to prevent septic complications. There is strong evidence that additional first postoperative day antimicrobial medication reduces even more the incidences of septic complications and, by co-estimating the duration of hospitalisation, it proves to be the most cost-effective treatment.

9,02

Information and Expectations Evaluation of Laparoscopic Cholecystectomy in two differents groups of patients:

*Prof. J. Diez**
*Lic. M. Broner de Taraciuk***
**Prof. Surgery, University Hospital, Buenos Aires University.*
***Psychology Chief, Mental Health Dept., University Hospital, Buenos Aires University.*

Aims: Evaluate different informations and expectations of two groups of patients submitted to laparoscopic cholecystectomy in 1992-1993 and 1994-1996.

Methods: Evaluation consisted of a structured interview; considering ilness reaction, information about laparoscopic cholecystectomy and expectations about operation's types and results. The stress psychosocial factors were catalogued according to the DSM III-R of The American Psychiatric Association. A total of 108 patients were studied, 52 in Group A (1992-1993) and 56 in Group B (1994-1996).

Results: Group A indication, of laparoscopic cholecystectomy was primary done by surgeons.
Patients had little information about the surgery, its risks and results. They expected an almost «magic»and quick recovery. At Group B, patients were refered to surgery by internists, relatives, etc. They were awre about laparoscopic cholecystectomy's risks and its results. Their expectations about post surgery recovery were more realistic.
Although there is a straigh forward relationship in between stress factors and ilness, we did not found in bouth groups any difference at all.

Conclutions: Patients's reaction, to new surgical technique was evident in Group A. Their information was poor, the indications were done mainly by surfeons and expectations were unreal. In Group B with the laparoscopic cholecystectomy growing popularity the indications for surgery were done by internists and patients had realistic expectations towards its results. These results are typical of the impact of new techniques in bouth medical doctors and patients.

9,03

DAY-CASE LAPAROSCOPIC CHOLECYSTECTOMY

BJ Ammori, D Davides, A Vezakis, M Larvin, IG Martin, MJ McMahon
Leeds Institute for Minimally Invasive Therapy (LIMIT), Wellcome Wing, The General Infirmary, Great George Street, Leeds LS1 3EX, UK

AIMS: Day-case laparoscopic cholecystectomy (LC) offers patient convenience and cost savings. This paper reviews our experience with day-case LC over a 6-year period to determine its applicability and safety, and patient satisfaction.
METHODS: Of 744 consecutive patients who underwent LC at our institution between 1992 and 1998, 140 (19%) were selected for day-case surgery. Selection criteria included American Society of Anesthesiologists (ASA) score of 1 or 2, absence of morbid obesity, low risk for common bile duct stones, and convenience. Age alone was not considered a limiting factor. Patient satisfaction with day-case surgery was assessed by questionnaire at 6 weeks follow-up.
RESULTS: The annual number of patients undergoing LC increased gradually, but the proportion of patients scheduled as day-case remained static (median 18.5%, range 16%-22%). 117 of 140 (84%) patients were discharged home on the same day of the operation. Two patients were re-admitted with abdominal pain; of which one underwent a negative re-laparoscopy. The reasons for an overnight hospital stay were anaesthetic in 12 (52%), surgical in 7 (30%), and social or logistic in 4 (18%) patients. There were no conversions. 99 of 105 patients (94%) who completed questionnaire were satisfied with day-case surgery.
CONCLUSION: In carefully selected patients, day-case LC is highly achievable and safe, and provides high patient satisfaction.

KARGER
Fax +41 61 306 12 34
E-Mail karger@karger.ch
www.karger.com

9,04

LEFT SIDED GALLBLADDER : A RARE POSITION ANOMALY

George Savanis , G. Velimezis , J. Antoniades , A. Entsev , P. Stavlas , E. Perrakis
Dept. of Surgery , Western Attica Gen. Hospital , Athens , Greece

INTRODUCTION

The left-sided gallbladder is a rare congenital anomaly . About 70 cases have been reported internationally .

PATIENTS AND METHODS - RESULTS

In the last 7 years three patients out of 2256 who underwent laparoscopic cholecystectomy in our dept. had a left-sided gallbladder . The patients admitted for recurrent abdominal pain in the right upper quadrant . U.S. revealed a multiple cholelithiasis without any reference to anomalous position of the gallbladder . Preoperative physical examination and laboratory data were normal . The procedure in these 3 cases was completed laparoscopically .

CONCLUSION

Current theories regarding the etiology of this rare anomaly are presented . Laparoscopic cholecystectomy is the method of choice at left-sided gallbladder cholelithiasis , even in the presence of situs inversus totalis . Accompanying anomalies of the bile ducts and hepatic vessels must be taken under consideration during the laparoscopic procedure .

9,05

PORT-SITE METASTASIS FROM UNSUSPECTED GALLBLADDER CARCINOMA AFTER LAPAROSCOPIC CHOLECYSTECTOMY

K.Toutouzas[1], G.Bonatsos[1,2], K.Birbas[2], N.Durakis[2], E.Leandros[1], G.Androulakis[1], B.Golematis[2]

[1]First Dept. of Propaedeutic Surgery, Athens University, Athens, Greece
[2]TYPET 'Hygeias Melathron', Athens, Greece

Background: One of the potential drawbacks of laparoscopic cholecystectomy (LC) in patients with unsuspected gallbladder malignancy is the increased risk of port site metastasis. The aim of this study was to examine the incidence of metastasis in the abdominal wall among six patients operated for cholelithiasis and synchronous unsuspected gallbladder carcinoma diagnosed either during laparoscopy or in the early postoperative period.

Patients: From November 1990 to November 1998, 3670 patients underwent laparoscopic cholecystectomy with a preoperative diagnosis of benign gallbladder disease. Synchronous gallbladder carcinoma was suspected during laparoscopy in 3 patients (0.08%) and frozen section confirmed the intra-operative diagnosis. The procedure converted to laparotomy and histologic examination of the gallbladder revealed the presence of an adenocarcinoma infiltrating the serosa in all patients (T3). Postoperative investigation revealed liver metastasis in two patients. One patient with intraoperatively diagnosed gallbladder carcinoma received adjuvant radiotherapy.
In three patients (0.08%) with gallbladder malignancy, the tumor was missed during laparoscopy and cholecystectomy completed laparoscopically. Microscopic examination of the specimen diagnosed an unsuspected in situ carcinoma in one patient and adenocarcinoma of the gallbladder infiltrating the serosa in two patients. All patients (n=6, 0.16%) were observed for 4 to 17 months following cholecystectomy.

Results: Four months after LC, one patient (16.7%) with postoperatively diagnosed gallbladder carcinoma presented with nodules at port sites. Biopsy proved to be adenocarcinoma and the patient underwent resection of the nodules and received adjuvant radiotherapy. The remaining five patients with gallbladder malignancy diagnosed during or early after LC were observed for 9 to 17 months (mean 11.1 months) without any sign suggestive of metastasis in the abdominal wall.

Conclusions: 1) Intraoperative diagnosis of gallbladder carcinoma is difficult and as much as 50% of tumors will be missed during laparoscopy. 2) The risk of tumor seeding of laparoscopic tracts exists and 3) Conversion of the operation is justified when gallbladder carcinoma is suspected during laparoscopic cholecystectomy.

9,06

LAPAROSCOPIC APPROACH FOR COMMON BILE DUCT STONES

M. Nichitaylo, O. Lytvynenko, P. Ogorodnik.

Department of Biliary Surgery
Institute of Clinical & Experimental Surgery, Kiyev, Ukraine

Aims: to evaluate results of laparoscopic approach in patients with common bile duct (CBD) stones.

Methods: The aim of the present study was to evaluate results of laparoscopic choledocholithotomy (LCLT) in 45 patients with CBD stones. 26 patients had undergone cholecystectomy before were subjected to LC after initial failure of endoscopic sphincterotomy (ES) In 19 patients with suspected CBD stones, LCLT followed laparoscopic cholecystectomy after diagnosis verification on intraoperative cholangiography. Choledochoscopy, placement of a T-tube, interrupted single-layer vicril sutures, and antiseptic washing of CBD completed the procedure.

Results: Early postoperative complications developed in 4 patients: wound infection (3) and subhepatic abscess (1). The latter was cured by ultrasound guided punction. Postoperative cholangiography demonstrated presense of small retained CBD stones in 5 patients. ES successfully treated all of them. There was no mortality. During the follow-up (1,5 - 3 years) all patients were symptom-free.

Conclusions: LCLT proved to be safe and effective procedure in patients with CBD stones.

9,07

LAPAROSCOPIC BILE DUCT INJURY: CHANGING REFERRAL PATTERN AND LONG TERM MANAGEMENT

Shah S.R., Mirza D.F., Afonso R., Olliff S., Mayer A.D., McMaster P., Buckels J.A.C.
The Liver and Hepatobiliary Unit, Queen Elizabeth Hospital, Birmingham B15 2TH, UK.

Aims: To evaluate the trend in referrals of laparoscopic cholecystectomy related bile duct injury and review management in a tertiary referral centre.
Methods: Between 1991 and Sept 1998, a cohort of 50 consecutive patients referred to the unit with laparoscopic cholecystectomy related bile duct injury were evaluated. Injuries were categorised based on cholangiography and operative findings. Management was tailored to individual needs.
Results: Patients operated after Jan 1996 had a shorter median interval to referral (14 vs 35 days, P < 0.05). Type E injuries now form a smaller proportion of referrals (56% vs 84%, p = 0.03), though number of referrals has increased. Of 28 patients re-operated before referral, 24 required further surgery. Management after referral included reconstructive surgery (29), T tube insertion (3), hemihepatectomy (2), biloma drainage (2), ERC stent (5), percutaneous balloon dilatation (6), percutaneous biloma drainage (2) and conservative management (6). Four patients died and 8 (all with complex injuries) have had subsequent cholangiitis over a median follow up of 34 months.
Conclusions: Laparoscopic bile duct injuries continue to be a complex management problem with risk of death and long term morbidity. There is a trend towards early referral to tertiary centres.

9.08

LAPAROSCOPIC BILE DUCT INJURIES - REFERAL PATTERNS AND MANAGEMENT AT A TERTIARY CARE CENTER

SS Sikora, A Kumar, NR Das, A Sarkari, R Saxena, VK Kapoor.
Department of Surgical Gastroenterology, SGPGIMS, Lucknow, India

INTRODUCTION

Laparoscopic cholecystectomy (LC) is perhaps associated with an increased incidence of bile duct injury than open cholecystectomy. We reviewed our experience of management of laparoscopic bile duct injuries.

PATIENTS AND METHODS

From October 1992-1998, 34 patients with bile duct injuries following LC were managed. 16 patients had an injury following LC at our center (0.01% incidence) whereas 18 patients were referred following injury. The mean injury-referral interval was 5.9 months (range 12 hours -31 months). Injuries were classified as per the Strasberg classification. The presentation, type of injury, management and outcome was analyzed in these patients.

RESULTS

Of the 16 patients who sustained injury at this center [types A (n=9), D (n=5) and E (n=2;)], fourteen were detected during LC, whereas two patients presented as postoperative bile leak. Patients with type A injuries were managed by laparoscopy (n=1), conversion and ligation of the subvesical duct (n=7) and endoscopic sphincterotomy in the postoperative period (n=1); those with type D by repair of lateral rent over a t-tube; and those with type E by conversion and hepaticojejunostomy (HJ). All patients had an excellent outcome at a mean follow up of 36.6 months (range 1.3-71.7).18 referred patients had external biliary fistula [EBF](n=9), biliary peritonitis (n=1) and benign biliary stricture[BBS] (n=8) on presentation. The type of injury were: B (n=1), D (n=2), E [14 (6 with EBF + 8 with BBS)] and not known (1). Four patients underwent early repair of the ductal injury before referral [repair over a t-tube (n=2) and HJ (n=2)] of which three developed restricture on presentation. One patient (type B injury) was referred within 12 hours, and had a successful repair over a t-tube. Two patients with early repair for lateral injury had excellent outcome. 11 patients had BBS and underwent repair with excellent (n=10) and fair (n=1) outcome at a mean follow up of 27.9 months (range 2.3-59.1). Four patients were lost to follow up.

CONCLUSIONS

The spectrum of injuries is different at a tertiary care training center as compared to that in a general surgical practice. Intraoperative recognition and repair at an experienced center gives the best results. Missed injuries and attempts at repair in inexperienced hands results in serious sequelae of stricture formation and long term morbidity.

9.09

EXPLANATIONS ON THE REASONS OF THE COMMON BILE DUCT INJURY DURING LAPAROSCOPIC CHOLECYSTECTOMY

D. Tsatzalos, V. Primikiris, P. Voulgaris, G.Papadopoulos, Th. Megas, M. Nikoliadis
2N° SURGICAL DEPARTMENT-"PENTELI" HOSPITAL OF ATHENS

Laparoscopic cholecystectomy has become routine procedure for surgicall treatment of gallbladdel lithiasis. One of the most significance complication is the injury of the common bile duct during the operation. In 1876 LC (1993-1998) we faced 30 cases of common bile duct injury. In two of them the duct had been cut. In 3 the duct injured due to dislocation of the metal clip. In 7 the trauma caused due to improper cutting of the cystic duct. The rest 18 were small injures resulting bile leakage. The complications treated surgically or conservatively. No patient died, and all are in good health up to now. We are going to discuss the reasons they led to the bile duct injuries and the best way, according to our opinion, to avoid them.

9.10

CONTEMPORARY MANAGEMENT OF MAJOR BILE DUCT INJURIES

CH Wakefield, J. Wigham, KK Madhavan and OJ Garden
University Department of Surgery, Royal Informary of Edinburgh, United Kingdom

Aim: Bile duct injury is a recognised and serious complication of cholecystectomy. This study examines one unit's experience in the management of iatrogeic bile duct injuries and the effect of the introduction of laparoscopic surgery.

Methods: A retrospective cohort study of patients referred to a tertiary hepatobiliary unit with bile duct injuries, over a 14 year period until November 1998.

Results: In the 75 patients, injuries were perpetrated at laparoscopic cholecystectomy (n=42), open cholecystectomy (n=30) and during gastroduodenal surgery (n=3). Their median age was 55(18-83) and women predominated (M:F, 27:48). Operative cholangiograms were peerformed in 16 (22%) of the biliary procedures. Nine were identified as being abnormal and initiated reconstructive procedures. In a further 18 patients, the injury was identified and repair peerformed at the index procedure. In all, 44 (59%) patients underwnt operative interventions and 24 (32%) radiological or endoscopic interventions prior to referral. Laparoscopic surgery was associated with injuries of greater severity than open cholecystectomy, Type I/II 39% vs 77%, Type III/IV 61% vs 23%, laparoscopic vs open (p=0.03, K2). Following referral (median delay 57 days) 70 patients underwent surgery, 51 hepaticojejunostomies, 7 revision of bilio-enteric anastomoses with hepaticojejunostomy, 2 right hepatectomies, 2 OLTm 3 peritoneal toilet and 5 lesser repairs. The 30 day mortality was %, the postoperative morbidity rat was 13% and median hospital stay was 10 days. The current median follow up interval is 14 months (0-120), during which 2 (3%) patients have experienced holangitis, and 8 (11%) have had an episode of cholestasis, leading to 3 further procedures (2 revisions of Roux limbs and 1 right hepatectomy).

Conclusions: Laparoscopic cholecystectomy related bile duct injuries are of a more severe type than those inflicted at open surgery. The successful masnagement of these injuries, with efficacious long-term results requires the full range of hepatobiliary procedures.

Dig Surg 1999; 16 (suppl 1): 34-36

Pancreas tumor III.

10,01

EVALUATION OF POSSUM SCORING SYSTEM FOR PANCREATO-DUODENECTOMY IN A SPECIALIST CENTRE

Khan AW., Agarwal AK., and Davidson BR.

Royal Free Hospital and UCL Medical School, Pond Street, London. U.K.

AIMS:Crude rates of morbidity and mortality can be misleading. POSSUM (Physiological and Operative Scoring System for enUmeration Morbidty and mortality) takes into account the preoperative as well as the operative criteria to provide a risk adjusted prediction of morbidity and mortality rates for comparative audit purposes over the whole range of general surgical operations. The risks of pancreatic surgery have significantly come down as it has come to be concentrated in specialist HPB centres. This pilot study was undertaken to assess POSSUM's usefulness for pancreatic resection in a specialist HPB centre in UK.

METHOD:Parameters that are assessed include 12 physiological variables which are: age, respiratory and cardiac history, blood pressure, pulse rate, Glasgow Coma Score, blood haemoglobin, WBC count, urea, Na, K, and ECG. Operative parameters are:operative severity, multiple procedures, total blood loss, peritoneal soiling, presence of malignancy and mode of surgery. Each variable is further graded into 4 to give a point value on an exponential score (1,2,4,8), which is then used in the equations for morbidity and mortality. 50 patients undergoing elective pancreato-duodenectomy at the Royal Free Hospital and School of Medicine, London over the last 10 years were evaluated in a retrospective study. POSSUM was used to assess the risk of operative morbidity and mortality for each patient and compared with the actual data recorded.

RESULTS: The average predicted operative morbidity was 91% and hospital mortality was 41% The actual operative morbidity was 42% and post-op hospital mortality was 4%.

CONCLUSIONS: This pilot study suggests that the POSSUM overpredicts the risk of morbidity and mortality for pancreato-duodenectomy in a specialist centre. This could be due to better operative and post-op care in such centres. Further work is needed to assess its usefulness over the whole spectrum of HPB surgery and perhaps modify the predictor equations.

10,02

PANCREATIC RESECTIONS-TO DRAIN OR NOT TO DRAIN

R. Dawson, NCA Puntis
University Hospital of Wales
Cardiff CF4 4XN, United Kingdom

Aim: To asses the usefulness of abdominal drainage in major , pancreatic resecrtional surgery.

Method: Retrospective analysis of 50 consecutive patients undergoing resections under the care of one surgeon.

Results: Meain patient age was 57.6 years (range 21-77). The procedures included 33 Pylorus preserving pancreatico duodenectomie, 7 Whipples, 4 Total pancreatectomies and 6 left sided resections. 34 resections were for malignant or highly dysplastic lesions, 9 for pancreatitis and 7 for other benign disease. All patients except one had a mean of 3 drains placed at surgery. Postoperative morbidity included 10 leaks (3 deaths), 3 cases of intra abdominal haemorrhage (1 death) and 1 case of intra abdominal sepsis. Anastamotic leak was revealed in the drain contents alone in 2 patients, by systemic signs and drain contents in 4, and by systemic signs lone in a further 4. Information obtained from drainage alone altered patient management in 2 cases and possibly affected the outcome in one.

Conclusions: The role of drains in abdominal surgery has been long debated. They cause complications including intra abdominal sepsis, haemorrhage and erosion into hollow viscus. In this series, drains possibly affected the outcome positively in one patient only. On the other hand many of the complications we had, some directly resulting in mortality, could have been contributed to or even caused by the drains themselves. The overall benefit is therefore uncertain.

These figures would suggest a cautious approach to the placement of drains after pancreatic resections. However only a prospective randomised trial can definitively answer the question as to whether they cause more trouble than they are worth.

10,03

BENEFITS OF HIGH HOSPITAL VOLUME IN PANCREATIC RESECTIONS

Pegan V., A. Tomažič

University Medical Centre Ljubljana Slovenia

Objective
To improve the postoperative results after pancreatic resections our aim was to gain experience by means of increasing the number of patients per surgical unit. Five years ago in Slovenia we have reached a consensus to concentrate the patients requiring pancreatic surgery in only two surgical units. This agreement resulted in reaching the »high volume« standards in our surgical departement.

Methods and patients
In 1995 and 1996 we have perfomed 23 pancreatic resections yearly and in 1997 and 1998 the number of patients increased slightly to 24 patients per year. The predominant diagnosis was cancer of the pancreatic head (33 patients) and in the four year period 72 pancreaticoduodenectomies were performed, 22 with the pylorus preserved. Out of 94 pancreatic resections 3 total pancreatectomies and 4 extended excisions for low grade malignancies of the Vaterian papilla were carried out.

Results
The postoperative morbidity after pancreatic resections in 1996 and 1997 (46 patients) was 41 %, disruption of the gastroenteroanastomosis and of the pancreatiocojejunal anstomosis being the most frequent cause (6 patients). The mortality due to surgical complications in this period was 10,8 %.
In the years 1997 an 1998 (48 patients) the morbidity has been lowered to 20.8 % and we have lost only one patient due to dehiscency of the pancreaticojejunal anastomosis (mortality = 2 %).

Conclusion
The retrospective analysis shows clearly the positive impact of "hospital volume" in the management of pancreatic cancer. The effect of regionalization was demonstrated in only few years after its implementation by significant lowering of the postoperative morbidity and in- hospital mortality.

KARGER
Fax +41 61 306 12 34
E-Mail karger@karger.ch
www.karger.com

10.04

HORMONAL NON-ACTIVE NEUROENDOCRINE PANCREATIC TUMORS. EXPERIENCE OF TREATMENT OF 31 PATIENTS

Buriev I., Fedorov V., Tsvirkun V., Karmazanovsky G., Guzeeva E., Akimova E., Demidova V., Savvina T., Vtiurin B.
A.V.Vishnevsky Institute of Surgery, Moscow, Russia

The course and prognosis of neuroendocrine pancreatic tumors differ the rest of tumors of the same localization. The most significant diagnostic and medical problems arise in hormonal non-active asymptomatic tumors. For 15 years the authors have studied the results of treatment of 31 patients with hormonal non-active neuroendocrine pancreatic tumors being 10,9% of all the patients with pancreatic tumors. The disease developed asymptomatically before the development of complications: jaundice (12), duodenal impassability (2), massive abdominal formations (6), hyperthermia (4). CT revealed typical symptoms: accurate tumor contours, slow growth with «pressing» of surrounding structures without the signs of infiltration, later - metastasing and quick stabilization of the process in combined treatment. In 68% of the cases increased Ca19-9 in low CEA level was revealed. Radical operations were performed in 28 patients, palliative - in 3 patients. Morphological tumor investigations revealed 7 types. As clinical-laboratorial data revealed no signs of tumor hormonal activity, electron microscopy showed specific secretorial granules in tumors cells of all the cases. Mortality was 9,6%. Recurrency - 3 cases, 3-5-year survival is 87,1% and 83,8% corr.

Neuroendocrine pancreatic tumors have specific clinical-morphological picture and more favourable prognosis. It defines the peculiarities of diagnostic and medical tactics for such patients.

10.05

SURGICAL TREATMENT OF 11 INSULINOMAS

E. Hadjiyannakis, P.Alfaras, S.Drakopoulos, A.Papakonstantinou, C.Stratopoulos, I.Terzis, F.Hadjidimitriou, A.Poultsidi, A.Katsas, A.Mitrakou, S.A.Raptis.
1st Surgical Dept –Transplant Unit, Gen Hospital "Evangelismos of Athens", Greece.

Aim: We present our experience from the surgical treatment of 11 insulinomas, ginen the difficulty in their preoperative localization and the problems concerning their surgical removal.
Methods : In the past 8 years, 11 patients with insulinoma (4 men and 7 women) were surgically treated. Patients' mean age was 47 years. In all cases Whipple's triad was present. Diagnosis was made with the combination of abdominal U/S, C/T and angiography.
The fasting pre and postoperative plasma glucose mean value was 2,8 nM/l and 4,9 nM/l respectively, while the pre and postoperative plasma insulin mean value was 282 pM/l and 72 pM/l respectively.
In all cases but one the tumor was precisely localized preoperatively.
Results : In 5 patients the tumor was enuclated, in 3 patients Whipple procedure was performed, while 2 patients underwent segmental pancreatectomy. In the eleventh patient who was previously operated twice (whipple procedure and enucleation of several insulinomas) a total pancreatectomy was performed. The size of the insulinomas was in 6 cases 1-1,9 cm, in 3 cases 2-2,9 cm and in 2 cases >2 cm.There was no postoperative death.The complications were 2 pancreatic fistulae which were treated with somatostatin and 2 wound infections. The case of two brothers that both had insoulinoma should be noted.
The first one who was surgically treated elsewhere twice (Whipple procedure and ecucleation), was reoperated in our Department and a total pancreatectomy was performed due to an additional insoulinoma in the tail of the pancreas. He is now a canditate for a pancreatic transplant.The other one underwent enucleation of two insoulinomas. The histologic diagnosis showed neuroendeocrine carcinomata of the pancreas. Two years postoperatively he is in a good condition, free from disease.
Conclusion : The surgical treatment of insoulinomas is the only radical therapeutic choice.

10.06

C. Pasquali, D. Miotto *, F. Meduri , S. Savastano *, G. Liessi #, C. Sperti, G. Casarrubea *, A. Maffei-Faccioli, S. Pedrazzoli.
Dept. of Medical and Surgical Sciences, Institute of Radiology *- University of Padova, and Radiology # Castelfranco V. Hospital, Italy.

INTRA-ARTERIAL CALCIUM INJECTION TEST AND VENOUS SAMPLING AS LOCALIZING PROCEDURE IN INSULINOMAS.

From November 1993, 14 patients (8 M/6 F) with hypoglycemic syndrome suspected to have an insulinoma underwent angiography and intra-arterial calcium injection (IACI) test as localizing procedure.
US scan, CT-scan and/or MRI were performed before the IACI test . Calcium (0.015-0.025 mEq/Kg b.w.) was injected in each arterial branch supplying the pancreas and Insulin was assayed in the blood collected for 2 min. from hepatic vein. Positive test was defined as a three-fold increase of insulin after calcium. Eleven patients had a positive IACI test. A peak of insulin secretion after injection of a single artery occurred in 10 cases while in one case we detected a peak of insulin after calcium injection in two arteries. All cases had a typical single adenoma (size < 1 cm. in six) found at surgery. Only 6/11 patients had a positive non invasive imaging before angiography. Angiography alone (positive in 8/11 cases) detected 3 more insulinomas, but it was negative in 3/6 cases with a small (< 1 cm) adenoma. Intraoperative ultrasound was positive in 8/9 cases investigated but negative in the single (0.8 cm adenoma) not felt or seen at surgical exploration, on the basis of angiography and the IACI test results.
In three of the original 14 cases investigated, the IACI test was not localizing. A slight Insulin rise following each of the artery injections occurred in a MEN 1 patient with a macroadenoma of the tail and diffuse nesidioblastosis. No insulin rise was seen in a malignant insulinoma with multiple liver metastases. Finally, no insulin rise was seen in a case later recognized to have hypoglycemia secondary to self administration of oral antidiabetics.
IACI test was found useful to provide correct information before surgery "regionalizing" the source of insulin hypersecretion in all cases with a typical single adenoma, including six cases with small adenoma., Caution is needed in evaluating negative tests, possibly related to extended disease or other uncommon causes of hypoglicemia.

10.07

OCCULT PANCREATIC NEUROENDOCRINOMAS

Markovic M., Kati} V., Basic H., Nikolic D.
Clinic of oncology, Nis Yugoslavia
Institute of pathology, Nis Yugoslavia

Aim: Pancreatic endocrine tumors are uncommon, frequent of small size or component of MEN I syndrome with multihormonal and ectopic hormone activity.

Methods and results: Having in the mind the pointed characteristics, we report the following four neuroendocrinomas, found during autopsies: PPoma, associated with secondary hyperparathyroidism, insulinoma, associated with corticotroph microadenoma of pituitary gland (MEN I), gastrinoma, which has induced recidivant ulcers after surgically treatment (Zollinger - Ellison - syndrome) and VIPoma, associated with WDHA syndrome (Werner - Morrison syndrome). Macroscopically, they are well demarcated, firm consistency and dark red in color. Their size ranged between 12 and 28mm and of benign nature. Precise diagnosis of these tumors was done using immunocytochemical analysis: NSE, Chromogranins and synaptophysin, as well as specific monoclonal antibodies.

Conclusions: The authors have concluded that pancreatic neuroendocrinomas represented complex biological systems displaying a high degree of phenotypic heterogeneity.

10.08

CYSTIC MUCINOUS TUMOR OF THE PANCREAS

Z. Sparchez[1], M. Tantau[1], B. Diaconu[1], T. Zaharia[2], C. Iancu[3]
[1] 3rd Medical Clinic, [2] Department of Pathology, [3] 3rd Surgical Clinic, University of Medicine Cluj-Napoca, Romania

We report the case of a 62 year old woman with a cystic mucinous tumor of the tale of the pancreas. She was admitted by emergency to the hospital for moderate epigastric pain irradiating to the left upper abdominal quadrant which occurred after a fat meal. In the past she had some episodes of abdominal pain which resemble the present one, episodes which lasted for a few hours, one day being most. She did not drink alcohol and her family history was not significant. Physical examination showed a patient with good nutritional status (60 kg weight at 160 cm height) and palpation revealed a tender epigastrum. All other data were within the normal.

Abdominal ultrasonography revealed a normal sized pancreas with slight inhomogenous structure, a dilataton of the main pancreatic duct.

The final diagnosis was made by ERCP which showed protrusion of the papilla into the duodenal lumen and mucin leaking from its dilated orifice, az uniformely dilated (9-10 mm) main pancretic duct. In the tale of the pancreas ERCP showed a cystic dilatation, lobulated in shape of the collateral ducts.

The cytological examination of the mucin sampled from the MPD showed mucosecretant benign columnar cells in an amourphous basophilic medium, probably mucin.

Surgical treatment was determined by the potentially malignant evolution of the tumor and consisted of distal pancreatectomy with splenectomy. The histological examination of the resected piece confirmed the diagnosis. A 6 months follow-up revealed neither symptoms nor recurrence of the tumor.

10.09

METASTATIC TUMORS OF THE PANCREAS. A CLINICOPATHOLOGICAL STUDY OF 62 CASES

Lampert K, Nemcsik J, Paál E.
2nd Department of Pathology, Semmelweis University of Medicine

Aims: Metastatic tumors of the pancreas occur rarely. The data in the literature about them is limited, and restricted mostly on case reports. The authors try to give a review on metastatic pancreas neoplasms.

Methods: We retrieved 60 cases from the archives of the 2nd Department of Pathology, Semmelweis University of Medicine for the period of Oct. 1988 to Oct. 1998, among the 7783 autopsy cases and 92571 surgical biopsies. The case documentation and histological slides were reviewed.

Results: Among the total number of pancreatic neoplasms 4.5% were of metastatic origin. Primary sites for those lesions were identified in 59 of 60 cases: the most frequent primary site was stomach (n=14), followed by lymphoid tissue (n=8), kidney (n=7), lung (n=6), esophagus (n=5), colon (n=4), skin, gall bladder, liver, retroperitoneum (n=3 each), breast, adrenal gland, urinary bladder (n=1 each). One metastasis originated from an unknown primary tumor.

On histology most of the tumors (n=43) were carcinomas: adenocarcinoma (n=21), hypernephroma (n=7), planocellular carcinoma (n=6), small cell carcinoma (n=4), hepatocellular carcinoma (n=2), and transitiocellular carcinoma, carcinoma NOS, anaplastic carcinoma (n=1 each). Among the non-epithelial tumors there were lymphomas (n=8), malignant melanomas (n=3), paragangliomas (n=2), and one each of neuroblastoma and leiomyosarcoma.

12 of the cases were symptomatic (causing jaundice, abdominal pain or hypoglycemia)

Conclusions: According to data in the literature hypernephroma and pulmonary carcinoma are the most frequent primary sites, giving metastasis into the pancreas. The largest series that has been published so far is reviewing of 47 cases. Our results are comparable to the ones published concerning the frequency of metastatic lesions of the pancreas. Excluding the cases involving the pancreas with direct spread from neighboring organs, the prevalence of the various metastatic tumors in the pancreas is similar to the data in the literature. No data were found about metastatic paraganglioma and transitiocellular carcinoma.

Dig Surg 1999; 16 (suppl 1): 37-38

Acute pancreatitis II.

11,01

Infected necrotising acute pancreatitis - long term results.

K. Bielecki, A. Włodarczyk, J. Sieklucki, A. Gajda
Department of General Surgery Medical Center for Postgraduate Education, Warsaw, Poland

Necrotizing acute pancreatitis (NAP) complicated by infection is a very serious disease resulting in malfunctioning of the other organs. It is still associated with a very high mortality.
The aim of study was the evaluation of late consequences of infected NAP (INAP) in patients treated with the „open abdomen" technique.
Patients and methods: From 1990 to 1997 thirty three patients (M-26, F-7) aged 30-56 years, with severe course of INAP were treated in our Department. All patients were treated with the „open abdomen" technique with repeated (from 2 to 12) peritoneal lavage and necrosectomy. Sixteen patients (48,5%) of this group survived. The follow-up was conducted from 1 to 7 years after the onset of disease. The follow-up included: 1. clinical examination and self-assessment according to Visick scale, 2. UGT panendoscopy, 3. biochemical analysis estimating the endocrine function of the pancreas, 4. exocrine function tests : faecal elastase-1 concentration and faecal chymotrypsin activity 5. abdominal CT scan, 6. Neuro-psychological assessment.
Results: clinical examination revealed normal body weight, good condition and in all patients abdominal wall herniation (3 pts were already operated due to this complication). All patients were classified as group I according to the Visick scale. Endoscopy showed gastric and/or duodenal mucosa inflammation in 8 (50%) pts. In 4 (25%) pts glucose levels in serum were elevated. Exocrine function tests did not reveal any significant abnormalities in all pts. CT abdominal scan showed no pathological changes in pancreas. Neuro-psychological tests did not reveal any significant abnormalities in all patients.
Conclusion: Patients who survived and recovered from infected acute necrotizing pancreatitis present only a minor, clinically non-significant psychological and pathophysiological abnormalities in long-term follow-up (1-7 years).

11,02

DATA OF SEPTICO-TOXIC CONDITION CAUSED BY NECROTIZING PANCREATITIS

Kovács G., Hallay J., Bakó A., Kovács Gy., Sipka S.[1], Sápy P.
2nd Department of Surgery, University Medical School of Debrecen
[1]3rd Department of Internal Medicine, University Medical School of Debrecen

42 patients were treated for acute pancreatitis in our clinic between 1997 and 1998. 25 of them were operated when wecrosis was found in the pancreas.

The indications of early operation (within one week) in patients with acute necrotizing pancreatitis (12%) were acute abdomen, MOF and deteriorating of the general condition (against intensive treatment). The mortality rate was high (66,67%) in this group.

Late or delayed operation (after a week) was performed in patients with pancreatic abscess, infected necrosis with serious condition. The mortality rate was 4,5% in this group.

In our treatment we applied antibiotics, enteral and parenteral feeding, ventilation therapy in the case of ARDS, H2 blockers for prevention of stress ulcer and etc. We followed up in last year the immunological state, body parameters and different of laboratory data of these patients.

Frequent and serious complications are characteristic in acute necritizing pancreatitis that demand careful intensive treatment including early feeding and using wide-spectrum antibiotics.

11,03

Secchi M.A; Sanchi W.; Tagliaferri E.; Nosti E.; Quadrelli L.; Rossi L.; Serra F.
Surgical Division, Hospital Italiano, Hospital Provincial and Hospital de Emergencias.
ROSARIO – ARGENTINA .

MORTALITY IN ACUTE PANCREATITIS. A LAST 20 TH CENTURY APPROACH.

INTRODUCTION: Mortality in patients with acute pancreatitis (AP) is different when we compare Mild and Severe cases at different periods of times. Before 1970 Mild cases had 10% of mortality and Severe cases 50%, but in the 1980´s it was 2% to 5% in mild and 40% in Severe. In the last years several reference centers had no mortality in Mild cases and less than 30% in Severe cases.

PATIENTS AND METHODS: In order to analyse mortality rates and causes of death we reviewed 431 cases of those patients having acute pancreatitis of any etiology from 1991 to date.
At admission patients were divided into two groups according to Atlanta Symposium. Etiology was determined by multidisciplinary approach and an individual treatment was adapted for each patient. Mortality referred to those hospitalized cases.

RESULTS: 383 patients had Mild AP and 48 had Severe AP on the first day of admission. There was no mortality in Mild cases (0%) and we had 15 patients who died from Severe cases (31%), but only 2 in the last years. From the 15 patients who died, 11 had multisystemic organ dysfunction (M.O.D) before 48 hs since the onset of the symptoms and were classified as Fulminant Pancreatitis (Mean Apache II: 26±3) and 4 as Severe with 1 or 2 organs disfunction (Mean Apache II: 20 ±3) ($p < 0.05$). The cause of mortality was: M.O.F during the first week in 7 patients, 1 P.T.E and 7 infected necrosis or abscesses.

DISCUSSION: Our mortality rate in AP is always related to severe cases. The prediction of mortality with a M.O.D evaluation system was the most appropriate because 73% of patients who died had failure of 3 or more organs on the first two days (Fulminant cases). But the end of this century a clinical definition based on the 1992 Atlanta Symposium was accepted. In a near future early MOD detection, selective use of antibiotics, progression in enteral and I.V. nutrition support, early detection of local complications by dynamic CT Scan and minimal invasive surgical procedures on biliary tract and pancreas are some of the main causes we expect result in lower mortality in those patients having AP.

KARGER
Fax +41 61 306 12 34
E-Mail karger@karger.ch
www.karger.com

11.04

PANCREATIC ABCESS – A 3 YEAR SURVEY OF AN INTENSIVE CARE UNIT

João Raposo; Jorge L.Correia; Henrique V.Dias; Mª Eugénia Alves; Aurélio Godinho; Ana M.Mouro, M J Queirós Medeiros.
Pulido Valente Hospital - Faculty of Medical Sciences - Lisbon - Portugal

INTRODUCTION – On receiving patients suffering from acute pancreatitis, our staff has usually used the criteria of severity defined by Ransom for the purpose of evaluation and management of the disease. This procedure is, however, not always possible due to the tardy arrival of some patients to the referral centre. A series of patients suffering from severe pancreatitis was analysed in order to obtain and early diagnosis of pancreatic abscess and to identify factors associated with mortality.
PATIENTS and METHODS – We have analysed a series of 47 patients with severe pancreatitis, referred to the I.C.U., in a three year period (1996 to 1998). There were 29 males (61.7%), and 18 females (38,3%), the mean age being 58 years. Aethiological factors were: alcohol ingestion (38.3%), gallstone (29.8%), post ERCP (19.2%); drugs (2,1%); miscellaneous (6.4 %); indeterminate (4.2%). The mean Ranson criteria at 48 hours was 3.1. The mean APACHE score in the first 24 hours in ICU was 11.4 (score > 8 = severe pancreatitis).
All patients had clinical, laboratory and contrast CAT scan evaluations, in order to detect early and worrying findings of a pancreatic abscess. We have analysed the surgical procedures (mainly debridement and external drainage) used to treat some complications and tried to establish the criteria more likely to lead to a good result. Nine (19.1%) patients were operated on in an emergency, 8 (17%) for pancreatic abscess and 1 for sterile pancreatic necrosis. In 2 of these cases reoperations were required. Another 6 patients underwent elective biliary tract surgery. Laparoscopic approach was used as the procedure of choice in the treatment of cholelithiasis before discharge. In this series the global mortality rate was 8.5% (4 out of 47 patients). The mortality rate in the emergency surgical group was 11.1% (1 out of 9 patients).
CONCLUSION – We have concluded that age and clinical situation based on the APACHE score are poor prognostic factors. The likelihood of infection in severe pancreatitis is significant. An early intervention to treat infected necrosis influences favourably the prognosis.

11.05

ACUTE PANCREATITIS-STRATEGY AND TREATMENT

Jeramov N., Vijachki IV., Petkov CHR., Vijachki D, Gachev N.

Clinic for Emergency Surgery, University Hospital "Queen Jiovanna", Medical University-Sofia, Bulgaria

Aims: In this retrospective trial we assess how acute pancreatitis patients respond to nonoperative therapy; operative methods and results after surgery for acute necrotizing pancreatitis

Methods: We present 738 acute pancreatitis patients, treated from 1987 to 1998 in our clinic. In all cases we start a nonoperative therapy comprising losses replacement, analgesics (including narcotic ones), spasmolytics, antibiotics, protease inhibitors-Contrical or Gordox (only during 1997 and 1998) and/or somatostatine (Sandostatin), H_2-blockers, naso-gastric tube. Monitoring of the main parameters as blood pressure and pulse rate, number of leukocytes, values of serum amylase, urea and creatinine is performed.

Results: 576 responded to this therapy and recovered. The ones who worsened-162 acute necrotizing pancreatitis patients-underwent surgery: necrectomy followed by postoperative prolonged local lavage in the area of pancreatic couch or laparostomy. This method contributes to a prolonged evacuation of biologically active substances and devitalized tissues. The average number of Ranson's Prognostic Criteria was 4.5. Furthermore, mortality is reduced to 19%. A mortality analysis is done. Surgery (cholecystectomy and bile duct exploration) is offered to patients who recovered from acute pancreatitis caused by cholelythiasis and/or choledocholythiasis.

Conclusions: The majority of patients respond to the nonoperative therapy. Despite the recent improvement in diagnostics and treatment of acute pancreatitis morbidity and mortality rates are still high.

11.06

TWO STAGED MARSUPIALISATION OF CAUL WITH SINISTRAL AIMED LUMBALISATION DURING PANCREANECROSIS

Cicala E.T., Botan I.A., Jacub V.A., Casian D.A., Popa G.I., Petrov D.G..
Medical University „N. Testemitsanu", Moldova

Aims: Development of optimal method of marsupialisation of caul, allowing executing repeated quality necrectomias at pancreanecrosis without executin time of ventrotomy is very relevant.

Methods: We offer method of marsupialisation, which consists in the following. During the first laparotomy (at 5-8 days after laparotomic drainage of abdominal cavity) is making a wide incision in ligament gastrocolic closer to transverse colon. Making sure in necessity of future repeated necrsecvestrectomias (haemorragic pancreanecrosis), we fixate ligament gastrocolic for long spread to abdominal wall using next way. Ends of incised ligament gastrocolic are fixing with capron sutures to abdominal wall in cross direction of projection of body. Ligament gastrocolic is fixating at the level of ventrotomy incision at it with creating of channel, following to pancreas. Laporotomy wound is sewing completely above and below. If will diagnose sequestration in four, five or nine days, using intravenous anaesthesia, we incise abdominal wall between ends of ligament gastrocolic, which was fixed to abdominal wall before. As result we get T-shaped access to pancreas.
In cases of unsatisfied drainage of trail-end pancreas area, we determine, using bimanual method, localization of maximal infiltration retroperitoneal space tissues and doing lumbotomia.

Results: There were six patients with necrotic-purulent pancreatitis, which were treated by this method. Average number of necrosequestroectomias were 6-8. One patient died.

Conclusions: Described method of access to pancreas has posibilities of more quality inspection of omental bursa during every procedure of necrosequestroectomia, it is low traumatic and low contingency of creation of fistulas of alimentary tract.

11.07

CARCINOID TUMOR OF THE COMMON BILE DUCT. CASE REPORT

A. Lombardi, G. Batignani, A. Amorosi°, G. Nesi°, E. Mazza*, A. Calabrò&, C. Surrenti& and F. Tonelli.
Unita di Chirurgia, Gastroenterologia& e Radiodiagnostica.* Anatomia ed Istologia Patologica° University of Florence.

We report a case of primary carcinoid tumor originating in the distal part of common bile duct. To our knowledge this is the 14th reported in the literature and the 2th of the distal common bile duct. The patient, a 30 years-old male, presented with a sudden diarrhea with pale stools and dark urine, mild jaudice, pruritus and weight loss. Laboratory evalutation revealed abnormal LFT's with signs of biliary obstruction. Abdominal U.S. showed a normal gallbladder without stones with mild dilatation of intra and extrahepatic biliary tree and with a 2 cm solid ipoechoic tumor in the head of the pancreas closed to distal bile duct. An helical CT confirmed these findings and showing an hyper- vascular pattern of the tumor. An Echo-Endoscopy confirmed the previous characteristics and showed the absence of infiltration of the distal bile duct. An multihormonal screening showed an increase in the plasma serotonin, 350 ng/ml (normal range: 90-180) and platelets serotonin 1470 ng/109 plt (normal range: 200-600) ; all other gastrointestinal hormons were within normal range. Tumor markers (CEA and CA 19-9) were not elevated. At operation the tumor was found arising in the common bile duct and seemed to infiltrate the head of pancreas. The patient underwent a standard pylorus-preserving pancreatoduodenectomy. Pathological examination of the specimen showed a neuroendocrine tumor (carcinoid) of the distal bile duct, infiltrating the wall, MIB-1 index was 6%. The resection margins were negative. The postoperative plasma serotonin went back to normal levels. One year later the patient was healthly, without evidence of recurrent disease.

Dig Surg 1999; 16 (suppl 1): 39-41

HPB clinical experience

12.01

EFFECTS OF CHEMOTHERAPEUTIC DRUGS ON GASTRONTESTI-NAL MOTILITY AND EMESIS, AND THEIR RELATIONSHIP

Qin XY Song LJ, Niu WX, WU ZG
Zhong Shan Hospital, Sanghai, P.R. China

Aims: To find out whether Chemotherapeutic drugs can result in seerious side-effects.
Methods: A perfusion system was used to dynally evaluate the variations in gastrointestinal motility and their relationship with vomiting in 18 patients (11 male, 7 female, age 41-57yr) who received chemotherapy after radical colorectal operation. Intraluminal pressure of the gastrointestinal tract was measured dynamically for 72 hours, during which the first day acted as a control. On the second day, the patient was given cisplatin and 5-FU. On the third day, the patient was given chemotherapy+ondansetron. 14 patients fulfilled the entire 3-day study 4 patients completed only a 2-day study period.
Results: A total of 159 migrating motor complexes (MMCS), 8.832. 33 in each subject, were recorded within 24 hours during the control peeriod, while a total of 236 MMC (13.113. 53 on average) were noted during chemotherapy, the difference was statistically significan (P<0.01). During chemotherapy+ondansetron, 183 MMCs were recorded in 14 patients, (13.073. 60 in each patient), compared with controls (9.142. 54 MMCs), statistical significance was prominent (P<0.01),but no significance was found when compared with chemotherapy alone (I 3.143. 96), P<0.05. Compared with the chemotherap stage, significance was found (P<0.05), suggesting that ondansetron blocked the vomiting reaction induced by chemotherapeutic drugs. Upper abdomen discomfort or nausea occurred I hour prior to vomiting in all patients. An average of 280 min (2802 5 m n x SD) was noted, from commercement of chemotherapy to the first vomiting episode.
Conclusions: Chemotherapeutic drugs increased gastrointestinal motility, manifested as shortened MMC cycle, increased MMC frequency, accelerated velocity of MMC propagation, and increased MMC III. Chemotherapy caused vomiting in patients. Ondansetron, a 5-HT3 receptor antagonist, suppressed gastrointestinal motility induced by chemotherapeutic drugs. It is hypothesized that increased gastrointestinal motility and emesis induced by chemotherapeutic drugs possibly arise from different mechanisms.

12.02

THE PREVALENCE OF HEPATOBILIARY DISORDERS IN PATIENTS WITH ULCERATIVE COLITIS

B. Radovanovic, T.Tasic, A. Nagorni, B. Bajagic, V. Dinic-Radovic
Clinic of Gastroenterology and Hepatology, University of Nis, Yugoslavia

Hepatobiliary disorders are sistemic complications or extraintestinal manifestations (EM) in inflamatory bowel diseases. EM are symptoms of the sistemic character of IBD. Although the association betwen hepatobiliary disorders and IBD is known, the pathogenesis and cause of hepatobiliary disorders in IBD are unknown.
Aim: The aim of this study was to analyse prevalence of hepatobiliary disorders and to investigate any correlation among the clinical stage of ulcerative colitis, the endoscopic grade of the disease, the extensiveness of colonic involvement and hepatobiliary disorders.
Methods: ninetytwo patients with ulcerative colitis were studied up from 1994 through 1998years.
Results: thirtysix of the patients were at grade III, thirty grade II, nineteen grade I, and seven grade 0, endoscopically. fortytwo patients had left sided colitis, thirtythree proctosigmoiditis, ll pancolitis and six proctitis. thirtythree patients had severe, fortyfive moderate and fourteen mild diseases. eight patients had elevated transaminase (ALT and AST) levels. Sonographically,fourteen patients had hepatosteatosis. But all of them had normal liver function tests. three patients had sclerosing cholangitis.eighteen patients had cholelithiasis.One patients had autoimuni hepatitis.
Conclusion: We did not find any correlation between hepatobiliary disturbances and endoscopic grade of colitis, extensiveness of colitis or clinical severity of disease.

12.03

The New Reference Center on Quality of Life in Oncology - Part of Quality Management in Modern Surgery

Küchler, Th., Kremer, B.

Dept. for General and Thoracic Surgery, University of Kiel, Germany

Intro: Quality of Life (QoL) has become one of the most important outcome variables in modern medicine. During the last ten years reliable measures of QoL especially in oncology have been developped. Today's challenge is to incorporate these measures in clinical quality assurance programs and to establish QoL-measures as clinical routine. Since 1998 the Deutsche Krebshilfe e. V. granted a "Referencecenter on Quality of life in oncology". Òverall aim of this center is the collection of information on any activity or study result relevant to QoL. Accordingly the scope of this center will be to support actively studies and activities on outcome research with focus on QoL and/or patients satisfaction.

Aims: The mandate of the reference center ranges from methodological counselling on how to assess QoL in a given setting, to participate in (multicenter) trials that incorporate QoL and to realize own specific research. The longterm aim of this project is to establish a databank on QoL for most tumor entities and in different treatment modalities, accessible for all care providers as well as for patients. Therefore the close cooperation with the German Cancer Society ("Deutsche Krebsgesellschaft") is mandatory

First Results: One year after being established the referencecenter is part of a total number of 42 studies, that focus as primary or secondary outcome on QoL. The scope of these studies ranges from small, very specific studies (for exaple QoL after struma surgery -developpment of a specific struma cancer questionnire) to large multicenter trials (i. e. the national kidney cancer project). Within thes studies a variety of specific instruments („modules") for specific tumorsites and treatment modalities that can be used in combination with a core instrument (i. e. the EORTC QLQ C-30) have been developped and are now available for the surgical community.
In this respect the Reference Center on Quality of Life is working constantly on the methods and prerequisites to establish QoL as a standard outcome measure in (surgical) oncology.

KARGER
Fax +41 61 306 12 34
E-Mail karger@karger.ch
www.karger.com

12,04

Percutaneous liver biopsy in patients high risk for bleeding. The protective role of fibrin glue.

T. Petsas(*), A.Apostolopoulou(**), G.Skroubis(**), C.Vagianos(**).

From the Departments of Radiology(*) and Surgery(**), University of Patras Medical School, Patras , Greece.

Aims: Liver biopsy represents the diagnostic procedure of choice for focal liver lesions. Although generally safe, it may be complicated by bleeding, particularly at the presence of coagulation disorders. We tried to evaluate the efficiency and safety of using the fibrin glue to seal the needle track, in hemorrhage-prone patients, who underwent percutaneous liver biopsy.
Methods: 42 patients, at high risk for hemorrhage were divided in three groups, according to the type of the disease and the bleeding diathesis (BD), as documented by increased PT, a-PTT or decreased platelet count. Group A (n=19) diffuse liver disease and (BD), Group B (n=13) focal liver lesions and BD and Group C (n=10), highly vascularised focal hepatic lesions without BD. Liver biopsies were obtained by using a Coaxial 18 Gauge, 10 T through length, 9 cm long Trocar Needle system (William Cook Europe A/S). At withdrawal, the needle track was occluded by injection of 1ml fibrin glue (Tissucol-Kit, Immuno GmbH Heidelberg, Germany), mixed with contrast agent. The deposition of the sealant was studied by C/T scan or ultrasonograghy after 24 h. Bleeding complications were recorded during the following 48h.
Results: The procedure was well tolerated. In three cases it had to be repeated due to inadequate tissue sampling. In all cases, diagnosis was achieved by histology. The sealant was shown to fill the needle track and tamponade the point of entry to the liver surface. A total of two serious complications were noted, all belonging to Group B. Treatment was conservative with blood transfusion (3 and 2 units). No further complication was recorded.
Conclusion: Our results show the diagnostic efficacy and safety of percutaneous liver biopsy, particularly when combined with obstruction of the needle track by fibrin glue injection. Fibrin glue reduces the bleeding complications of the method and is very useful when treating patients with coagulation disorders. who are at significant bleeding risk.

12,05

OUR EXPERIENCE IN TREATMENT OF CHOLESTATIC LIVER DISEASES

Joksimovic N, Serafimoski V, Neskovski M, Milosevski M.
Clinic of Gastroenterohepatology, Medical Faculty-Skopje. R. Macedonia.

Beneficial effect of ursodeoxycholic acid (UDCA) treatment in patients with cholestatic liver diseases has been reported. In this study we investigated the effect of UDCA in 65 patients with biochemical, ultrasoundly and histologically proven various cholestatic liver diseases. All patients were treated with UDCA 10 mg/kg/day.

Thirty one patients had fine needle biopsy proven compensated alcoholic hepatitis (AH) with or without HCV infection (16 HCV negative and 15 anti HCV positive); Chronic viral hepatitis (CH) in 19 pts.; Autoimmune hepatitis (AiH) 5 pts.; Primary biliary cirrhosis (PBC) 4 pts.; Secondary biliary cirrhosis (SBC) 4 pts., and Caroli's disease (CD) with cholestasis in 2 patients. Clinical, biochemical and histological parameters were followed for a period of one year. Clinical (jaundice, pruritus and fatigue), biochemical markers of cholestasis and hepatocellular damage (aminotransverases, alkaline phosphates and bilirubin) in 72% patients with PBC, in all patients with SBC and CD, 68% with CH, 63% with AH and 50% with AiH, were improved. The beneficial effect of UDCA on the liver histology was assessed in all patients after minimum of 6 mounts of therapy.

Our results suggest that UDCA leads to biochemical and clinical improvement in patients with cholestatic liver diseases. The use of UDCA in the treatment of chronic cholestatic liver diseases appears to be safe and without side effects.

12,06

EXPERIENCES ON INTERFERON TREATMENT OF PATIENTS WITH CHRONIC VIRAL HEPATITIS IN HUNGARY DURING A FIVE-YEAR PERIOD

A. Pár (co-ordinator) and the Hungarian Viral Hepatitis Study Group*
University Medical School, Pécs, Hungary.

Aim: to study the course of disease and evaluate the management of more than one thousand patients with chronic viral hepatitis diagnosed and treated by uniform criteria.

Patients and methods: 1122 patients (pts) were included and followed-up: 129 suffered from hepatitis B virus (HBV)-related liver disease, out of them 11 had HBV+Hepatitis Delta virus (HDV) and 24 had HBV+ hepatitis C virus (HCV) infection, while 993 pts had chronic hepatitis C. Interferon (IFN) alfa-2b (83%), IFN alfa-2a (16%) and natural leukocyte IFN (1%) were given at a weekly dose of 3x 3-5 MU for 6-12 months. In HCV hepatitis, non-responders were treated with ribavirin + IFN combination as well. A total of 826 pts have completed the therapy.

Results: In hepatitis B, IFN caused an end of treatment remission (ETR) in 46%, sustained response (SR) in 33%, HCV pts showed a 41% ETR, with 22% SR. In non-responder or relapsed HCV pts a combination therapy of ribavirin + IFN alpha 2b resulted in a 64% ETR and a 40% SR rate. IFN withdrawal was needed in 87 pts (11%), mostly due to non-compliance and side effects.

Conclusion: the efficacy of IFN in chronic viral hepatitis is suboptimal, thus new therapeutic modalities are needed. In chronic hepatitis C, a combination of IFN with ribavirin is promising as a therapy of choice.

* L.Dalmi, Gy.Weisz, (Debrecen), M.Abonyi, A.Csepregi, K.Dán, K. Dávid, J.Fehér, E. Ibrányi, G.Lengyel, M. Horányi, G. Horváth, E. Nemesánszky, I. Mihály, M. Pusztai,L. Rókusz, F. Szalay, L.Telegdy, Gy.Tolvaj,(Budapest), J.Gervain, A.Gógl (Székesfehérvár),I. Nagy, J.Lonovics, Zs.Ozsvár (Szeged), F. Schneider (Szombathely), P. Ribiczey (Zalaegerszeg), I. Rácz, I.Pete, L. Varga (Győr), Zs.Váczi, L.Csák, (Miskolc) A.Tusnádi (Szolnok), T. Várkonyi (Békéscsaba), .Gasztonyi, F. Pakodi, A.Pár, G.Pár (Pécs)
(Supported by grants from ETT 031/96 and OTKA T 023476).

12,07

PHASE II STUDY OF CPT-11 ADMINISTRATION IN PROGRESSIVE COLORECTAL CANCER PATIENTS AFTER SURGICAL TREATMENT FOLLOWED BY UNSUCCESSFUL THERAPY WITH 5-FU.

By
D. XYPOLYTAS, N. ZIRAS, G. KYRATZIS and V. SKOUNTZOS

From the 2nd Surgical department, General Peripheral Hospital "K.A.T.", 145 61 Kifisia, Hellas and 1st department of Agii Anargiri, Cancer Hospital Athens, Hellas.

AIM: The assessment of CPT-11, a camptophecin derivative, in colorectal cancer patients pretreated with surgery and 5-FU.
PATIENTS - METHOD: In this phase II Study 22 patients with colon and rectal adenocarcinomas were enrolled. Of those patients, 14 were males and 8 females, the age was ranged from 54-74 years and the performance status WHO≤2. The location of the metastasis was in the liver (12 patients), lungs (5 patients), or in both organs (5 patients). CPT 11 was given as a first line treatment in six patients with early relapse (less than 6months) after adjuvant treatment with 5-FU and as second line treatment after prior unsuccessful 5-FU treatment in sixteen patients. The dosage schedule of the drug was infusion of 350mgr./m^2, in 90 minutes, every 3 weeks and a total of 120 treatment cycles were given, which means 5.45 cycles per patient.
RESULTS: The observed responses were 2PR (9.1%) 3MR (13.6%), 12 SD (54,5%) and 5PD (22.7%). The medium time of progression was 6 months (ranged from 3-12 months). Twelve patients (55%) had a symptomatic improvement. Toxicity evaluated in all treatment cycles included acute cholinergic syndrome grade 1-2 in 48 patients over 120 patients (40%); late onset diarrhea grade 1-2 in 40 patients (33.3%) and grade 3-4, in 10 patients (8,.3%); vomiting 1-2 grade in 35 patients (29.1%); in cases of grade 3-4 neutropenia prophylactic support with G-CSF was given in the next cycles and in 53 cycles with G-CSF the observed neutropenia was only grade 1-2.

CONCLUSION: CPT-11 at a dose of 350mgr./m^2, every 3 weeks is well tolerated. Stabilization of the disease associated with a symptomatic relief was observed in this study, so that chemotherapeutic agents could be useful in the management of this disease.

12.08

IRINOTECAN (CPT 11) IN CYTOREDUCTIVE LIVER SURGERY. FIRST EXPERIENCE.

Severtsev A., Laptev V., Ivanova E., Sedova L., Remizov M., Smirnova N., Sukhanov A., Tupikova E.
MED CENTRE FOR RUSSIAN GOVERNMENT (Moscow; Russia): ① United Hospital & Policlinics ("Volynsky" Hospital), ② Postgraduate & Research Centre

Cytoreductive surgery is the treatment of choice for patients with advanced cancer (especially for colorectal cancer) with liver metastases. One of important parts of this strategy is chemotherapy (especially intraarterial regional chemotherapy). The most conventional drug for these purposes is 5-FU. Unfortunately, it has some serious side effects and complications during intraarterial infusions to the a.hepatica. On the other hand, the new anti – tumor drug, irinotecan is one of most effective drugs for advanced colorectal cancer during systemic treatment. In addition, according to known metabolism of this agent, it is active for regionar liver chemotherapy. References about the intraarterial intrahepatic use of irinotecan are absent.
The aim of this study was the development of the clinical treatment protocol for liver colorectal metastases with direct intraarterial regionar administration of irinotecan.
The study has been begun from June 1998. We have had 1 patient with complete course till December 1998.
Case report: Patient 54 years old, female had surgery two years ago for sigma cancer (resection with stoma, and closing the stoma 6 months later) in other hospital. She admitted to our hospital, because of 3 metastases in right lobe of liver. There were 3 large metastases (more then 2 cm in diameter) in the right lobe on the surgery and 5 additional small metastases in both lobes. The surgery was finished with the intraarterial port insertion (a. hepatica) for postoperative chemotherapy. In postoperative period patient had systemic and direct intrahepatic chemotherapy (2 sessions) with the use of 5-FU and cisplatin. After second session patient had symptoms of biliary tree damage. Next 4 sessions we used irinotecan (100 mg/sqm) with direct infusions into liver and systemic administration. We didn't have any serious side effects or complications (local or systemic) during this treatment. CT scan & US showed complete resorbtion of metastases.
Conclusion: Irinotecan could be used as anti – tumor drug for direct intraarterial administration into liver during advanced colorectal cancer with liver metastases (as an active part of cytoreductive surgery).

12.09

EARLY EXPERIENCE WITH LAPAROSCOPIC PANCREATECTOMY

Ammori BJ, Vezakis A, Davides D, Larvin M, McMahon MJ
Leeds Institute for Minimally Invasive Therapy (LIMIT), Wellcome Wing, The General Infirmary, Great George Street, Leeds LS1 3EX, UK

AIMS: To describe early results of laparoscopic pancreatectomy, and to discuss its limitations and future perspective.
METHODS: Between 1993 and 1998, 9 patients underwent laparoscopic distal pancreatectomy for endocrine tumours (n=4), cystadenoma (n=3), adenocarcinoma (n=1) and chronic pancreatitis (n=1).
RESULTS: There were seven females and three males. The median age of patients was 62 years (range 30-83 years). Distal pancreatectomy with splenic preservation was performed in 9 patients. The ultrasonic dissectors were utilised and facilitated dissection. Nonetheless, the procedure was converted to open pancreatectomy in two patients. The pancreas was divided with a linear stapler in 8 patients and with the harmonic scalpel in one. Median operative time was 300 minutes (range 240-360 minutes). Postoperative pancreatic fistula developed in two patients in whom the pancreatic stump was not sutured, and responded to radiological and supportive management. There were no postoperative deaths. Median postoperative hospital stay was 12 days (range 5-60 days). All laparoscopically treated patients remain well at a median follow up of 24 months (3-36).
CONCLUSION: Laparoscopic pancreatectomy is a technically demanding procedure, but appears feasible and safe. Oversewing of the divided pancreatic stump may reduce the risk of pancreatic fistula. The benefits of the laparoscopic approach remain to be demonstrated.

12.10

THE BASING OF LAPOROSCOPIC ACCESS TO PANCREAS

Dr. V. Sedov, Dr. M. Fishman, Dr. V. Yurlov
The department of facultative surgery of Pavlovls State Medical University
St. Petersburg, Russia

During of last decade the diseases of pancreas considerably increased, especially pancretitis, with the variety of hard complications, which often lethal outcome. In the most difficult cases the patients can be saved only with the help of urgent operation. The aim of our research is find out the safest way to reach the pancreas and the surrounding formations for the laparoscopic surgery. We conducted two kinds of rresearches: we examined copses end patients who got laparoscopic surgery. Such data were found the weight of the body, sex, age, the rib angle, the width of gastrocolic ligament, the distance from the xiphoid cartilage to belly button, the length of the cavity of the omentum bag with its borders, the place end extent of the diligence of transverse colon to the omentum bag, estimated the amount of gastrocolic-omentum arteries. After analyzing the literature and our own researches we came to the following conclusions. Only the left sections of gastrocolic ligament, transverse colon are always attached to the omentum beg. An access to the pancreas is best to perform rough gastrocolic ligament in the left sections, closer to the stomach, via the vessel free area with clipping the necessary gastrocolic-omentum vessels to the right. The first trocar should be introduced into the near belly area, the second trocar has to be introduced along medioclavicularis line in the middle of the distance between xiphoid cartilage end the belly button. The third trocar is introduced along the front underarm line in the left underrib, the fourth one-on the level of the belly button left down the third trocar. Additionally it is possibly to introduce the fifth trocar from the right along the front underarm line of the belly's level. It is able to introduce the laparoscope to the third point for more convenient observation of the entire part of the pancreas abjacent to the omentum begs.

Dig Surg 1999; 16 (suppl 1): 42-44

HPB Laparoscopy II.

13.01

ACUTE CHOLECYSTITIS IN THE LAPAROSCOPIC ERA

Sirinek KR., Schwesinger WH, Gross GWW*, Strodel WE, Departments of Surgery and Medicine*, The University of Texas Health Science Center at San Antonio, 7703 Floyd Curl Drive, San Antonio, TX, USA 78284.

AIMS: Early laparoscopic procedures were usually limited to patients with symptomatic but otherwise uncomplicated gallstone disease. As experience increased, the laparoscopic approach was extended to more difficult hepatobiliary problems. To assess the effects of this evolving surgical strategy, we analyzed our recent laparoscopic experience with acute cholecystitis (AC) and compared it with laparoscopy for non-acute cholelithiasis (NAC). METHODS: Between March 1991 and September 1997, a total of 3619 patients underwent cholecystectomy; 1224 for AC (34%) and 2395 for NAC (66%). There were 2077 women and 642 men with a mean age of 39 years. RESULTS: Overall, there were nine deaths (0.25%), seven of which occurred in men (78%) and in 5 (56%) with gangrenous cholecystitis. The number of AC patients in whom laparoscopic cholecystectomy (LC) was successfully completed increased 4-fold during the 78 months of the study. Thus, the fraction of AC patients treated with open cholecystectomy (OC), either as a primary procedure or secondary to a conversion from laparoscopy (7%), decreased from 58% (1992) to 19% (1997). Men comprised only 18% of all cholecystectomy patients but they represented 26% of all AC patients and 43% of AC patients who required conversion to OC. By contrast, the fraction of patients with NAC who were successfully treated with LC increased from 61% 1992 to 95% in 1997 with less than 3% of the latter group requiring conversion.

	ACUTE		NON-ACUTE	
	TOTAL	DEATHS (%)	TOTAL	DEATHS (%)
OC	373	5 (1.3%)	351	0
LC	739	1 (0.1%)	1958	2 (0.1%)
LC → OC	112	1 (0.9%)	86	0
TOTAL	1224	7 (0.6%)	2395	2 (0.1%)

CONCLUSIONS: (1) Nearly all patients with NAC (95%) and most patients with AC (81%) can be successfully managed laparoscopically. (2) Nevertheless, compared to NAC, patients with AC continue to have a substantially higher conversion rate (2.5 vs 7.0%) and postoperative mortality (0.1 vs 0.6%), especially in male patients with gangrenous cholecystitis. (3) Further improvements in outcome will depend on new therapeutic approaches and earlier therapeutic interventions.

13.02

DELAYED LAPAROSCOPIC CHOLECYSTECTOMY AFTER ACUTE CHOLECYSTITIS IS A DIFFICULT PROCEDURE

R.Aerts, E.Vandermeeren, A.D'Hoore, M.Miserez, L.Filez, F. Penninckx, UZ Gasthuisberg, Department of Abdominal Surgery, Catholic University of Leuven, Belgium.

Background. Laparoscopic cholecystectomy (LC) for acute cholecystitis is feasible, but difficult. Cooling off the inflammation for 6-8 weeks might result in an easier and safer operation.

Methods. In a consecutive series of 208 LC, the difficulty of delayed LC after acute cholecystitis (49 patients) was compared with that of early LC for acute cholecystitis (10 patients) and elective LC for colics (92 patients). Operating time, intraoperative difficulties, conversion rate, postoperative morbidity and hospital stay were analysed.

Results. The operation was significantly longer in the early and delayed LC group (87.5 and 75 minutes) than in the elective LC group (55 minutes). Intraoperative difficulties occurred significantly more frequently (50 and 47 %) than in elective LC for colics (9 %). Conversion rates were significantly higher, 10, 16.3 versus 1 %, respectively. No significant difference in postoperative complication rates was observed in this study. Preoperative hospitalization to cool off acute cholecystitis took 9.1 days on average. Postoperative hospital stay after early and delayed LC (3.5 and 4.3 days) was comparable with that after elective LC for colics (2.7 days).

Conclusion. There is no benefit in cooling off acute cholecystitis and delaying LC for 6-8 weeks. Delayed LC was found to be a difficult procedure, comparable with early LC.

13.03

FACTORS PREDICTING UNSUCCESSFUL LAPAROSCOPIC CHOLECYSTECTOMY FOR ACUTE CHOLECYSTITIS

Hammarström L-E, Mellander S, Rudström H
Dept of Surgery, Mälarsjukhuset, Eskilstuna, Sweden

Aims: Laparoscopic cholecystectomy (LC) was soon after its advent performed in patients with acute cholecystitis (AC). The need for conversion to open cholecystectomy (OC) varies greatly and is reportedly necessary in 0 to 75% of LCs for AC. In patients undergoing LC for gallstone disease, signs (ultrasonographic etc.) of acute gallbladder inflammation have been found predictive of increased rate of conversion to OC, as compared with patients with no or chronic inflammation of the gallbladder. However, among patients with AC, factors predicting the need for conversion of LC to OC have not been unanimously defined. In this study such factors were sought for.
Methods: A retrospective series from 1992 to 1997 comprising 65 and 78 patients with clinical, laboratory and ultrasonographic signs of acute calculous cholecystitis scheduled for LC or OC, respectively, and who did not undergo bile duct exploration. Among the 65 patients who had initial laparoscopic approach, 17 had successful LC and 48 were converted to OC (LCconv).
Results: Out of eleven preoperative parameters analyzed, four were found to differ between the LC and LCconv groups, namely age (46.8±4.1 vs. 63.5±2.2 years; $p=0.004$), C-reactive protein (43.7±12.1 vs. 117.4±13.6 mg/L; $p=0.007$), leucocyte count (9.9±1.0 vs. 14.0±0.6 x 10^9/L; $p=0.001$) and positive bile cultures (1/15 vs. 18/44; $p=0.03$) (values are means±sem), whereas seven factors (a history of cholecystits or jaundice, symptom duration before surgery, body temperature, ultrasonographic signs of gallbladder wall edema or thickening or perivesicular edema) were similar between the LC and LCconv groups. Total hospital stay was similar as well (median 5 and 6 days, respectively).
Conclusions: These findings suggest that superimposed bacterial infection in conjuction with AC might be of importance for unsuccessful LC.

KARGER
Fax +41 61 306 12 34
E-Mail karger@karger.ch
www.karger.com

13.04

SPILLED GALLSTONES DURING LAPAROSCOPIC CHOLECYSTECTOMY

Mrksic M.
Medical Center, General hospital, Surgical department, Senta, Yugoslavia

Aims: Laparoscopic cholecystectomy (LC) has become the treatment of choice in the management of calculus gallbladder disease. Gallbladder perforation/laceration during LC with spillage of its content - bile and gallstones, is not uncommon. According to literature data it occures in 10-40%. Often, the spilled stones are left unretrieved in abdominal cavity. Although, in majority of patients, retained gallstones are of no consequence, there are reports of complicationes such as intraperitoneal abscess, intrahepatic abscess,entero-biliary-cutaneous fistula, cutaneous sinuses, small bowel obstruction. The aim was to analyse the experience with gallstones spilled at LC.
Methods: Prospective study on 201 patients who underwent LC by a single surgeon in period : June1995.- October 1998. was done. Mean age in studied group was 46.5 years (range : 16-76). There were 151 women and 50 men (75.2%:24.8%).
Results: The mean operation time was 64 minutes (range :20-180 minutes). In two patients (1%) the operation was converted to open due to distorded anatomy, but never due to lost gallstones. There were no common bile duct injuries and no postoperative deaths. In 52 patients (25.2%) perforation or laceration of the gallbladder occured. In 18 (8.9%) the spillage of the gallstones occured. One to 109 stones were retrieved in consecutive cases. In 7 cases (3.5%) it could not be possible to retrieve the lost stones. All patients sustained gallbladder laceration received broad spectrum antibiotics for two to three days.Patients with unretrieved stones are regulary followed up clinicaly and by US: one, three and 6 months after operation. The mean follow up is currently 11.5 months (3-26 months). No major complications due to lost stones were observed. In, one patient sucutaneous abscess containing one lost stone 3 mm in diameter in trocar port site (drain site) was observed.
Conclusions: Gallblader perforation and stones spillage during LC is not uncommon . In case of stones spillage it is advisable to retrieve all or as many stones as possible and to irigate the peritoneum. Although in majority of patients unretrieved gallstones are of no consequence, complicationes may occure, and because of that follow up of such patients is advisable.According to this experience there is no need to convers LC , even if some stones are unretrieved.

13.05

LAPAROSCOPIC APPROACH FOR THE TREATMENT OF SYMPTOMATIC NON-PARASITIC LIVER CYSTS IS EFFECTIVE AND MINIMAL INVASIVE

Andriani O.; Grondona J.; Secchi M.; Bracco R.; Russi R.; Suhl A.; Diez J.
Unidad de Hígado de la Fundación Favaloro (Buenos Aires), Centro Médico Martin y Omar (San Isidro), Hospital Italiano (Rosario), Clínica Pueyrredon (Mar del Plata), Hospital Naval (Buenos Aires), Hospital Francés (Buenos Aires), Hospital de la Universidad de Buenos Aires. **Argentina**.

Aims: To evaluate the efficacy of laparoscopic approach for unroofing symptomatic non-parasitic liver cysts.
Methods: Seventeen patients with symptomatic non-parasitic liver cysts were treated by laparoscopic approach between June 1993 and August 1998. Cases of policystic and hydatic diseases were excluded. No patient had previous treatments. Surgical technique consisted in laparoscopic wide unroofing of the main or the symptomatic cysts. Analysis of morbidity and mortality, postoperative hospital stay, persistence or relief of symptoms and recurrence were evaluated as well.
Results: Eleven women and 6 men, with a mean age of 56 years (32-74) were included in the study. Twenty-two cysts were treated. Diameter ranged from 5 to 30 cm (mean 10.4 cm). Disease was unilobar in 11 cases (65%) and bilobar in 6 (35%). Eleven of the 22 cysts were located in the right lobe while another 11 were in the left. Main symptoms were pain in 12 (70%), discomfort and increasing size during surveillance in 6 cases (35%), and palpable mass in 6 (35%). Four trocars were mostly used (13 procedures) although 5 ports were used in 4 instances. In 2 cases of a huge cyst evolving the entire right lobe, a lateral approach was required. Haemorrhagic fluid was found in 4 cysts (18%). Omentoplasty was associated in 3 instances in order to avoid folding of the border of the cyst wall, fluid reacumulation and recurrence. Cholecystectomy was contemporarily performed in 8 patients: 6 for cholelitiasis and in 2 were mandatory because of the location of the cysts. A tubular drain within the residual cavity was left in 8 cases (57%). The mean time of its withdrawal was at the 2nd postoperative day. Conversion to open surgery was not required in any case. Mild omalgia was observed in 2 patients. Mean postoperative stay was 2 days (1-5) and all patients began their normal physical activity within the 20 postoperative days. Mortality was nil. Mean follow-up was 25 months (3-48). Two patients were lost. A solitary cyst located on segments 3-4, approached only from the right side of the falciform ligament, recurred 6 months later, and was successfully treated by laparoscopy. Another patient remained with a residual cavity, asymptomatic after 2 years of follow-up.
Conclusions: Laparoscopic approach for wide unroofing of symptomatic non-parasitic liver cysts is advised even for large cysts in the right lobe, since this procedure has demonstrated good results.

13.06

LAPAROSCOPIC APPROACH IN THE MANAGEMENT OF LIVER CYSTS

V. Sorin, P. Schechter, V. Katz-Shnir, S. Levi, A. Czerniak
Department of Surgery A. The E. Wolfson Medical Center, Tel-Aviv University, Holon, Israel

Aim: To evaluate the management of symptomatic liver cysts in the era of minimal invasive surgery.
Methods: Patients with symptomatic liver cysts diagnosed by CT-scan and US were managed surgically by the laparoscopic approach. Partial excision of the cyst was performed in instances of simple cyst, while partial excision and unroofing was performed in instances of polycystic liver disease. Surgery was aided and directed by laparoscopic ultasound (Sharplan Usight laparoscopic US system, Israel, 8 MHz laparoscopis US probe enabling verification of adequacy of excision and identification of additional deep lesions.
Results: Ten patients (3 male, 7 female, age range 29-78) with symptomatic solitary liver cysts (7) and polycystic liver (3) were operated. 9 patients underwent laparoscopic cyst excision and unroofing using the above method. In one case the procedure was converted to laparotomy because of the demonstration of a cystobiliary fistula. One patient with polycystic liver had recurrence of symptoms 5 months after laparoscopic unroofing and was reoperated. There were no other recurrence in a follow up period of 6 months to 2 years.
Conclusions: Minimal invasive surgery should be the first line of management of symptomatic liver cysts. The use of laparoscopis US assessment at operation optimizes treatment particularly in instances of polycystic liver disease.

13.07

MINIMALLY INVASIVE TECHNOLOGY IN THE TREATMENT OF LIVER ECHINOCOCCOSIS.

S.A.Dadvani, A.N.Lotov, G.H.Musaev, O.S.Schkrob, V.N.Avakian, S.A.Kondrashin, V.J.Zavodnov, V.R.Matevossian.
Moscow Medical Academy, Surgical Clinic N 1, Moscow, Russia

Aims: to assess the efficacy of invasive methods in the treatment of liver hydatid disease.
Materials and methods: In our surgical clinic from 1986 to 1998 59 patients with liver echinococcosis underwent treatment. In 44 (74,6%) patients cyst was solitary single-camer, in 3 (5,1%)-multiple single-camer and in 12 (20,3%)-solitary cysts in liver and spleen. In all patients was fulfilled percutaneous drainage of the cyst under ultrasound control. Cyst cavity was processing with 10.0-20.0% NaCl solution (up to 1996), now we use 50-86% glycerin. After microbiologically proven parasite destruction we destroy and aspirate chytinic membrane of the cyst under endoscopic control per dilated punction channel. In multiple liver cysts used simultaneous or step by step percutaneous drainage. In combined disease underwent surgery and percutaneous drainage. In the operative period patients underwent peroral therapy with Albendazol.
RESULTS: All patients were treated with good results without serious complications with mean drainage duration of 16±3 days. Clinical follow-up was from 4 months to 11 year. Follow-up in 4-7 months in 15 patients reveal residual cavity required percutaneous punction. In one patient in subcutaneous fat formatted new cyst after early drainage removal.

13.08

Combined Closed-Open method: A Safer technique of primary cannula insertion at Laparoscopy

Agarwal AK
Department of GI Surgery, G.B.Pant Hospital, New Delhi, INDIA

Background : Laparoscopy has a risk of rare but serious and often fatal injuries during insertion of the primary trocar. Injuries due to Verres needle are much rarer and trivial on most occasions, which seal spontaneously.

Aims: To make Laparoscopy safer, the technique of first cannula insertion was modified, combining the advantages of both the closed & the open methods using the Verres needle and the blunt cannula and avoid the use of the sharp first trocar.

Methods (Technique): The technique consists of 3 steps: creation of pneumoperitoneum using a verres needle, incision of the peritoneum and a blunt cannula insertion. Pneumoperitoneum can be created using verres needle with reasonable safety. This lifts the anterior abdominal wall away from the intra-abdominal contents, making the superficial knife incision safer and easier for gaining an entry into the abdominal cavity using a blunt cannula or a blunt exchange rod.

RESULTS: We have safely used this technique over the last three years.

CONCLUSION: The described technique is a simple and cheap modification, which can be used by all laparoscopists without the need for any specialized training.

13.09

END RESULTS OF TROCARS INSERTION DURING ABDOMINAL LAPAROSCOPIC PROCEDURES

Diez JA, Gutiérrez Maxwel VG, Arozamena C, Oria MA., Napolitano AF
Buenos Aires University, Buenos Aires Argentina

AIMS: To evaluate the incidence and course of incissional hernias related to trocars insertion during laparoscopic procedures.
METHODS: 4603 incissions were performed as a result of 1183 laparoscopic procedures, from march 1991 to february 1998. These procedures included 1095 laparoscopic cholecystectomies and 88 diagnostic laparoscopies or tumoral stagings.The procedures were done by two different surgical teams with a different approach to the umbilical incision. One group used a 20mm. trocar and posterior aponeurotic closure for the gallbladder extraction on 345 patients. The other group performed the extraction of the gallbladder through a 10mm. incission with no aponeurotic closure in 710 patients, widening and incissional closure in 191 patients as a result of difficulties in gallbladder extraction, and in 37 patients wideningof the incission according to Hassan´s technique because of previous surgeries involving the periumbilical region. The remaining 5mm. incissions (n= 2278) and 10mm. incissions (n=1142) on the different abdominal quadrants were treated without aponeurotic closure. Patients follow up was from 8 months to 8 years.
RESULTS: Among 1183 laparoscopic procedures, an incissional hernia was diagnosed in 8 patients (1.1%). Five of them developped on 10 mm. umbililical incissions with no widening or posterior aponeurotic closure. Two patients presented an umbilical incissional hernia after the procedure on incissions with widening and closure.The remaining patient developped a herniation on a lateral 10 mm incission. No complications developped on 5 mm incissions.
CONCLUSIONS : The incidence of incissional hernias after a laparoscopic abdominal procedure is low. Lateral 10 mm incissions and umbilical wounds with no aponeurotic closure are at highest risk of developping an incissional hernia. Predisposing conditions include : incissional location and length, and posterior aponeurotic closure. The latter being the most relevant as most of the incissional hernias occurred in non-closed wounds.

Dig Surg 1999; 16 (suppl 1) 45-47

Biliary I.

14,01

CHOLECYSTECTOMY AND COMMON BILE DUCT EXPLORATION IN PATIENTS WITH CIRRHOSIS. a RETROSPECTIVE STUDY

N. Economou, A. Karkaletsis, P. Karydakis, A. Kyriakidis, V. Argitis, D. Papagoras, D. Pinialidis, N. Neofytou, G. Antsaklis

Data collected retrospectively from patients with cirrhosis who underwent cholecystectomy with common bile duct exploration or simple cholecystectomy. This study includes 26 patients which were hospitalized between Dec. '95 and Dec. '98.
Chid's criteria were used for the classification of the cirrhosis of the patients. Patients with child-C stage cirrhosis appeared to have the highest incidence of intraoperative bleeding and other major postoperative complications. The degree of bleeding in these patients varied.
In patients with child-A and child-B stages who underwent emergency or planned operative procedures had fewer intraoperative problems as well as postoperative complications. These groups were considered to be safe for any operation conducted on the bile duct system.
Conclusions: Any operation regarding the gallblader and bile duct system in patients with child-A and child-B stag cirrhosis can be performed with safety. On the contrary the child-C group carried a major risk in intraoperative and postoperative complications, so for this group of patients we recommend conservative - if possible - treatment.

14,02

PARTICULARITY OF ERCP AND SPHINCTEROTOMY IN THE CASES OF ANATOMICAL ABNORMALITIES

Danch A. V.
Department of Surgery "N.Anestiadi", University of Medicine and Pharmacy "N.Testemitsanu", Kishinev, Republic of Moldova

Aims: The present study was performed in order to evaluate optimal technique of endoscopic retrograde cholangiopancreatography (ERCP) and endoscopic sphincterotomy (ES) in the cases of anatomical abnormalities.
Methods: From 1992 to 1998, a total of 684 consecutive patients underwent endoscopic procedures were included in the study. There were 132 men and 530 women with an average age of 48 years (ranged from 6 to 88 years). Indications for endoscopic procedures were: jaundice, common bile duct stones, chronic pancreatitis, stricture of bile and pancreatic duct, etc.
The next endoscopic operations were performed: ERCP (n=582), ES (n=588), stone extraction (n=372), ES + Wirsungotomy (n=18), ES + nasobiliary decompression (n=38), placement of a biliary (n=16) and pancreatic (n=3) stents. Difficult situations (n=96) – 14% for ERCP and ES were considered in the following cases: (1) non-typical localization of papilla of Vater -5(0.73%), (2) juxtapapillary diverticulum - 37(5.4%) and (3) longer (>1cm) papillary stenosis. In four cases (localization of papilla of Vater in D-I or pylorus) ERCP was performed with a combined using of gastroscope and duodenoscope. We preferred a combination of papillotome devices, ES on the endoprothesis or nasobiliary decompression tube in difficult situations (juxtapapillary diverticulum or/and longer papillary stenosis). In high-risk cases, determinated by anatomical abnormalities, the ERCP and ES were performed in repeated endoscopic session: two-stage - 16(2.3%) cases, three-stage - 6(0.87%) cases and more then three - 3(0.43%). In 12 cases the ERCP and ES were performed with original endoscopic sphincterotome device.
Results: ERCP and ES were successfully accomplished in 656 (95.6%) patients, but in the group with anatomical abnormalities - in 68 (70.8%). The procedure-related mortality in high-risk group for ERCP and ES was 2.1%. Overall mortality after ES - 0.29%.
Conclusion: Our study suggest that (1) anatomical abnormalities of ampula of Vater reduce the successful rate of ERCP - ES and increase the procedure-related mortality; (2) in this situation is more preferable to use the papillotome devices combination and repeated endoscopic sessions.

14,03

IS RADICAL SURGERY IN ADVANCED GALLBLADDER CARCINOMA JUSTIFIED ?

Broering DC., Hillert C, Bloechle C, Gundlach M, Izbicki JR, Rogiers X.

Dep. of Hepatobiliary Surgery, University of Hamburg, Germany

Aims: Advanced gallbladder carcinoma, defined as stage II, III or IV tumor is associated with a poor long-term prognosis. Radical surgery including resection of adjacent liver and regional lymphadenectomy (LA) has been advocated to improve survival.
Methods: In the present study we evaluated the course of 77 patients, that underwent surgery for advanced gallbladder carcinoma. 4% of the patients had stage II, 22% stage III, and 74% stage IV tumors. R0 tumor resection was achieved in 33 (43%) patients. 9 patients underwent cholecystectomy (CHE) and LA. 15 patients underwent CHE combined with segment IV/V liver resection (LR) and LA of the hepatoduodenal ligament. 9 patients underwent right extended hemihepatectomy (EHH). 44 patients underwent operative exploration or palliative by-pass procedure. In surviving patients mean follow-up was 13,6 months ranging from 2 to 90 months.
Results: The mortality rate was in the LR and EHH-group with 6% lower than the overall perioperative mortality with 7,7%. The morbidity was 20% overall. In R0 resections Kaplan-Meier-analysis revealed a mean survival of 10, 24, and 16,2 months of the patients, who underwent CHE + LA, CHE combined with segment IV/V LR and regional LA, and EHH, respectively. In patients with palliative by-pass procedure or opertive exploration, mean survival was 6,6 months. After 24 months 28,4% of the patients with R0 resection were still alive compared to only one patient in the palliative treated group. In the patients with R0 resection no difference in survival was detected when N0 status was compared with N1.
Conclusions: If complete resection of advanced gallbladder carcinoma is achieved, radical surgery procedures including segment IV/V liver resection or EHH combined with regional lymphadenectomy even in T2 tumors provide a significant increase in survival with an acceptable mortality and morbidity.

KARGER
Fax +41 61 306 12 34
E-Mail karger@karger.ch
www.karger.com

14.04

PALLIATIVE SURGERY FOR THE TREATMENT OF JAUNDICE CAUSED BY TUMOROUS EXTRAHEPATIC BILE DUCT OBSTRUCTIONS

Balogh Á, Varga L, Mohos G, Palásthy Zs.
Albert Szent-Györgyi Medical University Department of Surgery, Szeged, Hungary

Authors report 93 surgically treated patients operated on for jaundice caused by primary extrahepatic bile duct cancer. 16 of our patients (17%) underwent a resective procedure, 23 patients (25%) explorative laparotomy, and 53 of them (57%) palliative surgery following unsuccessful or recurrent jaundice after non-surgical palliation. The previously applied palliative methods have been transpapillary stenting, endoscopic pig-tail drainage, percutaneous transhepatic drainage and/or dilatation. 23 of the 53 surgically treated patients underwent an exploration of the bile duct and some kind of external drainage was inserted. 30 of our 53 patients were operated on by hepato- or hepatico-jejunal by-pass. For this purpose, we used a 50 cm long Roux-en-Y jejunal loop. A comparison of drainage procedures to biliodigestive by-pass operations showed that the time of desicterisation, the rate of postoperative complications, the mortality and the postoperative quality of life were superior in the group of patients undergone biliojejunal anastomosis. Our conclusion is, that palliative surgery for jaundice, caused by tumours of the extrahepatic bile ducts is justified in cases with a previous unsuccessful attempt for endoscopic stenting or occlusion, or dislocation of endoscopic placed endoprosthesis. A bilio-digestive by-pass with a Roux-en-Y jejunal loop yields a superior quality of life, less complication rate, faster desicterisation and disappearance of cholangitis than external drainage procedures.

14.05

PALLIATIVE TREATMENT OF MALIGNANT OBSTRUCTIVE JAUNDICE

ŞİMŞEK A., KAYMAKÇIOĞLU N., YAKUT M., PEKER Y., ÇETİNER S., ŞEN D.
Gülhane Military Medical Academy Gen.Surg.Dept. Etlik/ANKARA

Palliation of malignant biliary tract obstruction is still associated with significant complications. Many techniques for the palliative management of patients with malignant obstructive jaundice have been developed, including endo-prosthesis, operative transtumor stenting and biliary-enteric by-pass, but the general prognosis remains poor. We review our experience with emphasis on therapeutic options.

From 1993 to 1998, 60 patients with malignant obstructive jaundice unsuitable for curative patients were treated in our unit. There were 34 men (56%) and 26 women (43 %). With median age 61 years (44-82), 29 patients (48 %) had associated diseases. Diagnosis was based on ultrasound and computed tomography, supplemented when necessary by direct cholangiography and citology. Clinical aspects, method of management, complications and mortality were assessed.

The principal sites of the lesion were the periampullary region in 29 patients (48%) and the upper/third/ hilus in 10 (16%) the middle-third in 9 (15%) the lower-third in 10 (16%) and diffüse in 2 (3.3%) patients. Surgical treatment was employed in 25 (41%) cases, radiological in 35 (58%) cases. Surgical therapy included hepaticojejunostomy and choledochojejunostomy and in 7 patients (11%) an associated gastro-jejunostomy was done. Radiological treatment included percutaneously endo-prosthesis, transtumor stending by CT or US guided. Univariate analysis was performed to discriminate variables in relation to morbidity and mortality. The median hospital stay was 16 days. 13 patients (21%) had complications and 6 (10%) died. The morbidity was associated mainly with pulmonary complications. The main causes of death were renal dysfunction, sepsis and multiple organ failure, peritonitis. The median survival of the patients available was 10 months with 5% of the patients alive at 2 years.

These results show that while short-term palliation is reasonable morbidity and mortality are high. The only significant factor influencing mortality was the pretreatment bilirubin level. Surgery for biliary tract obstruction is still associated with significant morbidity and mortality.

14.06

PRIMARY CARCINOID TUMOR OF THE COMMON BILE DUCT. CASE REPORT.

A.Lombardi , G.Batignani , A.Amorosi° , G.Neşi° , E.Mazza* , A.Calabrò[&] , C. Surrenti[&] and F.Tonelli .
Unità di Chirurgia , Gastroenterologia[&] e Radiodiagnostica* del Dipartimento di Fisiopatologia clinica. Anatomia ed Istologia Patologica° .
University of Florence.

Carcinoid tumors of extrahepatic biliary tree are reported exceedingly rare .
We report a case of primary carcinoid tumor originating in the distal part of common bile duct . To our knowledge this is the 14th reported in the literature and the 2th of the distal common bile duct . The patient , a 30 years-old male , presented with a sudden diarrhea with pale stools and dark urine , mild jaudice, pruritus and weight loss . Laboratory evalutation revealed abnormal LFT's with signs of biliary obstruction . Abdominal U.S. showed a normal gallbladder without stones with mild dilatation of intra and extrahepatic biliary tree and with a 2 cm solid ipoechoic tumor in the head of the pancreas closed to distal bile duct . An helical CT confirmed these findings and showing an hyper-vascular pattern of the tumor. An Echo-Endoscopy confirmed the previous characteristics and showed the absence of infiltration of the distal bile duct . An multihormonal screening showed an increase in the plasma serotonin, 350 ng/ml (normal range: 90-180) and platelets serotonin 1470 ng/10^9 plt (normal range: 200-600) ; all other gastrointestinal hormons were within normal range. Tumor markers (CEA and CA 19-9) were not elevated . At operation the tumor was found arising in the common bile duct and seemed to infiltrate the head of pancreas . The patient underwent a standard pylorus-preserving pancreatoduodenectomy . Pathological examination of the specimen showed a neuroendocrine tumor (carcinoid) of the distal bile duct , infiltrating the wall , MIB-1 index was 6% . The resection margins were negative . The postoperative plasma serotonin went back to normal levels . One year later the patient was healthly , without evidence of recurrent disease.
CONCLUSION : Carcinoid tumors of the biliary tree are rare (0.2-2% of the carcinoid); in literature , only one case treated by means of pancreatoduodenectomy . We advocate aggressive operative extirpation , realizing that this tumor , like to previous reports in literature , is associated with slow progression so a radical resection .

14.07

JATROGENIC INJURIES OF BILE DUCTS AFTER OPEN AND LAPAROSCOPIC CHOLECYSTECTOMIES

Prof. W. Jedrzejczyk MD PhD, M.Jackowski, M. Zalucki*, K. Leksowski**
*Clinic of General, Gastroenterological and Oncological Surgery in Torun, ** Surgical Clinic of the Military Hospital in Bydgoszcz

Aim: The aim of the study was to estimate early and longtrm results of surgery in jatrogenic injuries in bile ducts.
Material and method: In our Clinics between 1978 and 1992, 3940 typical cholecystectomies were performed. After these operations we have found injuries of common bile duct in 18 patients. We decided to reoperate them. In 14 cases we performed operation Roux-en-Y, 4 times we sutured the injured bile duct with the use of T-tube. Since 1993 w haven't noticed this type of complication after open cholecystectomy.

In both Clinics 3150 laparoscopic cholecystectomies were performed within last 5 years. In 8 cases the postoperative bile duct injury was diagnosed. 4 of the patients were operated with the Roux-en-Y method, I with the Rodney-Smith metod and 3 times we sutured the bile duct on the T-tube.
Results: The best results we noticed after the Roux-en-Y operation. 1 patient died becouse of the haemorrhagic shock (haemobilia) after the Rodney-Smith operation. In 2 cases the secondary bile duct stenosis was diagnosed and patients had to be operated once more.

We have to emphasise that 7 of 8 of the complications after laparoscopy occured during the first year of introducing the method in our clinic.

Dig Surg 1999; 16 (suppl 1): 48-50

Liver tumor I.

15,01

HEPATIC SURGERY AND TRANSPLANTATION FOR CYSTIC LIVER DISEASE

Jenkins BL, Lim PCM, Ammori BJ, Prasad KR, Pollard SG, Lodge JPA
Department of Hepatobiliary Surgery and Transplantation, St James's University Hospital, Leeds L59 7TF, UK

AIMS: To describe our experience with hepatic surgery and orthotopic liver transplantation for cystic liver disease.

METHODS: Between 1992-1998 we treated 46 patients with cystic disease of the liver. They were classified as follows: hydatid disease, cystadenoma, cystadenocarcinoma, simple solitary cyst, multiple simple cysts, and polycystic liver disease. Investigation in all cases was by CT or MRI, hydatid serology and tumour markers. Indications for surgery were pain, distension, vomiting and failure of aspiration therapy, or evidence hydatid disease, cystadenoma or cystadenocarcinoma on imaging or serology.

RESULTS: Hydatid disease was uncommon (n=3), reflecting U.K. practice. Two patients have been treated by formal hepatic resection: 1 left hepatectomy, 1 right hepatectomy. One patient is currently undergoing assessment. Cystadenoma (n=4) and cystadenocarcinoma (n=2) have also been treated by surgical resection.
Cystadenoma patients underwent hepatic resection (segmental 2, hepatic lobectomy 2). Only one patient with cystadenocarcinoma was operable at presentation (right trisegmentectomy). Simple solitary cyst (n=17), multiple simple cysts (n=6), polycystic (n=1 4) disease was managed conservatively in 21 cases. Radiological drainage was carried out in 5. Laparoscopic surgery was used in 6 patients (fenestration 4, left hepatectomy 1, right hepatectomy 1). Open resection was used in 3 patients (left hepatectomy 1, right hepatectomy 1, right trisegmentectomy 1). Liver transplantation was performed for intractable pain in 4 cases, 2 combined with kidney. There were four deaths (operative 3). Laparoscopic treatment failed in three patients.

CONCLUSIONS: The seriousness of cystic disease of the liver is often underestimated. Although conservative management was possible in 57% of benign cystic disease, the rest required surgery. Accurate diagnosis by complex imaging is important to look for hydatid cysts and tumour. Transplantation has a small but significant part to play in management of this group of patients, accounting for 8.7% of the patients and 19.0% of the surgical cases in this series.

15,02

OPTIONS ON SURGICAL METHODS IN THE TREATMENT OF HYDATID CYST OF THE LIVER.

Authors: Niculescu D., Plesa C.,Tircoveanu E., Ene D., - First Surgical Clinic "Sf. Spiridon" Hospital - Iasi - Romania

Aims : Evaluation of the results obtained by different surgical methods used in management of the hepatic hydatid cyst (HHC), as an argument to choise an apropriate method to treat the various tophographic and clinical situation of hydatid hepatic desease.
Methods: Retrospective study of 195 cases (104 female, 91 male) treated in The First Surgical Clinic Iasi Romania, between 1986 - 1997. 140 of them had a single cyst, 27 had double cyst and 28 had multiple localisation. Predominant affected was the VIIth and VIIIth hepatic segments. There was 98 cases uncomplicated cysts, 39 cases ruptured in a biliary ducts, 18 ruptured in peritoneum, 28 with supuration of the cyst and 12 with other complications. Most of them was treated by conservative surgical methods (cystotomy 14 cases, less or more large pericystectomy 174 cases). It was only 7 resection: ideal cystectomy - 4,segmentectomy - 2,atipic hepatectomy - 1. Omentoplasty was succesfull used 19 cases as a treatment of the restant cavity. Some complications was treated by a surgical procedure on extra hepatic biliary ducts: colecystectomy - 48 cases and 23 Kehr coledocothomy.
Results: The average postoperative hospital stage was 26 days. There was no postoperative complications in 151 cases and 28 reinterventions (immediate - 2, early - 2, late - 15, very late - 9). There was no postoperative death.
Conclusions: Better results in management of HHC can be obtained by using a surgical method apropiate to each one of the different anatomo - clinical situation.

15,03

OBSTRUCTIVE JAUNDICE CAUSED BY RUPTURE OF HYDATID CYSTS OF THE LIVER INTO BILIARY DUCTS. SURGICAL MANAGEMENT.

Daskalakis K, Tsepetis E, Papoutsas D, Karachristos A, Giaglaras A, Diamantopoulos G.

3rd Surgical Department, Evangelismos Hospital, Athens, Hellas.

Aims: The aim of this study is to present the problems in the management of obstructive jaundice caused by rupture of hydatid cysts of the lives into biliary ducts.
Methods: During the last 12 years (1986 – 1997), 113 patients with hepatic hydatidosis underwent surgery. Sixty-three were males and sixty females, 17-76 years in age. The majority of the patients operated on electively.
Twenty-two patients (19,4%) with rupture of the cyst into the bile ducts, obstructed jaundice and cholangitis, operated on in emergency basis.
In all patients with rupture of the cyst, common bile duct was explored, the daughter cysts were removed and T- tube or bilio-enteric anastomosis was made.
Partial cystectomy, suture of the intracyst peripheral bile ducts and omentoplasty was performed in all of these patients.
Results: No serious complications were in this series. There were 4 biliary fistulas. Two of these, headed spontaneously after 2 months and 2 needed an endoscopic sphincterotomy. There were no postoperative deaths. The mean hospital stay was 16,2 days.
Conclusions: The rapture of the cyst into bile ducts, needs CBD exploration and cleaning, suture of the communications and management of the hydatid cyst.
Partial cystectomy and omentoplasty is the procedure, which is applicable in the majority of patients, with excellent results.

KARGER
Fax +41 61 306 12 34
E-Mail karger@karger.ch
www.karger.com

15,04

CHALLENGING COMPLICATIONS OF HYDATID DISEASE

Yılmaz ÖZEN MD, Özkan YÖNÜK MD, Halil BİLGEL MD.

Uludağ Univ. School of Medicine General Surgery Dept, Turkey.

Aims :Instead of the improvements in Liver Surgery, hydatid disease and it's complications are still difficult problems of surgery in endemic areas of the world. Because there is no effective medical therapy, surgery remains the only radical method of treatment. Several methods with self advantages and disadvantages generally effect and sometimes defines the outcome.

Methods:The data from consecutive series of 242 patients operated on for liver hydatid disease between September 1987 and September 1998 were analysed. There were 98 men (%40.5) and 144 women (%59.5) aged 16 to 83(mean 42 years). 6 patients were admitted to emergency cervice with acute allergic condition due to rupture of the cyst into peritoneal cavity. The localisation of 149 single cysts (%61.6) was in right lobe, 57 single cysts (%23.3) in left lobe, and 14 multiple cysts (%5.1) in both lobes, and 22 multiple cysts (%9.5) both in liver and in other parenchymal organs and abdominal cavity. 38 cases were recurrent hydatidoses (%15.7). The Surgical procedures that applied to the cysts were, partial cystectony-drainage in 204 cases (%84.5), total cyst excision in 23 cases (%9.6), Liver resection in 7 cases (%2.7), percutancous drainage in 8 cases (%3,2) who had type I, II or some III cysts.

Results :Postoperative compl cations were as follows: İntra operative collapse in 2 cases, biliary fistula in 21 cases, hemobilia in one case, obstructive jaundice in 4 cases, broncho-biliary fistula in one case, cysto-cutancous fistula in one case, sclerosing cholangitis in one case, abscess formation in the residual cyst cavity in 13 cases. One patient died due to spontaneous massive bleeding during the evacuation of a big calcified cyst which eroded the vena cava. No recurrence or remarkable complications occurred after liver rescetions, total closed cyst excision and percutaneous drainage procedures.

Conclusions : The cysto-biliary connections and recurrences are the most challenging complications. Preoperative precise evaluation, desicion making and meticulous surgery are the gold standards of management. Percutaneous drainage is the best conservative method in suitable cases and total cyst excision and liver resection in complicated cases give the best results in experienced centers.

15,05

SURGICAL TREATMENT OF HEPATIC HYDATID DISEASE

Acarlı K., Demirel S., Tekant Y., Bilge O., Alper A., Emre A., Arıoğul O.
Istanbul Faculty of Medicine, Hepatopancreatobiliary Surgery Unit, Istanbul, Turkey.

Hydatid disease continues to be a major health problem in Turkey. Twenty-one years' data from a hepatopancreatobiliary unit were reviewed to assess the effectiveness of the operative treatment of hepatic hydatidosis.

Between January 1977 and May 1998, 571 patients with hepatic hydatid disease were operated on in the Hepatopancreatobiliary Surgery Unit of the Istanbul Faculty of Medicine in Istanbul, Turkey. Three hundred and thirty-two patients were female and 239 male, with a mean age of 40 years (range 18-83). Sixty-three percent of the patients had a single cyst while 37 % had more than one cyst. Cysts were located in the right lobe of the liver in 60% of the cases, in the left lobe in 19% and bilobar in 21%. Cysts were complicated in 30% of the patients (biliary communication, infection, etc.). Operative modalities used ranged from simple drainage and unroofing (35.6%) to cavity management techniques such as introflexion and omentoplasty (21.2%) and resectional procedures such as pericystectomy and liver resections (9.1%). In 126 patients with multiple cysts (22.1%), more than one surgical modality was employed. As an alternative to open surgery, laparoscopic treatment (8.6%) and percutaneous drainage (3.3%) were used in carefully selected patients. Biliary exploration and/or biliodigestive anastomosis was performed in 16% of the patients in complicated cysts.

Two patients died (0.4%) in the early postoperative period. Sixty percent of the patients could be followed up for a mean period of 4,5 years (range 8 months – 156 months). The recurrence rate was 11%.

In conclusion; after 20 years' experience, surgery remains to be the gold standard in the treatment of hepatic hydatid disease, offering the only chance for cure. But there is still no standard surgical modality for every cyst ! Surgical approach should be tailored to the individual patient.

15,06

Diagnosis and Treatment of liver echinococcosis. Radical versus conservative treatment

V. Skountzos, G. Kyratzis, V. Gougoutas and S. Karakalos.

Second department of General Surgery, General Peripheral Hospital "K.A.T.", 145 61 Kifisia, Hellas.

Materials and Methods: Between 1970 and 1998 a total of 42 patients treated surgically for liver hydatid cysts. The average age was 45.2 years with a male / female ration 1:1. Although we are favored of radical surgical procedures, they were applied in only 14 patients and more conservative treatment in 28 patients.

Results: A total of 49 cysts in 42 patients with liver echinococcal cysts were treated surgically. Radical surgery was done in 14 patients (capsulectomy was performed in 5 cysts, partial hepatectomy in 3 cysts); conservative surgery was performed in 28 patients (in all cysts, cystectomy was included; omentoplasty was added in 3 cysts, unroofing and omentoplasty in 12 cysts, unroofing and marsipulazition in 7 cysts, intubation only in 5 cysts and unroofing with intubation of the remaining cavity in 4 cysts).
The postoperative morbidity was 5% and there was only one death in a patient with multiple echinococcosis underwent a big surgical procedure. From the 42 patients only 30 of them we were able to followed up and they had remained free of recurences up to now.

Conclusion: Although we are favored of radical resection on liver echinococcosis, radical excision was not attempted in many cases (28 out of the 42 patients). Liver echinococcosis is a benign disease and our aim shall be to cure the patient from the disease, avoiding also, if it is possible, a major operation carrying more post operative morbidity and mortality in complicated cases.

15,07

EVOLUTION OF THE SURGICAL TREATMENT OF LIVER HYDATIDOSIS. REETROSPECTIVE MONOCENTRIC STUDY

M. Jeremic, M. Stojiljkovic, M. Stojanovic, P. Stojanovic, Lj. Jeremic, S. Jeremic
Surgical Clinic, Clinical Center Nis, Yugoslavia

Aims: Liver hidratic echinococcosis (LHE) is an endemic disease in Yugoslavia like in the ofter Mediterranean countries (3.8 per 100.000 inhabitants). We looked out our experience in this pathology over the last forty yers (1957-1977 and 1977-1997).

Methods: In the first period (1957-1977) 103 patients were operated on. In the second period (197-1997) 146 patients were surgically treated. Demographic characteristic is male/female ratio 72/177, with average age of 44.1 years.

Results: Cysts localization's were as follows: right lobe (167 pts or 67.06%), left lobe (52 pts or 20.88%), bilobar cysts (30 pts or 12.04 %). Basic diagnostic methods were scintigraphy and arteriography in the first period and ultrasonography and computer tomography in the recent period. Total sensitivity and specificity rat of diagnostic procedures was 72.69%. In the first period the most common operations were conservative (74.75%), associated with high recurrence (1.60%) and complication (19.41%). Total pericystectomy was performed in 16.50%, liveer resection in 8.73%. In the recent period 32.87% total pericystectomy and 10.27% liveer resection have been performed with lower complication rate (10,95 and without recidives). The most common complication has been biliary fistula: 7.76% in the first period and 4.79% in the second. Mortality rate has been 1.60%. Postoperative hospitalization has been 26 (first series) and 12.4 days in the recent Seri.

Conclusions: Radical surgical approach results with the lower complication rate and eliminates the recurrence. However, partially pericystectomy with omentoplasty is very good solution, without surgical risqué, especially in the treatment of „problematic" cysts (adhered to VCI or hepatic veins or centrally localized).

15.08

OMENTOPLASTY :REPORT OF 186 CASES

Muftuoglu T, Koksal N, Kurt R, Uzun MA, Günerhan Y, Alptekin A.
Haydarpasa Numune Hospital, Istanbul, Turkey

Aim: Hydatosis is still endemic in Mediterranean region.The incidence of hydatic disease of the liver in this area has remained high during the last 25 years. There are many alternatives in the surgical management of hepatic hydatic disease. Our choice to management of cystic cavity has been omentoplasty for a long period. The aim of this retrospective study is to present outcomes of omentoplasty.

Patients and methods:
We analyzed retrospectively 211 patients with hepatic hydatid disease admitted between 1990 and 1998 in Department of General Surgical Clinics. Ultrasonography was used in big majority of the cases (88.5%) in diagnosis. The right lobe (70%), left lobe (18%) and right and left lobe (12%) were involved.
Twenty four patients were found intrabiliary ruptured hydatid cyst (13%) and six patients were treated for free perforation into abdomen (4%). Others were uncomplicated hepatic hydatic cyst. One hundred and eighty six patients 88 percent) were treated with omentoplasty after drainage of cystic cavity.

Results: Mortality rate was 1 per cent of all cases. 0n trabadominal abscess were developed in two patients (1%) and one managed with percutaneous drainage and other underwent open surgery. Bile fistula were found in twelve patients (6%) in postoperative period and closed spontaneously. The average of postoperative stay in hospital was 9.2 days. Twelve patients who underwent omentoplasty were admitted with presenting recurence of hydatid disease (6.4%).

Conclusion:
Omentoplasty is safe, effective and reliable procedure in management of cystic cavity because of lower mortality, morbidity and recurence rates compared with other techniques.

15.09

SURGICAL TREATMENT FOR SPLENIC HYDATIDOSIS: SPLENECTOMY OR ORGAN-PRESERVING PROCEDURE?

***Pavliuc G V**, Tsybyrne K A, Mishin I V*
Dept. of Surgery, Laboratory of Liver Surgery, Medical University "N.Testemitsanu",
Kishinev, Republic of Moldova.

Introduction: Splenic echinococcosis (SE) is rare, even in areas where hydatid disease is endemic. The use of organ-preserving or radical surgical procedures (splenectomy) in the management of SE is controversial. In this study, we have retrospectively evaluated the results of different surgical procedure for SE.
Materials and Methods: From 1985 to 1998 a total of 364 consecutive patients with abdominal hydatid disease were treated surgically in our department. In 23 of these patients (6.3%) hydatid cyst were located in the spleen (SE): in 5 - only in spleen and 18 patients had associated liver hydatid cysts (5) and peritoneal echinoccocosis (13).
Preoperative diagnosis of PE was established using ultrasonography, CT scan, immunologic test and X-ray. Solitary cyst in the spleen were found in 16 (69.5%), and multiply cysts in 7 (30.5%). The size of the splenic hydatid cysts ranged from 8 to 25cm, complications took place in 8 (34.7%) patients: cyst supuration (6) and calcification of the cyst (2).
In all cases a median supraumbilical incision was used. Partial excision of splenic cysts with omentoplasty was performed in 10 cases and splenectomy in 13 cases. During organ-preserving procedure, noncommercial fibrin tissue sealant (with low concentration of thrombin - 50-100 U/ml) was used as supplement to surgical technique for hemostasis and fibrinadhesive omentoplasty. Concomitant liver hydatid disease or multiple peritoneal cysts were managed surgically at the same time.
Results: Two patient with disseminated peritoneal echinoccocosis died during the early postoperative period due MOF (mortality rate 8.6%), and one patients had minor complications. Recurrence of SE was occurred in two cases after partial incision of splenic cysts and need splenectomy.
Conclusion: Surgery remains the treatment of choice for splenic hydatidosis. Partial incision of the splenic cyst with omentoplasty may be used only for solitary and superficial hidatid cyst. Splenectomy remains the therapeutic procedure of choice for multiply and complicated hytatid cysts.

Dig Surg 1999; 16 (suppl 1): 51-53

Biliary II.

16,01

GALLBLADDER CANCER IN LAPAROSCOPIC OPERATION?

V. PRIMIKIRIS, D. TSANTZALOS, P. VOULGARIS, G. PAPADOPOULOS, S. TSOUPANOS, M. NIKOLAIDIS.
2"° DEPARTMENT OF SURGERY - 1ST HOSPITAL H□A - °□PENTELI" - ATHENS

Laparoscopic surgical procedure, is now a days, an acceptable method in treatment of gallstone's disease. A serious contraindication to the above concept is the presense of gallbladder cancer.

Considerable numbers of cases, of gallbladder cancer, in general have as a first appearance feature the symptoms of acute cholocystitis. The incidence of unsuspected cancer that is faced during current cholocystectomy is about 0,4 %.

We present, here, our experience in 1570 LC that have taken place from Jan 1991 to Aug I 997 and in which we encountered 9 cases of gallbladder cancer. In three of them we found out cancer "in situ" after routine histopathologic examination. The patients had submitted only cholocystectomy and remained under six months supervisory follow up. So far all the three are alive without indications of local recurrence or metastases. The other two had developed hepatic metastases by the time of operation. In these patients we inserted a stendt tube through the ERCP procedure. Both of them died 4 and 8 months after operation, respectively.

Surgeons who operate using laparoscopic procedures must be acquaint with the idea of facing a malignancy in gallbladder and they must have prepared their selves in proceeding a biopsy if any suspicion exists, even in the slightest case. The big dilemma is whether the operation must be continued as an open one or not.

In our series three stages with cancer "in situ" had good results, up to now, without proceeding an open laparotomy. Nevertheless the issue remains controversial. We believe that in case of facing the suspicion of malignancy, it is wise to proceed a biopsy from the lesion and the suspected area in order to confirm the diagnosis of cancer and its stage and then an open laparotomy must be performed. The laparotomy could take place the same time or in a few days depending on the specific conditions.

16,02

SPONTANEUS INTERNAL BILLIARY FISTULAE (REPORT OF 26 CASES)

Djordjevic R, Kitanovic A., Zajic S.

Surgical Department Health Center Kruševac

The purpose of this article is to present all cases of biliodigestive and biliobilia-ris fistulas diagnosed and operated in our department.

From 1988 to 1997 we were operated 26 patients with biliodigestive (20) and biliobiliaris (6) fistulae. The factors which we analyzed were: symptoms, diagno-stic procedure, treatment, morbidity and mortality, sex, age and staying in hospital.

There were 20 biliodigestive fistulae, all cholecysto-duodenal, without chara-cteristic symtoms. Preoperative diagnostic corectly perfomed in 2 patients (x-rays examination and US). Surgical treatment in all of them were cholecystectomy and suture of duodenum. In second group we had got 6 patients with bilio-biliaris fistulae (Sy Mirizzi type-II). The base sign in all patients was obstructive jaundice. The diagnostic was performed intraoperativly with cholangiography. In three cases we performed cholecystectomy and hepatico-jejunostomy sec. Roux en Y, and in three cases we performed cholecystectomy and suture existing defect of hepatico-choledochus with T-tube.

There were 20 women and 6 men, with a mean age of 68 years old. We had 3 cases with wound infections, and we were not registrated lethal outcomes.

Spontaneus internal biliary fistula is an anusual disease most frequently in elderly patients with long term cholelythiasis.

16,03

THE ROLE OF EARLY INTERVENTION IN ACUTE BILIARY PANCREATITIS

Kalahanis N., Delis S., Pikoulis E., Tsigris C., Papalambros E., Bastounis E.
First Department of Surgery, University of Athens, Medical School, Athens, Greece

Aims: The purpose of our study is to evaluate and document the morbidity and mortality after early surgical intervention in mild and severe forms of gallstone pancreatitis.
Methods: 146 patients admitted to the author's surgical service over a 5year period with clinical diagnosis of gallstone pancreatitis. There were 86 male and 60 female patients ranging in age from 35 to 72 years. Ranson's prognostic signs were used to classify all patients. All patients operated on early (less than 72 hours after admission). The operation includes the performance of open cholecystectomy via a subcostal incision with or without intraoperative cholangiograma.
Results: There were 8 patients with operative findings of hemorrhage, 102 patients with edematous and 36 patients with normal pancreas. Impacted ampullary stones were found in 28 patients. The common duct stones were noted more after among those patients older than 50.
In 120 patients a cholangiogram was obtained and 28 patients underwent common bile duct exploration. The 108 patients with mild pancreatitis had 5.5% morbidity and 3.7% mortality. In the 38 patients with severe pancreatitis the morbidity and mortality rates were 21.05% and 15.7% respectively.
Conclusion: The morbidity and mortality with early surgical intervention in our study was low and without significant difference with the morbidity and mortality of late intervention from the literature. It also deminishes the length of stay and the incidence of recurrent gallstone pancreatitis.

KARGER
Fax +41 61 306 12 34
E-Mail karger@karger.ch
www.karger.com

16,04

THE PREVALENCE OF UPPER GASTROINTESTINAL ABNORMALITIES BEFORE AGE OF 40 MAY ENCHANCE THE RISK OF GALLSTONE DISEASE

Sipos P., Szabó Á., Jakab I., Turcsányi G., Faller J.

Semmelweis University of Medicine, Kútvölgyi Clinic, II. Dept. of Surgery, Budapest

The functional and pathological correlation between the diseases of upper gastrointestinal tract and the formation of gallstones in a similar aged population is still unclear and needs more identification, but some statistical data may draw attention to certain findings.

The aim of this study is to discuss whether the upper gastrointestinal abnormalities discovered during routine gastroscopy performed prior to laparosocpic cholecystectomy may arise the prevalence of gallstone disease or not. 422 gastroscopy performed before the laparoscopic cholecystectomy discovered in 55% of the patients gastrointestinal abnormalities.

In some studies (e.g.: Multicenter Italian Study) association were found between gallstone disease and peptic ulcer. Portincasa and coworkers showed out existence of multiple functional defects of the upper gastrointestinal tract in gallstone disease.

According to the data in the literature and our data the prevalence of gallstone disease and gastritis rised linearly with age. The prevalence of gastritis in Hungary according to epidemiological data was the following: 20-29 yrs=42%, 30-39 yrs. =58%, 40-49 yrs.= 75%, 50-59 yrs= 80%. The prevalence of gastritis in patients with gallstones was the following: 20-29 yrs.= 71%, 30-39 yrs.= 73%, 40-49 yrs.= 45%, 50-59 yrs.= 56%, 60-70yrs.= 61%.

Our result shows that before the age of 40 the prevalence of gastritis and upper GI abnormalities may enhance the risk of formation of gallstone disease.

16,05

SUBHEPATIC BILOMA CAUSED BY PERMEABLE EXTRAHEPATIC BILE DUCTS

Ondrejka P., Sugár I., Szabó M., Vajda V., Bognár G., István G., Faller J.
2nd Deparment of Surgery, Semmelweis University Medical School, Budapest, Hungary

Introduction: Spontaneous extrahepatic biloma associated with a constricted and stoneless gallbladder is an uncommon clinical finding.
Patient and methods: A 84 year old female patient was admitted to our department with right subcostal pain and tenderness. She had obstructive jaundice. The urgent abdominal ultrasound examination showed a markedly dilated common bile duct, but could not verify gallbladder. Because of the poor general condition of the patient we started conservative treatment, and non surgical solutions were planed. After initial improvement the right subcostal tenderness increased after two days, and local peritonitis developed. The controll US examination demonstrated a subhepatic fluid collection, so we decided to carrie out an operation.
Results: During the operation we found a biloma under the left hepatic lobe containing aproximately 300 ml of bile. The common bile duct was extremly dilated, and the gallbladder proved to be constricted, stoneless and obstructed. We carried out cholecystectomy and choledochotomy. The common bile duct was full of smaller-bigger stones and sludge. Perforation on the gallbladder or on the extrahepatic bile ducts was not found. Because of the bad general condition of the old patient we were forced to do the minimal solution, which was the washing out of the bile ducts and an insertion of a Kehr T tube. In the postoperativ period the patient's general condition was acceptable. After a week we carried out control cholangiography through the T tube, which demonstrated several residual small stones in the choledochus. Then an endoscopic billiary clearence was performed succesfully, after which the patient became stone free.
Conclusions: Subhepatic biloma owing to a permeable common bile duct caused by gallstones is a rare event. The emptying of the biloma and the clearence of the choledochus are essential as treatment in a case like this. In elderly patients for these purposes the minimal surgical solutions are madatory.

16,06

MICROLAPAROTOMY CHOLECYSTECTOMY

Rozsos I., Szira P.
Moritz Kaposi Medical Centre, Kaposvár, Hungary

Aims: The microlaparotomy cholecystectomy is not a widespread procedure yet.
Methods: I order to further elaborate on the procedure and to demonstrate its value, 2400 micro- and minilaparotomy cholecystectomies, without exclusion or selection, were analysed.
Results: The operations were completed with microlaparotomy (less than 4 cm incisions) in 2241 cases (93,38 percent) with modern minilaparotomies (4-6 cm) in 146 cases (6.08 percent), with conventional minilaparotomies (6-8 cm) 6 cases (0.25 percent). Only 7 cases (0.29 percent) required longer than 8 cm incision. In 133 ceses (5.5 percent) stone was removed from the common bile duct through less than 6 cm incisions. The mortality rate was 0.12 percent and 210 patients (0.41 percent) underwent reoperation.
Conclusion: Comparing with laparoscopic cholecystectomy the advantages of microlaparotomy cholecystectomy are the less expensive instrumentation and the surgeon's 3-dimensional vision to operating field. The postoperative pain and recovery was similar to those of the patients with laparoscopic procedure. Our experiences show that cholecystectomies performed by micro- and modern minilaparotomy are realistic alternatives to the conventional and laparoscopic cholecystectomies.

16,07

Biliary injuries as a result of blunt abdominal trauma

Márkus B.[1], Döbrönte Z.[2], Gog T.[1]
Markusovszky Teaching Hospital, Szombathely, Hungary
Department of General Surgery[1]
2nd Medical Department[2]

The authors review the diagnostic and therapeutic problems of the rare extrahepatic biliary duct injuries as a result of blunt abdominal trauma in connection with a presentation of a case report.
A 47 year old man was admitted to the surgical department with jaundice, 95 days after sustaining a blunt abdominal injury following a 5 meter fall having been readmitted to 5 different departments. At operation an extent necrosis of the extrahepatic biliary ducts were found along with subhepatic collection of bile. The necrotic gall bladder was removed, the bile collection was drained and the bile sludge was flushed. Continuity of the bile flow was restored by a Roux-en-Y hepaticojejunostomy. The patient had an uneventful recovery.
The authors discuss the possible mechanisms of injuries.The signs and symptoms can sometimes be obvious, making early diagnosis easy, but more often - as in the authors' case - this can be difficult and delayed by several days. Ultrasonograhy, CT, hepatobiliary scan, ERCP and peritoneal lavage can aid the diagnosis. The authors discuss the choice of operation and its influencing factors (patient's general condition, other injuries, site of biliary duct injury, extent of the injury) together with the anatomy of the blood supply of the extrahepatic biliary ducts. Definitive repair or resection is performed in patients whose condition is stable, with the option chosen based on the extent of the ductal injury, namely, transection without loss of tissue, extensive defect in the wall or segmental loss of ductal tissue.
In summary they state that the diagnosis and treatment of biliary duct injuries as a result of blunt abdominal trauma can often necessitate surgical experience in hepato-pancreatico-biliary surgery.

16.08

PITFALLS OF TRAUMATIC BILE DUCT INJURIES IN PAEDIATRIC AGE GROUP

[1]El-Sefi Talaat, [1]Marwan I., [1]Shawki A., [2]El-Ebeidi G., [3]Fawzy A.T., [4]Abdel-Ghaffar T., [4*]El-Naggar O., [5]Rashed M.Y.T., [5*]El-Dessouky M.
Depts. of Surgery: [1]Liver Institute and [3]Faculty of Medicine, University, and [2]Mansoura University. Depts. of [4]Paedia [4*]Paediatric Surgery, Ain-Shams University. Depts. of [5]Mec [5*]Paediatric Surgery, Alexandria University.

Traumatic bile duct injury in children is rare and responsible for morbidity and mortality because of diagnostic delays.

Aims: To analyze the pitfalls in the diagnosis and manageme injuries.
Methods: Ten children sustained bile duct injury due to blunt tı and penetrating injury in one were studied.
Results: They were divided into 3 groups according to the time presentation after the trauma Group A (n=3) presented immed trauma with acute abdomen (live injury). On exploration, asso duct injury was detected in 2, but missed in one (33.3% subsequently was confirmed by endoscopic retrograde cholaı (ERC). Group B (n=3) presented 1-2 weeks after trauma with pain, distention, jaundice and fever. Exploration failed to localize bile duct injury in all. Postexploratory ERC identified the site of ı Group C (n=4) presented 6-36 months after trauma with recurren cholangitis due to bile duct strictura in all an choledochoduodena one. Two of them were found to have secondary biliary cirrhosis. management were found to have secondary biliary cirrhosis. management included primary repair, controlled, external c (endoscopic stenting) biliary drainage, and Roux-en-Y hepaticojej
Conclusion: Early diagnosis of bile duct injury in children is ve even during exploration. Repeated ultrasonography after bluı intraoperative cholangiography (in cases of liver injury) and E high suspicion arises) are essential to establish an early Management must be individualized according to the extent of and the time of the diagnosis. Biliary decompression (external c appears to be an effective modality for the management of partia injury.

Dig Surg 1999; 16: 54-56

Biliary III.

17.01

EARLY RESULTS OF SURGERY FOR BILE DUCT INJURY AND BENIGN STRICTURES

0

J P A Lodge, B J Ammori, T Mahmood, K R Prasad
Departments of Hepatobiliary Surgery, St. James's University Hospital, Beckett Street, Leeds LS9 7TF, UK

AIMS: Iatrogenic bile duct injuries and benign strictures may complicate laparoscopic and open cholecystectomy, gastric, pancreatic and hepatic surgery. Reconstruction with a Roux-en-Y biliary-enteric hepaticojejunostomy offers the best surgical treatment. This paper describes our early results of surgery for high bile duct injuries and benign strictures.

METHODS: Between October 1993 and August 1998, 31 patients underwent surgical revision of biliary injury (*n*=7) or benign biliary stricture (*n*=24) in our Hepatobiliary Unit. All surgery was carried out or supervised by the senior author (JPAL) using a Roux-en-Y hepaticojejunostomy. There were 8 males and 23 females, with a mean age of 57 years (range 25-79 years). Previous biliary surgery, including reconstructions (12 patients) preceded definitive repair in 28 patients. Biliary strictures were of Bismuth's types 2-4 in 65% of patients. Mean follow-up was 23 months (range 3-62 months).

RESULTS: Complications developed in eight patients (25.8%), of whom seven underwent previous reconstruction. Five patients (16%) required further surgical intervention (bleeding; 2, bile leak; 2). There were two in-hospital deaths (6.5%) at 19 and 113 days postoperatively. Symptomatic and radiological resolution were achieved in all survivors. There has been no clinical, biochemical or radiological indication of recurrence of biliary strictures to date.

CONCLUSIONS: Early results of bile duct reconstruction for injury or stricture are satisfactory. However, the operative risk in patients with previous bile duct reconstruction remains considerable. Long-term follow-up is required to determine the re-stricture rate.

17.02

OUR EXPERIENCES WITH SINGLE-LAYER BILIODIGESTIVE ANASTOMOSIS

Kelemen D, Csontos Zs, Horváth ÖP
1st Surgical Clinic of Medical University of Pécs, Pécs, Hungary

Aims: Even now there is no definite standpoint, whether the single or double-layer biliodigestive anastomosis is the better? The authors detailed their results with the single-layer technique.

Methods: The authors performed single-layer biliodigestive anastomosis in 153 patients between 1993 and 1998. In 96 cases the diagnosis was tumor, while the others were benign. Among the operative procedure there were pancreatoduodenectomy, pancreatic head resection, decompression, GEA and in small percentage of the cases other procedures. Hepatico- or choledochojejunostomy was twice as much as cholecystojejunostomy. 88,2% of the anastomoses was done with continuous suture technique, mainly with 4/0 PDS.

Results: There was complication in 45% of the cases, from which the rate of biliary fistula was 3,9%. The conservative therapy always healed these fistulas. Reoperation was in 7,1%, the operative mortality was 9,8%. Preoperatively 77,1% of the patients had cholestasis, which improved in all cases postoperatively. During the late follow-up period recurrent cholestasis was not found and the other results correlated with the literary data.

Conclusions: The authors offer the single-layer technique in the case of biliodigestive anastomosis. It is an effective and safe method with low complication rate.

17.03

CHOLANGIO-DUODENAL INTERPOSITION OF AN ISOLATED JEJUNAL SEGMENT (CDI) AFTER BILE DUCT RESECTION

Kremer B, Reibe F, Vogel I, Grimm H, Henne-Bruns D

Dept. for General and Thoracic Surgery, University of Kiel, Germany

Aims: The bilio-intestinal reconstruction after bile duct resection is routinely performed by an Roux-en-Y-loop. Interposition of an isolated jejunal segment (CDI) offers the advantage of endoscopic control and intervention during follow-up of these patients.

Methods: Between 1989 and 1998 in 55 patients (bile duct carcinoma n=38, benign strictures or choledochal cysts n=17) an interposition of an 10 to 25cm jejunal segment was performed after bile-duct resection.

Results: In 35 of these patients (63.7%) no cholangitis was observed during follow-up (6-92 months). In 8 patients (14.5%) cholangitis was already treated perioperatively, in 4 patients (7.2%) once a year. In 2 patients (3.6%) up to three episodes and in only 3 patients (3.6%) more than 3 infections per year were observed. Three patients were lost during the follow up period.
Diagnostic endoscopy could be performed in 22 cases before dischargement and in 11 cases the endoscopy was incomplete due to the kinking of the jejunal segment.
During the follow up time in 19 cases a diagnostic endoscopy could be performed. 26 patients died due to extrahepatic tumor recurrence.
In none of the patients with bile duct carcinoma therapeutic endoscopic intervention was necessary. Due to cholestatic problems after iatrogenic bile duct injury and CDI reconstruction therapeutic endoscopy was successfully performed in 3 cases (stent implantation n=2, removement of intrahepatic stones n=1); one patient had to be treated by PTCD.

Conclusion:
1. If a CDI is performed a short segment (less than 15 cm) should be used.
2. CDI should be restricted to patients in whom anastomotic re-stenosis or local tumor recurrence are expected to be the main problem during follow up.

KARGER
Fax +41 61 306 12 34
E-Mail karger@karger.ch
www.karger.com

17.04

COMMON BILE DUCT EXPLORATION. IS T – TUBE DRAINAGE ALWAYS NECESSARY?

Daskalakis K, Papoutsas D, Tsepetis E, Bursinos V, Papadopoulos A, Diamantopoulos G.

3rd Surgical Department, Evangelismos Hospital, Athens, Hellas.

Aims: The aim of this paper is to suggest that the use of T- tube drainage is not always necessary after common bile duct exploration.

Methods: from 1987 to 1998 (11 years), 412 patients with choledocholithiasis underwent CBD exploration.

Group A: Seventy-four patients (31 males, mean age 68,6 years and 43 females, mean age 61,6 years) were managed with primary closure of the CBD (17,9%). Group B: One hundred ninety seven patients (89 males mean age 66,8 years and 108 females mean age 63,3 years) were managed with T – tube insertion (47,8%).

Intraoperative cholangiogram was performed in all patients of both groups pre and post CBD exploration.

Surgical technique of primary closure is described in the paper.

Results: Main complications: Group A: Bile leakage from the drain for 3-4 days: 3 patients (4%) and residual stones in 2 patients (2,7%). Group B: Bile leakage in 14 patients (701%), residual stones in 12 (6%), biliary fistula in 3 (1,5%), CDB stricture in 3 (1,5%), acute pancreatitis 5 (2,5%) and bile peritonitis after T – tube removal in 3 patients (1,5%). Mortality rate was nil in group A and 1% (2 patients) in group B. Mean hospital stay was 6,3 days in group A and 15,3 days in group B.

Conclusions: We conclude that if indicated, primary closure of the common bile duct after choledochotomy for choledocholithiasis, is a safe and cost – effective procedure.

17.05

INJURIES AND BENIGN STRICTURES OF THE MAIN BILE DUCTS

Tsohataridis E., Beis I., Ziakas M., Evangelou G.
2nd Dept. of Surgery, NIMTS Hospital, Athens, Greece.

Aims: We present our experience on the management of injuries and benign strictures of the main bile ducts.

Methods: From 1992 through 1998 we managed 7 patients with injuries or benign strictures of the main bile duct. These patients may be classified into four groups: (I) Two patients had an injury of the main bile duct (Bismuth 1 and 2), after a difficult open cholecystectomy, found during the initial operation. Hepatico-jejunostocy (H-J) with a Roux-en-Y loop performed in both cases. (II) Two patients developed a benign stricture after a previous H-J performed 13 and 6 months before for Ca of the head of the pancreas, without local recurrence. One of the patients was managed with a new H-J and the other with the insertion of a stent via a percutaneous transhepatic cholangiography. (III) One patient developed a benign stenosis of the distal bile duct after manipulations with instruments for choledocholithiasis. He was managed with the insertion of a stent via endoscopic retrograde cholangiopancreatography. (IV) Two patients admitted with strictures of the main bile duct (Bismuth 1-2) after laparoscopic cholecystectomy performed in other Institutions. They both were managed with H-J.

Results: The patients were followed from 3 to 44 months. There were not deaths during the operations. There were a few crises of mild cholangitis in the patients managed with the insertion of stents. The results were very satisfactory in the patients with H-J.

Conclusions: H-J is the operation of choice in most of the cases with injuries or benign strictures of the main bile duct.

17.06

LONGTERM RESULTS OF BENIGN BILIARY STRICTURES RECONSTRUCTION

R. Čolović, D. Bilanović, M. Jovanović, S. Zogović
First Surgical University Hospital, Institute of Digestive Diseases, Clinical Center of Serbia, Belgrade, Yugoslavia

Over 25 year period (1974-1998), 137 pts were operated for benign bile duct strictures. There were 90 female (65,7%) and 47 male (34,3%) patients. The everage age was 50,2 years (from 16 to 84). Two pts had congenital stricture, 6 stricture due to chronic pancreatitis, one posttraumatic and 128 postoperative bile duct stricture (116 after cholecystectomy, 8 after distal gastrectomy for duodenal ulcer, 4 after hydatid cyst operations). According to Bismuth's classification, there were 26 (18,9%) strictures type I, 38 (28,0%) type II, 46 (33,5%) type III, 26 (18,9) type IV and one (0,7%) type V. A number of preoperative complications were registered in our pts: intrahepatic lythiasis (49), liver fibrosis or cirrhosis (16), atrophy/hypertrophy complex (7 pts), liver abscess (10), incisional hernia (13), biliodigestive fistula (7), colonic fistula (2), gastrojejunal fistula (1), supurative pericarditis (1), retroperitoneal biloma (1), portal vein thrombosis (1), perihepatic abscess (1), subphrenic abscess (1), biliary peritonitis (4), varices CBD (1) and a number of minor complications like inadequate Roux-en-Y anastomosis in 40 pts and so on. In 80 pts, one to six previous attempts of reconstruction were performed elsewhere. In two pts reconstruction was technically impossible due to portal vein thrombosis in one and due to inaccessible bile duct in the other. In 135 pts 136 reconstruction were carried out (one pt was reoperated one year after previous reconstruction). In 129 pts hepaticojejunostomy with 75 cm long Roux-en-Y limb, in 3 choledochoduodenostomy and in 3 a choledochoplasty were carried out.Three pts died in the early postoperative course (two in whom the reconstruction was impossible and one with previous renal insufficiency). Five pts died later, two due to variceal bleeding, one due to myocardial infarction, one due to pancreatic carcinoma and one due to cerebrovascular infarction. Nine pts were lost from follow up. The rest of 124 pts were followed up from 6 months to 27 years (median 7,5 years). Good results of reconstruction were achieved in 99 out of 124 reconstructed pts (79,2%), satisfactory in 23 (18,4%) and unsatisfactory in 3 (2,4%). We conclude that satisfactory results of reconstruction of benign bile duct strictures could be achived in a majority of patients provided that the proper reconstruction is not performed too late.

17.07

TREATMENT OF THE STRICTURE OF HEPATICOJEJUNOSTOMY

Keleti G.,Molnár P.,Hollós G.
St Laszlo Hospital.Budapest.Hungary

Aims: The authors review the treatment and outcome of the patients with strictur of hepaticojejunostomy (HJ).

Methods: 28 patients were treated with strictured HJ. at the St. Laszlo Hospital between 1992 and 1997.In the majority of the patients the HJ. was performed after laparoscopic injury -22 cases- and open cholecystectomy – 2 cases-.In two cases the stricture of HJ occurred after pancreaticoduodenectomy.There were 23 females and 3 males at the mean age of 43 years. The most common symptoms were jaundice and pruritus. The time elapsed between the HJ. and our treatment was 16.2 months.

Results: There were a strictly correlation between the number of the operations after the LC injury and the level of the biliary obstruction.The more operation were performed ,at higher level developed the stricture. Six patients were treated with percutan balloon dilation and 22 cases had operative treatment.

Transhepatic U tube with or without resection(4 cases) resection of the strictures HJ (4 cases) ,Hepp-Couinaud procedure (13 cases),Soupault-Couinaud procedure (1 case) .

The percutan ballon dilation was succesful in 3 cases.

In the operative group 1 patient died in the early postoperative period (4.5% op. mortality).The morbidity rate was 36.4%.The late results of the operative treatment seems to be very good. 21 patients have been alive, the majority of them without any postoperative problems.

Conclusions: The best results can be achieved with Hepp-Couinaud procedure in the cases with strictured HJ. after LC injuries. The percutan ballon dilation should be used only in the preoperative period.

17.08

REMOVAL OF THE IMPACTED STONES IN THE PAPILLA REGION UNDER VISUAL CONTROLL WITH FLEXIBLE CHOLEDOCHOSCOPE

CSENGERI A., ZWICK M., TAKACS GY.
DEPARTMENT OF SURGERY
GENERAL HOSPITAL SUBOTICA YUGOSLAVIA

AIM: THE AIM OF THE STUDY IS TO EVALUATE THE SUCCCESS RATE OF INTERVENTIONAL INTRAOPERATIVE CHOLEDOCHOSCOPY IN REMOVEING IMPACTED STONES IN THE PAPILLA OF VATER, THUS PREVENTING OPERATIVE MANIPULATIONS ON THE ODDI'S SPHINCTER.

METHODS: REVIEWING OUR OPERATIVE MATERIAL OF FIVE YEARS AND FOLLOW UP CASES IN WHOM THE INTERVENTION WAS PERFORMED.

RESULTS: SINCE 1993, WHEN WE STARTED WITH CHOLEDOCHOSCOPIES, 183 CHOLEDOCHOTOMIES WERE PERFORMED FOR CHOLEDOCHOLITHIASIS. INTRAOPERATIVE CONTROL OF THE BILE DUCTS WITH OLYMPUS T-20 FIBERCHOLEDOCHOSCOPE WAS DONE IN 43 CASES. IMPACTED STONES IN THE PAPILLA OF VATHER, NOT REMOVABLE WITH FORCEPSES WAS FOUND IN 26 CASES (14 %). CHOLEDOCHOSCOPY WAS PERFORMED IN 11 OF THESE PATIENTS. THE STONE WAS SUCCESSFULLY EVACUATED FROM 10 (91%). IN 13 CASES TRANSDUODENAL SPHINCTEROTOMY, IN 7 CHOLEDOCHO-DUODENOSTOMY WAS PERFORMED. INTRAOPERATIVE CHOLEDOCHOSCOPY WAS PERFORMED IN 5 CASES OF THE SPHINCTEROTOMY AND ANASTOMOSIS GROUP. EXTRACTION OF CALCULI WAS UNSUCCESFULL IN 1 CASE ONLY. IN 4 CASES AFTER REMOVAL OF THE STONE, BECAUSE OF STENOSIS, TRANSDUODENAL INTERVENTION ON THE PAPILLA HED TO BE DONE. WE MOST FREQUENTLY USED DORMIA BASKET OR FOGARTHY CATHETER THROUGH THE WORKING CHANEL. RETROJET DEVICE WAS LESS EFFECTIVE.

CONCLUSIONS: IN DIFFICULT CASES OF STONE IMPACTATION, FLEXIBILE CHOLEDOCHOSCOPE WITH ITS DEVICES MAY BE HELPFUL IN DESOBLITERATION OF THE PAPILLA AND IT MAY REDUCE THE RATE OF OPERATIVE SPHINCTEROTOMIES. EXPERIENCE IN BILIARY ENDOSCOPY IS RECOMENDED FOR THE SUCCESS.

Dig Surg 1999; 16 (suppl 1): 57-58

Liver tumor II.

18,01

PATHOLOGIC FEATURES AND PATIENT SURVIVAL IN PRIMARY LIVER CARCINOMA IN RELATION TO AGE.

Trotovsek B, Gadzijev EM.
Dep. of abdominal surgery, University medical centre, Ljubljana, Slovenia.

Aims: For primary liver carcinoma (PLC), the peak age of patients is at the sixth decade. However, the influence of age on the tumor biologic behavior and long-term patient survival is controversial.
Methods: We retrospectively studied 56 patients whose PLC were surgically resected and analyzed the pathologic and clinical features of the tumors and patient survival in relation to age. Clinical characteristics were noted including age, sex, history of alcohol abuse, hepatitis B and/or C positivity, TNM staging, macroscopic and microscopic tumour characteristics, treatment received and ultimate survival from the beginning of treatment. The patients were divided into two groups, younger than 60 years of age and older than 60 years.
Results: Twenty -nine patients were 60 years of age or under, and 27 were older than 60 years. The mean age was estimated at 54.2 +/. 4.2 years (p<0.05). The younger patients had: more frequent hepatitis B surface antigen positivity (p = 0.047), less cirrhosis (p = 0.034), less tumor encapsulation (p = ns). No correlation was observed between vascular invasion, tumour diameter, TNM stage, operative mortality and age of the patients. In univariate analysis was age more than 60 years associated with improved mean survival of 48 months compared to 26 months in younger group (LogRank =0.0149).
Conclusions: Less frequently associated cirrhosis in younger group did not compensate the difference in survival rates between the two groups. The treatment policy in the older group should not differ from that in the younger group and when ever possible we should try to radically treat older patients. We found that older patients tolerate procedures as good as younger and the biologic behavior of tumors is less aggressive in older group.

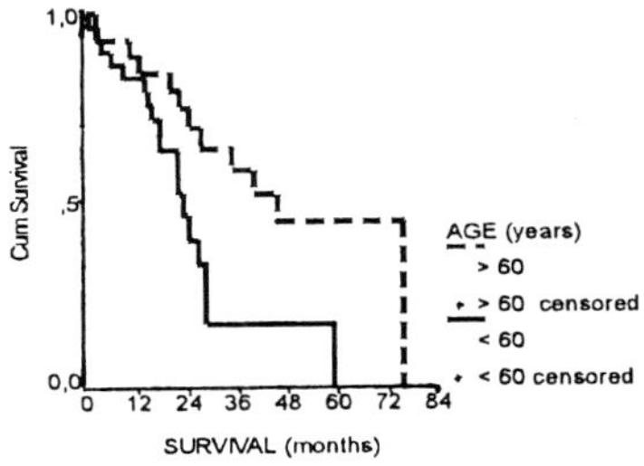

18,02

ROLE OF DIAGNOSTIC LAPAROTOMY IN THE ASSESSMENT OF FOCAL DISEASE OF THE LIVER

D. Görög, V. Weszelits, Z. Máthé, A. Tóth, F. Perner
Semmelweis University of Medicine Transplantation and Surgical Clinic, Budapest Hungary

Aim of the study was to evaluate the need of diagnostic laparotomy performed for nodular diseases of the liver in the era of widespread availability of imaging techniques.
Methods: Data of patients who were admitted in our institute for suspicion of focal liver disease were reviewed. All patients underwent on investigation that included ultrasound scan (US), computed tomography and/or magnetic resosnance imaging furthermore in selected cases radio-nucleide scan was done. Investigation toward primary tumour was considered in suspicion of liver metastases. When the diagnosis was uncertain US guided percutaneous liver biopsy was performed. Explorative laparotomy was indicated in case of unsuccesful diagnostic procedure that did not reveal the nature of focal liver disease. The intraoperative examination included ultrasound scanning and liver biopsy with frozen section. The present study does not evaluate those laparotomies which aimed the staging of a preoperatively known malignant tumour.
Results: 295 patients with focal liver disease were admitted between 1994 and 1998. During this period 19 diagnostic laparotomies (6,4 %) were performed which revealed benign lesion in 12 patients, primary liver malignancy in 3 cases and metastases in 4 patients. Among patients with benign focal disease (n=71) the rate of diagnostic laparotomy was higher /17 %/ than those with primary liver tumour (n=59) or metastases (n=165) /5 % and 2,5 %/. The yearly rate of laparotomy was the following, 1994 - 6 %, 1995 - 0 %, 1996 - 6,5 %, 1997 - 12 %, 1998 - 6,5 %. Only diagnostic laparotomy was done in 11 patients while further intervention followed it in 8 cases. One patients who presented bleeding from biopsy site and needed relaparotomy and bleeding controll died under sepsis.
Conclusions: Despite availability of imaging techniques the diagnostic laparotomy seems to be an important tool in assessment of nodular liver diseases in "difficult cases" (differentiation between benign and primary malignant lesions) even if it is not a procedure without risk. Considering the tumour seeding as a disadvantage of percutaneous liver biopsy the rate of explorative laparotomy can rise although the diagnostic laparoscopy that is proposed recently can take it unnecessary in selected cases.

18,03

INTRAHEPATIC FOCAL LESIONS (IFL) EVALUATION

Ditoiu A.V.*, Motoi O*, Stoica V**, Hortopan M***,
Fundeni Hospital,*Medical clinic,***Department of Pathology,
**Cantacuzino Hospital, Medical clinic, Bucharest Romania

Aim: histological examination of liver specimens from patients with suspicion of IFL, in order to establish the origin, the celular and histological type, the differentiation grade and the perilesional hepatic tissue status.
Methods: The study was performed on 58 hepatic tissue specimens (one or more samples from each patient), obtained through liver neddle biopsy or surgery, from patients with IFL (with suspicion of malignancy) addmited in Fundeni and Cantacuzino Hospitals between 1.01-30.09.1997.Histological examination was made in the ours Departments of Pathology.
Results: Sex ratio: 2:1 (M=68.96% / F = 31.04%), average age = 54.47 ± 16,21years (M = 58.57 yrs,F=48.05yrs). Besides liver cancer, which was found in 44 cases (75.86%) there were:normal hepatic tissue-4 cases, cavernous hemangioma - 3 cases, nonhodgkinina limphoma -1 case, liver abscesess -1 case, nodular focal hyperplasia -1 case, liver cyst-1 case,"white biopsy"-1 case. As histological types of liver cancers, we noted: hepatocelular carcinoma- 88.65% (with different subtypes) different sarcomas(s) - 9.08% (leiomios, hemangioendothelios, lipos, fibros, each with 2.27%), melanoma -2.27%. As differentiation grade (G): G1=25%, G2=45.45%, G3=9.09% G4=2.27%. Sourrounding hepatic tissue was affected in 25% cases (liver steatosis - 11.36%, liver cirrhosis-4.54%, chronic hepatitis - 2.27%). The suspected primary site based on the histological examination was: digestive tract - 1.36%, pulmonar-4.54%, melanoma -2.27%, vascular - 2.27%. Surgical exploration in 21 cases, detected metastatic nodes in 19% cases and reactive changes in other 19 cases.
Conclusions: Our data confirm those from literature in regard to the carcinomatous origin of 90% of liver neoplasms. We underline the much more frequent association of othe liver diseases like cirrhosis and chronic hepatitis (25% cases),a possible explanation may be the abstention of surgical or bioptical interventions in this patients.The relatively low prevalence of node metastasis, sugests the possibility of limited hepatic resection ,if there is a sufficient remaining functional hepatic mass.

KARGER
Fax +41 61 306 12 34
E-Mail karger@karger.ch
www.karger.com

18,04

ADENOMA AND ADENOMATOSIS: AN EMERGING LIVER PATHOLOGY

Zanus G. - Tedeschi U. - Cillo U. - Boccagni P. - Brolese A. - Bassanello M. - Bonariol L. - Urbani L. - Montin U. - Gringeri E. - Veroux M. - D'Amico D.F.
DEPARTMENT OF GASTROENTEROLOGICAL AND SURGICAL SCIENCES - PADOVA (ITALY).

Introduction. Current advances in imaging techniques and their capillary diffusion have induced a striking increase in early diagnosis of benign hepatic lesions. Liver adenoma has raised a great deal of interest not only in relation to its etiology, given the causative association with the use of oral contraceptives and anabolic steroids, but also because its diagnostic and therapeutic implications. Mandatory surgical management includes a broad range of interventions from tumor excision to liver transplantation.
Patients and Methods. 315 liver resections have been performed at the "Istituto di Clinica Chirurgica 1°" of the University of Padua from 1984 to 1998. 26 resections were carried out for liver adenoma. The patients, aged between 10 and 46 years (mean age 32 years) were mainly females (94%) and had an adenomatous lesion ranging from 4 to 15 cm in size. 65% of patients were symptomatic, in the remaining 35% the adenoma was detected incidentally. Preoperative work up included ultrasound guided cytology in 90% of patients. Preoperative cytology was not conclusive in 20% of cases, requiring histologic examination of the surgical specimen. Surgical procedures consisted of 11 segmentectomies, 3 bi-segmentectomies, 1 extended left hepatectomy, 4 sub-segmentectomies and 7 wedge resections. We did not experience post-operative hepatic failure nor liver transplantation in our series.
Results. Postoperative course was uneventful with no relevant complications (2 pleural effusions were treated conservatively). Mean hospital stay was 12 days without intra-perioperative nor late mortality. In 2 cases (7.7%) malignant transformation was incidentally found. Surgical treatment proved to be radical with no evidence of recurrence at 3-year follow up.
Conclusions. Hepatic adenoma, due to the high risk of malignant transformation, intratumoral hemorrhagic necrosis and diagnostic uncertainty even after histologic/cytologic examination, calls for a mandatory resective treatment including, whenever required, elective or urgent liver transplantation (massive intraabdominal bleeding secondary to rupture of the adenoma) as reported by Starzl.

18,05

HORISONTAL LIVER RESECTION

F. Jakab, P. Nagy, Gy. Kőszegi, E. Kádár
Departments of Vascular and General Surgery, Uzsoki Teaching Hospital, Budapest, Hungary

The segmental anatomy of the liver meant a great evolution in liver surgery. The significance of fissurae, hepatic vessels and sheets appeared in numerous new, technically more feasible surgical procedures. Recently the segmentectomy became the basic elements of our liver surgery aiming manly the fulfillment of oncological purposes. A new procedure has been worked out on the basis of segmental anatomy, called in our practice: **horisontal liver resection.**

Since January 1. 1995 reviewing 8321 interventions, the liver were involved in 292 patients. 4 out of 292 patient with liver surgery have been treated by **horisontal liver resection**. The main indication fields are as follows:
1.Surgery for gallbladder cancer (T1, T2),
2. Surgery for metastases of liver,
3. Surgery for primary tumours in segment 4B, 5, 6.

The horisontal liver resection means the removal of segment 4B, 5, and 6 alongside the horisontal plane. The procedure in vascular exclusion has been proved to be safe, quick, bloodless interventions in four patients. The average operating time: 1h 20', exclusion time: 19', blood need 0 units. Perioperativ morbidity: 3%, mortality=0 has been observed respectively.

In conclusion: The horisontal liver resection can be regarded as a kind of plurisegmentectomy, utilizing the existing anatomical property of liver.
The main indications are as follows: gallbladder cancer, primary or secondary tumours of segment 4B, 5, and 6. The quick and safe procedure has the benefit of bloodless and parenchyma saving liver resection.

18,06

IMPROVEMENT OF MORBIDITY AND MORTALITY RATES IN LIVER TRAUMA.

By
G. KYRATZIS, D. XYPOLYTAS, V. SKOUNTZOS.

From the 2nd Surgical department, General Peripheral Hospital "K.A.T.", 145 61 Kifisia, Hellas.

The treatment of hepatic injuries is a major surgical problem. Morbidity and mortality rates still remain high in complex liver trauma, but a reasonable improvement is recorded the last two decades.

An analysis of 620 patients with liver trauma admitted to the hospital, from 1963 to 1998 was done, 413 patients were males and 207 were females. The causative factor in the majority of patients was blunt abdominal injuries due to traffic accidents.

A comparison of morbidity and mortality rates in this series between two times period was attempted. The first period includes patients admitted to the hospital from 1963 to 1973 (total 88 patients) and the second period from 1974 till 1998 (total 532 patients). In the first period morbidity rates of 14% and mortality of 18% was recorded and in the second period the morbidity was 11% and the mortality was 8%, comparatively lower than previously.

Main factors influencing on those improvement rates were:
1. Better support of trauma patients prior to hospital admission.
2. Shortening of the time in evaluation and treatment of those trauma patients in the Emergency Room.
3. Appropriate surgery by surgeons familiar with liver trauma surgery, and
4. Post operative I.C.U. treatment in order to minimize complications because some of them, as it is well known, may become lethal.

18,07

EXTENDED HEPATIC RESECTIONS IN THE TREATMENT OF SEVERE LIVER TRAUMA.

L.Papastamatiou, L.Lapidakis, G.Kyratzis.
Dep. of Surgery, Apostle Paul Hosp.-KAT, Athens, HELLAS

The first historical report to hepatic trauma is from the Troyan war, described by Homer, according to which Ipsinor died after massive bleeding following open liver injury 3000 years ago. Hepatic injuries account for about 30% of all abdominal traumata and their severity is classified into 6 grades (revised Liver Injury Scale, 1994). According to this system the higher grades V and VI include Complex Liver Injuries. As such are described severe parenchymal damages (extended disruptions-avulsions) associated with trauma at the porta hepatis (laceration-rupture of the vena porta, hepatic artery-ducts) and or at the juxtahepatic venous system. The main charachteristic point of those injuries is, indisputably, their extremely high mortality and therefore they remain the greatest challenge even for the most experienced trauma surgeon.

Treating liver trauma, limited peripheral resectional debridement of devitalized hepatic parenchyma are often. In the contrary extended liver resections are rare, less than 5%, performed only if necessitated from the type of the injury. Three are the main causes obliging to such a procedure:
a) Multiple starlike deep ruptures (explosion type injury)
b) Almost total hepatic division, followed by doubtful vascularization of the smaller part of the liver.
c) Mandatory sacrifice of healthy liver tissue, required for control of bleeding, from the juxtahepatic venous system.
From a total of 708 blunt and penetrating liver injuries 184 have been classified in the 2 higher degrees. In 108 cases limited resectional debridement was performed, while extended resections were necessitated in 37 cases (5,2%). All but three resections were atypical, achieved by the use of the finger fracture technique. From the total of the 37 multi-injured patients, 22 died (mortality rate 59,5%) but 14 deaths were attributed to the liver trauma (37,8%), mostly due to irreversible haemorrhagic shock.

It is concluded that extended hepatic resection is a borderline procedure, aiming either to secure haemostasis or to removal of non viable large hepatic fragments.

Dig Surg 1999; 16 (suppl 1): 59-61

Hepatic metastases

19,01

STAGING LAPAROSCOPY FOR HEPATOBILIARY AND PANCREATIC (HBP) MALIGNANCY.

Rai R, El-Wash M, Youssef F, Davidson BR.

Universuty Department Of Surgery
Hepato pancreatic biliary Surgery and Liver Transplantation Unit
The Royal Free Hospital, London, UK.

Aims: The role of laparoscopy in the staging of intra-abdominal malignancies is controversial. We have examined its role in group of patients with hepatobiliary and pancreatic malignancies.
Methods :Over a period of 4 years (September 94- September 98), 89 patients with suspected HBP malignancies underwent staging laparoscopy under one consultant. All patients were considered to have resectable tumors as determined by radiological investigations. Most common malignancies were adenocarcinoma head of pancreas (n=24), Hepatocellular carcinoma (n=15), Cholangiocarcinoma (n=14).
Radiological investigations included dynamic contrast enhanced CT scan in all patients, angiography for 66 (74%), CTAP for 29 (32.5%) patients, MRI for 17 (19%) and post lipoidal CT for 17 (19%) patients. Patients found resectable on laparoscopy proceeded to laparatomy.
Results: Laparoscopy was successful in 86 (95%) patients. Dense adhesion from previous surgery prevented access for pneumoperitoneum in 2 and limited complete examination in other. In 2 patient laparoscopy detected irresectable disease in 14 (16%) patients and missed metastatic disease in 10 (11%) patients out of which 3 had vascular involvement, which was found after trial resection. Laparoscopy avoided unnecessary laparatomy in 14 (54%) patients with irresectable disease. Over all sensitivity of laparoscopy was 58% specificity was 100% and accuracy was 92%. Laparoscopy had similar sensitivity in cholangio and pancreatic carcinomas but laparoscopy was 100% sensitive in case of hepatocellular carcinomas. There was no mortality associated with the procedure and there were 3 minor complications.
Conclusions: Staging laparoscopy is safe , it decreases the non therapeutic laparatomy rate and increases the resectability rate of those proceeding to laparotomy. Staging laparoscopy is poor at detecting vascular invasion. Laparoscopy should precede laparotomy in patients with HPB malignancy.

19,02

STAGING LAPAROSCOPY IN THE EVALUATION OF COLORECTAL LIVER METASTASES

F.Youssef, F. Khan, S. Farahat , D.Vougiouklakis, B.R Davidson
HepatoBilliary and Pancreatic Surgery. Royal Free and University College Medical School, Pond Street, London NW3 2QG. UK=20

Aims: Laparoscopy has been shown to be useful in the staging of abdominal malignancies. Its value in patients with previous major abdominal surgery is controversial. The aim of this study is to evaluate the use of staging laparoscopy for patients with colorectal liver metastases.

Methods: 15 patients with colorectal liver metastases technically resectable on conventional imaging (Triple phase CT of chest and abdomen, MRI, Bone scan, CTArterio-portography and dual vessel Angiogram) underwent laparoscopy before proceeding to liver resection. None of the patients had any clinical or radiological evidence of local recurrence or other distal metastases. The site of the establishing pneumoperitoneum was in the periumbilical area in 6 patients and alternative sites were used in rest of the patients depending on the site of the previous colectomy incision. =20

Results: Laparoscopy was successfully completed in 14 patients. It was not successful in one patient because of dense adhesions. The procedure added 14=B18 minutes to the operation time. There were no procedure-related complications. The findings were similar to the radiology in 6 patients. Additional findings were seen in 8 patients; peritoneal lesions were found and confirmed on frozen sections in 2 patients, precluding resection in them; in 7 patients additional liver lesions were found precluding resection in 1 patient, but the resection was done for the other six patients.

Conclusion (1). Laparoscopic evaluation for colorectal liver metastases is safe (2). Adequate visualisation of the liver and abdominal cavity were obtained in 75% of patients (3). Spared unnecessary laparotomy in 20% of patients. (4). A larger study needs to be done before staging laparoscopy can be recommended as a routine for every patient considered for liver resection for colorectal metastases.

19,03

EX-VIVO AND IN-SITU RESECTION OF INFERIOR VENA CAVA FOR HEPATIC COLORECTAL METASTASES: HIGH RISK BUT WORTHWHILE

B J Ammori, K R Prasad, M C Bellamy[1], J P A Lodge
Departments of Hepatobiliary Surgery and Anaesthesia[1], St. James's University Hospital, Beckett Street, Leeds LS9 7TF, UK

AIMS Involvement of the IVC by hepatic tumours, albeit rare, is considered inoperable by standard resection techniques. Concomitant hepatic and IVC resection is required to achieve adequate tumour clearance. The aims of this paper are to describe the operative techniques and early results of inferior vena cava (IVC) resection in patients with advanced liver tumours.
METHODS: Between 1995 and 1998, 181 patients underwent hepatic resection in our unit. Six patients, aged 42-80 years (mean 61 years), with hepatic metastases from colorectal cancer underwent concomitant resection of the IVC and 4-6 hepatic segments. Resections were carried out under total hepatic vascular exclusion in four patients, and *ex-vivo* in two patients. Between 30°-360° of the intrahepatic IVC was resected and replaced with autogenous vein graft (n=1), Dacron tube graft (n=1) or patch (n=3), or repaired by primary suturing (n=1).
RESULTS: There were two early deaths due to multiple organ failure. One patient survived for 30 months following *ex-vivo* resection, but died from renal cell carcinoma. The remaining three patients remain alive at one, six and seven months postoperatively, with no signs of hepatic failure or venous obstruction. One patient developed pulmonary metastases at seven months postoperatively. Non-thrombotic occlusion of the neo-cava occurred in one patient, and was stented successfully.
CONCLUSIONS: Whilst concomitant hepatic and IVC resection is associated with a considerable operative risk, this aggressive surgical approach offers hope for patients with hepatic tumours involving the IVC, who are otherwise destined to a dismal prognosis. This surgery can be made feasible by the adoption of total hepatic vascular exclusion, with or without venovenous bypass, and by *ex-vivo* bench resection.

KARGER
Fax +41 61 306 12 34
E-Mail karger@karger.ch
www.karger.com

19,04

SURVIVAL AFTER REPEAT HEPATIC RESECTION FOR RECURRENT COLORECTAL METASTASES.

Staudacher C, Chiappa A, Zbar AP, Biella F, Bertani E, Crotti C*
Dept. of Emergency Surgery-University of Milan-ITALY
S. Raffaele Scientific Institute
**Imperial Medical College-Hammersmith Hospital-London-UK*

Aims: This is a retrospective clinical study done to examine survival of patients undergoing repeat hepatic resection for recurrent colorectal metastases.
Methods: The records of 41 patients undergoing hepatic resection for metastatic colorectal cancer were reviewed. Sixteen (39%) experienced recurrences confined to the liver. Ten (24%) of them underwent resection and make up the study population.
Results: The four women and six men had a mean age of 62 years (range: 44-82 years). In 60% of patients recurrent cancers involved both the same area near the resection line and remote sites from the first hepatic resection. In 30% of patients recurrent cancers were at sites remote from the first liver resection. In only one patient (10%) recurrent cancers was in the same area as the original hepatic resection. Three anatomical hepatic resections and seven non-anatomical wedge resections were performed. Average blood loss was 900 cc (range: 100-2700 cc); average hospital stay was 19 days (range: 8-34 days). Perioperative mortality was nil. Morbidity was 20%. Four patients died of recurrent disease, with a mean disease-free survival of 13 months (range: 5-21 months). Six patients experienced intrahepatic recurrence after the second hepatic resection. Of these, two patients underwent a third hepatic resection for intrahepatic recurrence 10 months and 24 months, respectively after the second hepatic resection. One of these patients experienced recurrence in the liver 9 months after the third hepatic resection. The tumour was resected, and the patient is still alive 31 months after the last liver resection with no evidence of disease. Six patients are alive and four of them disease-free, with a mean follow-up time of 34 months (range: 22-64 months). Actuarial 4-year survival was 44% and 4-year actuarial disease-free survival was 18%.
Conclusions: In properly selected patients mortality, morbidity, and survival after repeat hepatic resection are similar to those after initial resection.

19,05

DOES THE SUB-SPECIALITY OF THE SURGEON PERFORMING PRIMARY COLONIC RESECTION INFLUENCE THE OUTCOME OF PATIENTS WITH HEPATIC METASTASES REFERRED FOR RESECTION?

S. J. Wigmore, D. C. C. Bartolo, K. K. Madhavan, E. J. Currie, O. J. Garden
University Department of Surgery, Royal Infirmary of Edinburgh,
United Kingdom

Aim: This study attempts to establish whether the sub-speciality interest of the surgeon performing primary surgery for colon cancer influences resection rates and outcome of patients referred for consideration of resection of hepatic metastases.

Methods: Data have been collected prospectively on 230 patients with hepatic metastases arising from colorectal tumours referred to a single centre for consideration of resection. The patients were divided into those referred by colorectal specialists (CRS) (n=122) or general surgeons with other sub-speciality interests (GS) (n=108). The principal outcome measures studied were resectability of metastases, frequency and pattern of recurrence following resection and survival.

Results: No significant differences were observed between the two groups of patients with respect to age, sex, tumour stage, site of primary tumour or the frequency of synchronous or metachronous metastases. Technically resectable disease was identified in 84 patients (46% of the total patients referred by CRS and 26% of those referred by GS Cho Sq=9,1, p<0.01). Tumour recurrence occurred in 45% of patients referred by CRS and 75% of patients referred by GS (Chi Sq=6.5, P<0.05). Tumour recurrence involving bowel or lymph nodes accounted for 21% of all recurrences in patients referred by CRS compared with 50% in patients referred by GS. Overall the median survival was 24 months for patients referred by CRS and 15 months for patients referred by GS versus (Log rank - 13.1, p<0.0001).

Conclusions: Patients referred by GS are less likely to have resectable disease and if they do undergo surgery they are more likely to develop recurrent tumour and have a worse overall outcome compared with patients referred by surgeons with a sub-speciality interest in coloproctology.

19,06

IS IT JUSTIFIED TO RESECT BILOBAR COLORECTAL LIVER METASTASES?

Ercolani G, Mazziotti A, Grazi GL, Cescon M, Del Gaudio M, Ravaioli M, Cavallari A.
Dept of Surgery and Transplantation, Sant'Orsola Hospital, University of Bologna, Bologna, Italy

Aim: The role of liver resection for the treatment of bilobar hepatic metastases is still controversial. We evaluated the results in the resected patients with bilobar metastases compared to patients with unilobar single and unilobar multiple metastases.
Methods: Two hundreds and twenty-four liver resections for colorectal liver metastases were performed since 1984. In 130 patients (58%) there was a single lesion, in 55 patients (24.5%) there were multiple unilobar lesions, in 39 patients (17.5%) bilobar lesions. No differences in age and sex were among the 3 groups.
Results: The overall mortality was 0.8% (2/224 patients). No postoperative mortality occurred in the group with bilobar metastases. The global actuarial survival rate at 5 years was 40% in patients with single lesion, 23% in patients with multiple unilobar lesions, and 18% in patients with bilobar lesions respectively. Since 1991, with the introduction of some technical innovations like the routine use of anatomical segmentectomies, avoiding blood transfusion, and strictly respecting the surgical margin, the 5-year survival was 70%, 42% and 41% in the 3 groups, respectively. No significant difference was found in the survival between patients with multiple unilobar or bilobar metastases. The 5-year recurrence rate was 48.2%, 62.3% and 67.6% in the 3 groups and the difference between unilobar multiple and bilobar metastases was not statistically significant. In the group with bilobar metastases, 21 liver resections (56.7%) were performed without the need for blood transfusion and in 18 patients (48.6%) without the need for pedicular clamping. Mean postoperative stay was 9.5 days. In 4 patients with bilobar metastases two stage liver resection was performed with a mean waiting time of 40 days between the 1st and the 2nd hepatectomy. Two patients of them are still alive without recurrence 9 and 28 months after the 2nd resections, respectively. In the other 2 cases, the recurrence developed 6 and 9 months after the 2nd hepatectomy.
Conclusions: Liver resection is the best treatment for colorectal liver metastases. Long term results (nearly 20%) with low mortality and morbidity can be achieved even in patients with bilobar liver metastases, which should not be considered a contraindication to surgery.

19,07

EXPERIENCE WITH RADIO-IMMUNOTHERAPY (CI^{131} IF023C5) AFTER CURATIVE RESECTION OF COLORECTAL LIVER METASTASIS

Aims: The most effective therapy of colorectal metastasis is a curative resection (R0). Nevertheless, a high tumor recurrence is today reported. Is the use of new therapeutical approaches such as radio-immunotherapy helpfully to improve this situation?
Methods: We analized retrospectively 27 patients (18 men and 9 women) who underwent curative resections. Mean age was 46 years (range 58.2-78). Sole liver resections were performed in 16 patients, in 11 patients was combined with radio-immunotherapy (CI^{131} IF023C5). In 7/11 cases was as adjuvant and in 4/11 as a rescue.
Results: Overall survival rate was 21.1 months (21.9 resection vs. 21.7 resection + radio-immunotherapy). Survival rates were after 12 months 80.0% (24 patients), 24 months 46.3% (11 patients) and 36 months 23.3% (6 patients). In the resection group (n= 16) four patients died after 8.5 (range1-22) months, three of them showed a tumor progression. 7/11 patients of the resection group + radio-immunotherapy (adjuvant) are alive after 14.5 (range 9-19) months, while 4/11 patient of the same group (rescue) died after 12.2 (range 9-19) months.
Conclusion: The use of radio-immunotherapy did not improve the survival rate. However, the fact that patients who underwent resection combined with CI^{131} IF023C5 as adjuvant therapy are alive, may be considered as a beneficial effect. Further studies are requiered for the confirmation of this approach.

19,08

OUR EXPERIENCE WITH THE REGIONAL CHEMOTHERAPY OF LIVER METASTASES OF COLORECTAL CANCER

*Rahóty P., *Sulyok Z., *Köves I., *Besznyák I., *Dubecz S., **Láng I., **Pápay Zs., *** Bodrogi I., *** Baki M., Horváth Zs., ***Gyergyay F.,
*Department of Surgery, Department of Chemotherapy **B, ***C
National Institute of Oncology
1122 Budapest, Ráth Gy. u. 7-9.

In the case of solitary metastases of rectal malignancies surgical resection, in multiple metastatic tumours regional intraarterial chemotherapy provides more favourable therapeutic results.
Between January 1, 1983 and December 31, 1997 resection was performed in 1905 patients with colorectal cancer. In 59 cases simultaneously with primary surgery or postsurgically upon onset of liver metastasis for regional therapy Port-A-Cath implantation into the hepatic artery took place. Through the cannula 5-FU, Leukovorin or according to Aigner's scheme Mitomycin-C, 5-FU were administered. Treatment was applied in 5-day schedule, repeated on 5 to 8 occasions, at 3-week intervals.
Results: Partial remission occurred in 34 patients (57.6%), of them 14 patients (23.7%) developed PR <50% while 20 patients (33.9%) PR >50% for a duration of 6 to 15 months. In 21 patients (35.5%) despite therapy a slow progression or metastatic tumour development at other organ sites could be detected. In the PR and CR group 38 patients (76.4%) reported on considerable subjective improvement and better quality of life.
In selected cases regional chemotherapy is recommended as a therapeutic alternative for the management of liver metastases of colorectal cancer.

19,09

METASTASIS IS LESS COMMON TO CIRRHOTIC THAN NORMAL LIVER: A SYSTEMATIC REVIEW AND META-ANALYSIS OF POST MORTEM STUDIES

Mr K. Seymour FRCS, Mr R. M. Charnley DM.
Department of Surgery, Freeman Hospital, High Heaton, Newcastle Upon Tyne NE7 7DN, UK.

Aim: To examine the evidence of the hypothesis that the cirrhotic liver is afforded protection against metastasis and to review the plausibility of such a phenomenon.

Methods: Systematic literature review and analysis of combined data from post-mortem case-control studies.

Results: Overall, the crude rate of metastasis to normal liver was 37.3%, whilst the rate to cirrhotic liver was 23.7%. The Mantel-Haenszel (MH) fixed effects estimate of the odds ratio was 0.47, 95% confidence intervals (CI) 0.41-0.53, χ^2=68.2, p<0.001. The DerSimonian-Laird (DL) random effects estimation of the odds ratio was 0.42, 95% CI 0.31-0.58, χ^2=30 (df=1), p<0.001.
For tumours arising within the distribution of the portal vein, the crude rate of metastasis to normal liver was 47.6% whilst the rate to cirrhotic liver was 29.8%. The MH estimate of the odds ratio was 0.45, 95% confidence intervals 0.37-0.54, χ^2=68.2, p<0.001. The DL pooled odds ratio was 0.44, 95% CI 0.28-0.7, χ^2=12.3 (df=1), p<0.001
The MH and DL pooled estimate of the odds ratio were similar for groups of patients from the East (Japan) and West (Europe and the USA),

Conclusions: The evidence reviewed suggests that the likelihood of metastasis to the cirrhotic liver is lower than that to normal liver. The difference is highly significant. The degree of protection for tumours arising from within the distribution of the portal vein is neither greater or less than overall. The Eastern and Western hemispheres exhibit a similar degree of risk reduction. Potential mechanisms of hepatic protection are discussed.

19,10

COLORECTAL LIVER METASTASES OF GENNARI STAGES II AND III (CLM): SURGICAL AND TRANSCATHETER TREATMENT.

A.M.Granov, P.G.Tarazov, A.A.Polykarpov, D.A.Granov, V.V.Borovik
Research Institute of Roentgenology & Radiation Therapy, St.Petersburg.
St.Petersburg Medical University, Russia

Aim: To evaluate effectiveness of hepatic artery infusion (HAI), hepatic arterial chemoembolization (HACE), and hepatic resection for liver CLM.

Methods: Our prospective study included 161 pts with Genari's stage II and III of CLM. HAI with 5-7 g 5-FU and/or 30-50 mg Doxorubicin in Lipiodol was performed in 54 pts. HACE with 30-100 mg Doxorubicin - in - iodized oil plus gelatin sponge was carried out in 46 pts. In cases of hypovascular CLM, HACE was supplemented by transhepatic portal vein injection of 30 mg Doxorubicin in 10 ml Lipiodol. Every therapy was performed 2 to 4 times yearly. Curative hepatic resection was made in 41 remaining pts.

Results: Partial tumor response was seen in 6 (11%) and 31 (68%) pts after HAI and HACE, respectively. Mean survival rates were 8.0± 4.6 mo for HAI and 21.8± 10.3 mo for HACE (p<0.001). After hepatic resection, the survival was 22.6±11.4 (p<0.001 with HAI and non significant with HACE).

Conclusion: In our series, both the HACE and hepatic resection were more effective, than HAI for CLM. However, there was non significant difference of survival of pts between these treatments.

19,11

HEPATIC ARTERY INFUSION (HAI) AND CHEMOEMBOLIZATION (CE) IN NON-COLORECTAL LIVER METASTASES (Mts)

P.G.Tarazov, D.A.Granov, A.A.Zeadeh
St.Petersburg Medical University, St.Petersburg Research Institute of Roentgenology, St.Petersburg, Russia

Purpose. To determine effectiveness of HAI and CE in liver metastases from non-colorectal cancer.
Materials and Methods. Between 1986 and 1998, we treated 70 patients with unresectable liver metastases. The previously resected primary tumors were: gastric cancer (28), ovarial (9), renal cell (9), pancreatic (6), mammarial (4) carcinoma, cancer of the lung (4), other tumors (10). According to Gennari classification, 8 patients had stage I, 21 stage II, 38 stage III, 3 stage IVA liver Mts. HAI was performed through the angiographically placed catheter using 5-FU, doxorubicin, cisplatin. CE was made by hepatic arterial injection chemotherapeutic drug-in-iodized oil (13-30 mg liposoluble cytostatic Dioxadet or 30-80 mg Doxorubicin) and following arterial occlusion by gelatin sponge.
Results. In 1 month after the treatment, complete and partial responses were detected in 5% and 15% of patients, respectively. The rate of stabilization was 39%, while tumor progression was seen in 41% of patients. The survival was higher in Mts from gastric (15 mo) and ovarian (18 mo) carcinoma. Patients with Mts from renal cell carcinoma, mammarial cancer, carcinoma of the pancreas, and cancer of the lung showed short mean survival (8, 6, 4, and 4 mo, respectively).
Conclusion. HAI and CE are relatively effective in liver Mts from gastric and ovarian carcinoma and are ineffective in most patients with liver Mts from other primary non-colorectal tumors.

Dig Surg 1999; 16 (suppl 1): 62-64

Liver Transplantation I.

20,01

Liver transplant program in Prague

Results of consecutive 115 liver transplants

Ryska M, Trunecka P, Belina F, Spicák J, Peregrin J, Filip K, Vitko S et al.

Institute for clinical and experimental medicine (IKEM)
Prague, Czech Republic

Liver transplant program was commenced in IKEM in April 1995 within the institution already operating kidney, heart as well as pancreas transplant program with close cooperation of Professor P Neuhaus, Surgery department, Virchow University, Berlin.
Material and methods: Since January 1999 110 patients underwent 115 orthotopic liver transplantation (OLTx): cholestatic liver disease was indication in 17 patients, HCV in 15 and ETOH in 14 patients, others indications are analysed. Preoperative management with SBD and ATB prophylaxis, hepatectomy with IVC segment resection, VVS selectively, CHDCHDA in the first 50 transplants side-to-side with T-tube converted to end-to-end without T-tube, in immunosuppression ATG, CyA, AZA and MP, CMV prophylaxis postoperatively.
4 patients underwent re – OLTx, 1 underwent the third transplantation. Mean age of recipients was 44,4 years (3 – 64). In 111 transplants full – size liver graft was used, one graft reduction, 1 split in situ and 1 split ex vivo was provided.
Results: One year survival as well as cumulative survival is 92,7 %. CIT in average reached 7 hours, blood loss 8 units Biliary complication was appeared in 33 patients: in 70 % was treated by transduodenal endoscopicaly or transhepatic transcutaneously. The cause of death in 9 patients: aspergilosis, pseudomonas pneumonia, toxoplasmosis in 4 patients in late postoperative period, pneumocystis pnemumonia with lymphoproliferative disease in 1 patients, MOF in 2 patients and PNF in 2 patients in early postoperative period and cerebral bleeding in 1 patient. Causes of complications and death are analysed by authors.
Conclusions: Our promising results encouraged us to believe that a liver transplantation program can started safely under several cautions: experience in organ procurement and surgery, close cooperation with well-established liver transplant program.

20,02

ELDERLY DONORS: UTILIZATION STRATEGY AND POSTOPERATIVE OUTCOME

E. Andorno, A, Antonucci, G. Paraluppi, R. Mondello, R. Valente, A. Genzone, F. Panaro, N. Morelli, G. Dardano, F. Emili, L. Saltalamacchia, P. Grondona, M. Pittaluga, C. Bottino and Z. Valente
Department of Transplantation, S. Martino Hospital, Genoa

Purpose: Aim of this paper is to show how older donors (age <60 years) could be safely used, to improve liver supply as to reduce waiting list mortality rate.
Methods and Patients: From 1th Jan 1998 to 11th Dec 1998, 44 LT were performed at our centre, 3 of which using donors older than 60 years (63, 67, 84). Donor selection criteria: weight (<90 kg), sepsis, steatosis (30%macro), ICU (<7days), anuric hypotensive episodes (none). Donors under any of these conditions were excluded. Liver function tests (ALT, (GT, PT) were considered in evaluation but never as exclusion criteria.
Harvesting was performed with classical technique, using UW solution via aorta.
Recipients: Tab below

Donor-recipient matching: Low risk and short life span recipients were matched with the higher risk donors.
OL T technique: PiggyBack technique and early arterialization were adopted in all cases.
Data about cold ischemic time
(CIT) and warm ischemic time
(WIT) are shown aside

Results: Data about graft functional recovery and patient outcome are shown in Tab.
Conclusions: Aged livers can be safely used following the following steps: donor and graft evaluation, specific donor-recipient matching and early arterialization.

20,03

THE EVALUATION OF VENO-VENOUS BY-PASS IN LIVER TRANSPLANTATION BY MEASURING THE CEREBRAL OXYGENATION USING THE NEAR INFRARED SPECTROSCOPY (NIRS)

F.A Youssef, A.M. Seifalian, A. El-Desoky, K Rolles, B.R Davidson
Department of Surgery, Liver Transplant Unit
Royal Free Hospital and School of Medicine, London NW3 2QG. UK

Aims: The aim of the study was to evaluate the role of Veno-venous bypass (VVB) in preventing severe changes in cerebral oxygenation especially during the anhepatic phase of the liver transplantation using the Near Infrared Spectroscopy (NIRS). (VVB) is used in liver transplantation either as a routine for all the patients or under special indications aiming to prevent the severe alterations in the circulation, which might affect the cardiac function and consequently cerebral blood flow and cerebral oxygenation.
Methods: The NIRS was used to measure the cerebral oxygenation (HbO_2) during liver transplantation and for 24 Hours in the postoperative period in patients with or without VVB. Between December 1997 and August 1998, 35 patients were included the patients were in two groups. Group (1) fifteen Patients who had (VVB) the indications were cardiac in 10, renal 2, renal and cardiac in 1 and acute liver failure 2, and Group (2) twenty patients who did not have VVB. The period of monitoring was divided into operative (dissection D, anhepatic AH early and end, reperfusion RP) and postoperative (early 4 Hours and late, end of the monitoring) The other cardiovascular monitoring (Blood Hb, CVP, PCO_2, HR, BP) were also taken during the same period.
Results: The results are shown in the table:

HbO_2

μ mol/l	D	AH early	AH end	RP	PO early	PO late
+vvb	0.23±0.9	-2.73±1.5	-5.15±2.9	4.82±2.6	5.11± 1.7	4.95±2.4
-vvb	0.46±1.1	-4.82±1.7	-4.13±2.7	5.91± 3.5	5.37±2.3	5.02± 2.2

There was no significant correlation (r= 0.35, P= 0.25) between the changes in HbO_2 and the changes in the cardiovascular monitoring.
Conclusion: The measurement of the cerebral oxygenation in the study did not show any significant different between the two groups (P=0.5) and the VVB did not prevent the decrease in cerebral HbO_2 during the AH phase.

KARGER
Fax +41 61 306 12 34
E-Mail karger@karger.ch
www.karger.com

20,04

LONG TERM CONSEQUENCES OF ACUTE LIVER ALLOGRAFT REJECTION

Abou El-Ella Khaled, Shokouh-Amiri, Hathaway Donna, and Gaber A Osama.
Transplant Division, Department of Surgery, University of Tennessee – Memphis – U.S.A.

Aims : While the consequences of acute rejection on chronic kidney allograft function have been well established, because of liver's ability to regenerate, the rule that acute liver rejection may have in predisposing to chronic liver damage has been largely disputed.

Methods : We reviewed the outcome of 98 adult transplants performed between 1990 – 1994 using cyclosporine, prednisone immuno suppression. We divided the patients based upon the occurrence of rejection episodes into three groups, those without any acute rejection (NoRej = 19), those with rejections reversed by steroids (StSen = 31), and those with steroid resistant rejection requiring antibody rescue therapy (StRes = 48).

Results : All groups were demographically similar except for age (NoRej = 47.2 vs 42.4 and 4 .1 years respectively; P ≤ 0.05). There were also no differences in cold ischemia time, rate and quality of immediate function, or in incidence of hepatitis C recurrence. All groups had a similar mean follow-up of 29.7 months. At the last yearly follow-up, mean values for liver function differed between the three groups, median values were also different for liver enzymes and albumin (P ≤ 0.05). Histologically, chronic rejection (ChRej) was defined on routine yearly follow-up biopsy as chronic bile duct damage, ductopenia, or vascular changes (ChRej = 1 in NoRej, 2 in StSen, and 17 in StRes). Radiographic evidence of intrahepatic biliary strictures (IHBS) was zero in NoRej group, 1 in StSen and 11 in StRes group with P ≤ 0.05.

Conclusions: Development of features of chronic rejection on protocol biopsies appears to be more common in patients with histologically severe acute rejection, recurrent acute rejection and steroid resistant rejection. Patients with mild or steroid sensitive rejection do not progress to chronic rejection. Patients with steroid resistant rejection have a greater propensity to develop intrahepatic biliary strictures and an increased likelihood of transplant failure. We conclude that although complete recovery can follow milder steroid-sensitive rejection, damage invoked by severe & steroid-resistant rejection have consequences on structure and long-term fuction of liver allograft.

20,05

LIMIT OF AGE IN LIVER TRANSPLANTATION

Bilbao I., Lázaro J., Murio E., Charco R., Hidalgo E., Margarit C.
Liver Transplant. Unit. Hospital Vall d'Hebrón, Barcelona

The limit of age is one of the main controversies in the selection of liver transplant (LT) candidats. At the begining the limit was 55 years old, but later 60years was luniversally accepted.

Objective: The aim of this study is to analyse the 1 year outcome of LT in patients (pts) older than 60 years old.

Material and methods: From 1988 to 1997 225 LT have been performed in 208 pts. Sixty were older than 60 years. Variables from candidate, donor and operation have been analysed in order to asses if there are any difference in this group of patients comparing to the rest of the patients. Morbi-mortality at three months and 1 year have been also analysed.

Results: Pts<60 years differed from younger pts in the indiction to transplantation (more HCC and less retransplants and cholostatic disease, p=0.0001). UNOS status and Child-Pugh score were also less severe for older group with difference statistically significant. Older group also differed in the technique of the anhepatic phase (IVCP) and the biliary anastomosis performed (CC-TT without Kehr) due to changes of operative strategies along the time. Most of the aged candidates belonged to the last 5 years of our study period. During surgery, aged pts needed less transfusion and less drug support with differences statistically significant.

Postoperative results	< 60y(N=165)	< 60y(N=60)	p
Patient mort (3 months)	21 (17%)	8 (16.3%)	ns
Patient mort at 1 year	50 (32%)	17 (29%)	ns
Hospital stay (days)	33.5 ± 29	31 ± 45	ns
ICU stay (days)	14 ± 19	13 ± 17	ns
Biliary complications	29 (18.6%)	4 (6.9%)	.02
Rejections at ly	88 (57%)	27 (47%)	ns
Mean steroid bolus (g)	2.6 ± 2	1.8 ± 1.1	.02
Refractory rejections	20 (25.6%)	4 (19%)	.07
Infections at ly	130 (83.3%)	47 (81%)	ns
Renal insufficiency	84 (53.5%)	31 (53.4%)	ns
Cardiovascular compl.	43 (27%)	20 (34%)	ns
Neurological compl.	62 (39%)	21 (36%)	ns
Diabetes Mellitus	38 (24%)	17 (30%)	ns
Osteomuscular compl.	15 (12%)	10 (20.4%)	ns

Conclusions: Pts <60 years require a thorough examination of their cardiovascular and neuropsyquiatry status to be accepted as candidates. Taking into account these factors and with the new advances in surgical skills and postoperative treatments, outcome and results are similar than in younger pts.

20,06

RISK FACTORS FOR MORBIMORTALITY DURING THE FIRST THREE MONTHS AFTER LIVER TRANSPLANTATION (LT)

Bilbao I, Lázaro JL, Charco R, Murio E, Hidalgo E and Margarit C
Hospital Vall d'Hebrón. Liver transplant Unit. Barcelona. Spain

The majority of complications occur during the first three months after liver transplantation . Mortality is an obvious index factor to compare results among centers. However morbidity is more dificult to report because a lack of universal definition for each complication.

OBJECTIVE: The aim of this study was to analyse mortality and morbidity during the first three months post-transplant, as well as risk factors leading to mortality in this period.

MATERIAL AND METHODS:We have reweded 225 LT performed in 211 patients, from 1988 to 1996. All the events ocurring during the first 3 months post-transplant have been analysed and graded according to severity : Grade-I were complications easily controlled with usual medication. Grade-II were complications resulting in ICU stay > 5 days or hospital stays > 4 weeks but resolved with drug therapy. Grade-III complication was similar to Grade-II but requiring therapeutic invasive interventions. Grade-IV were complication with lasting disability but no evidence to progression. Grade-V was similar to grade-IV but with evidence to progression and Grade VI were complications leading to retransplantation or death. A total of 230 variables from donor, recipient and operation were analysed in order to considered risk factors leading to morbi-mortality during the first three months after transplantation.

RESULTS : Mortality at 3 months post-transplant was 18%. Causes of death were cardiopulmonary complications in 39% , infections in 30%, multiorgan failure in 18%, technical complications in 8%, PNF in 2.5% , refractary acute rejection in 2.5%. Risk factors leading to mortality were : advanced Child-Pugh score (p<.001), UNOS Status I-II (p=0.001), fulminant hepatitis (p=0.014), pre-transplant renal insufficiency (p=0.012), Na < 130 meq/l (p=0.014), intraoperative transfusion of > 10 RBC Units (p=0.004), > 10 plasma units (p=0.013), > 12 Units of platelets (p=0.04) and the need for intraoperative dobutamine (p=0.015) and furosemide (p=0.007). Dead patients presented more hemodynamic inestability during the first 5 days post-transplant (p=0.002), hemorrhagic complications leading to reinterventions (p=0.004), more incidence of hepatic artery thrombosis (p=0.025), early acute rejection < 10 days (p=0.039) and refractory acute rejection needing OKT3 and high doses of steroids(p=0.004), early severe infections (p<0.001) and post-transplant renal insufficiency (p=0.0001). Mean number of complications for death and surviving groups were statistically significant for grade III, IV and V complications.

CONCLUSION : The combination of advanced Child-Pugh score, with high UNOS status and renal insuficiency in a candidate that requires intraoperative politransfusion and suffers from postoperative hemorrhage, early and severe rejections and infections is usually fatal in the early outcome. None of the donor variables has been significant, regarding the adecuacy in the selection of donors.

20,07

H.-G. Marks, H. Kraemer-Hansen, J. Lüttges*), B. Kremer, D. Henne-Bruns
Department of Surgery, Christian-Albrecht-University Kiel, Germany, *)
Department of Pathology, Christian-Albrecht-University Kiel, Germany

Recurrent disease after orthotopic liver transplantation in patients with primary biliary cirrhosis

End stage primary biliary cirrhosis is a well accepted indication for orthotopic liver transplantation (tx).

Aim: Aim of this study was to investigate the problem of recurrence of PBC after Tx.

Methods: Between 02/84 and 09/98 21 patients (20 female, 1 male) underwent liver transplantation by our team at the Universities of Hamburg and Kiel. The primary immunosuppression was performed with CSA and prednison (n=7), CSA, prednison and azathioprine (n=7) or FK 506 and pednison (n=1).

Results: 4 patients died within 12 months after transplantation due to sepsis (3 pat.) or vanishing bile duct syndrom (1 pat.). Another 2 patients died 9,5 years and 11,5 years after tx (cholangiosepsis - metastases caused by an ovarian neoplasm). 15 patients caould be followed now between 9 and 142 months (mean 94 months, median 101 months). 6 pat. developed an isolated increase of IgM immunoglobulines, another 5 patients showed an increase of IgM and IgG during the follow up. Antimitochondrial antibodies were present in all 15 patients within 12 months after tx. 10 of the 15 patients developed PBC associated diseases 3 - 45 months after transplantation (Immunthyreopathy n=7, Myositis-Syndrome n=4, Polyarthritis n=3, Sicca-Syndrome n=2, Raynaud-Syndrome n=2).

During the follow up period in 5 cases the liver biopsy was suspicious of a recurrent disease of PBC (6 - 68 months after LTX). In 3 cases a typical granuloma was detected. Meanwhile the mean follow up period of these 5 patients is 8 years (5,5-11 years). None of them developed liver cirrhosis or showed a significant reduction of liver function.

Conclusions: We conclude that transplantation probably will not cure the basic immunological desease but it offers a significant prolongation of survival time with a good quality of life for patients with end stage primary biliary cirrhosis.

20,08

COMPARISON OF LAMIVUDINE AND FAMCICLOVIR FOR HEPATITIS B INFECTION AFTER LIVER TRANSPLANTATION

N Rayes, D Seehofer, AR Müller, WO Bechstein, T Berg, R Neuhaus, P Neuhaus

Department of Surgery, Charité, Campus Virchow, Berlin, Germany

Aims: Reinfection or de novo infection with hepatitis B after liver transplantation cause a decreased patient and organ survival. During the last years, the new nucleosid analoga famciclovir and lamivudine have shown promising results. We compared the long term efficacy of both drugs in a retrospective analysis.
Patients and methods: Between 11/93 and 8/98 we treated 31 HBV-infected liver transplant recipients with famciclovir (group A) and 35 patients with lamivudine (group B). HBV-infection was diagnosed in case of positive HBs-Ag and HBV-DNA. In group A, 25 patients had developed reinfection despite prophylaxis with hepatitis B-hyperimmunoglobulin, 6 patients had a de novo-infection. Group B consisted of 28 patients with reinfection and 7 with de novo infection. All patients from group A were primarily treated with famciclovir. In group B 9 patients had lamivudine as first line treatment, 23 patients were switched to lamivudine after failure of famciclovir therapy. The success of treatment was controlled by ALAT activity and HBV-DNA.
Results: In both groups most patients responded well to treatment as shown in the table. Suppression of viral replication could be demonstrated only for 2 to 18 months in most cases. Afterwards, HBV-.DNA increased again but this relapse was only accompanied by a mild hepatitis and low ALAT activity. Both drugs were well tolerated and no severe side effects were noted.
Conclusion: Famciclovir and lamivudine are effective in the treatment of HBV-infection after liver transplantation. Lamivudine could achieve a better suppression of viral replication even after failure of famciclovir therapy. After prolonged treatment resistance formation against both drugs occurs in most cases. Therefore, combination therapy may be useful.

group	Ø HBV-DNA [pg/ml]			best HBV-DNA result (n=)		
(n)	0 mo	2 mo	12 mo	neg	lowered	same
A (31)	2283	518	1475	4 (13%)	26 (84%)	1 (3%)
B (35)	1436	108	1246	27 (77%)	6 (17%)	2 (6%)

20,09

ANTIVIRAL COMBINATION THERAPY FOR LAMIVUDINE RESISTANT HEPATITIS B REINFECTION AFTER LIVER TRANSPLANTATION

Seehofer D, Rayes N, Neuhaus R, Berg T, Müller AR, Bechstein WO, Neuhaus P

Department of Surgery and Gastroenterology, Charité Campus Virchow, Humboldt University of Berlin, Germany

Aims: Nucleoside analogues like lamivudine and famciclovir have expanded therapeutical options for HBV infection after liver transplantation. The major problem is a relatively fast resistance formation during treatment which could be overcome with antiviral combination therapy. The following data are first preliminary observations for this combination therapy after liver trans-plantation.
Patients and methods: Eight patients after liver transplantation for chronic hepatitis B infection were enrolled into this preliminary study. All had reinfection of the graft and breakthrough of HBV during consecutive famciclovir and lamivudine monotherapy. Subsequently a combination therapy of lamivudine and interferon α 2a (group I, n=4) or lamivudine and famciclovir (group II, n=4) was initiated. The dosage of lamivudine was 150 mg od, of famciclovir 500 to 1500 mg daily. Interferon α was applicated 3 million units three times a week.
Results: Combination therapy was started 61 months (group I) and 25 months (group II) after liver transplantation. It markedly reduced viral replication rate in all patients despite lamivudine resistance. In group I three of four patients became HBV-DNA negative, in group II two of four patients. No patient became HBsAg negative or lost HbeAg during any of the antiviral therapies. All patients showed a prompt and significant reduction of ALT and AST levels after initiation of combination therapy. No severe complications, and especially no rejection episodes occurred during interferon application.
Conclusion: Lamivudine in combination with other antiviral agents, especially interferon α, might be a therapeutic option for hepatitis B reinfection after liver transplantation. Suppression of virus replication up to undetectable values is possible even in patients with lamivudine resistant virus mutations who failed to respond to antiviral monotherapy with lamivudine or famciclovir.

Dig Surg 1999; 16 (suppl 1): 65-67

Liver tumor III.

21,01

PRE TRANSPLANTATION DETECTION OF HEPATOCELLULAR CARCINOMA IN PATIENTS WITH END STAGE LIVER DISEASE: THE ROLE OF CT AND MRI.

Ben Haim M, Roayaie S, Likholatnikov D, Emre S, Fishbein T, Sheiner P, Miller CM and Schwartz ME. The Recanati / Miller Transplantation Institute, The Mount Sinai Hospital of the Mount Sinai--NYU Medical Center and Health System, New York.

Aims: Cirrhotic patients with end-stage liver disease (ESLD) are at risk for hepatocellular carcinoma (HCC). Routine screening is based on alpha feto-protein (AFP) blood level and liver ultrasonography (US). However, there is still a significant percentage of "incidental" HCCs in liver transplantation (LTx) explants. We evaluated the diagnostic value of AFP, CT and MRI.

Methods: We retrospectively compared clinico-pathological and radiologic findings in 198 LTx patients in whom HCC was found in the explants. Within 3 months prior to LTx, 38 patients had had CT scan, 38 had MRI, and the other 122 had no studies or only US.

Results: The clinico-pathological characteristics were:

	CT group	MRI group	No study or US
N	38	38	122
Median age (range) – years	56 (33-75)	57 (16-76)	58 (19-72)
Median AFP level -	393	143	10.1
Normal AFP level (%)	6 (15%)	11 (28%)	70 (57%)
Size – cm, median (range)	4.5 (1.1-13.5)	4.4 (1.1-15)	2.5 (0.5-15)
Size - <1 cm (%)	0	0	11 (9%)
Size – 1-2 cm (%)	6 (10%)	2 (5%)	22 (18%)

HCC was detected in 36/38 CT scans (94%), 36/38 MRIs (94%) but only in 37/122 (30%) in patients who had US or no studies. In 87/198 (43%) patients, AFP levels were normal. Most CTs and MRIs were performed in the later period of our program's activity. Rates of incidental HCCs over the years were:

Years	Incidental HCCs / all HCCs	CT or MRI / all HCCs
1988-1993	32/47 (68%)	6/47 (12%)
1994-1996	39/80 (48%)	23/80 (28%)
1997-1999	18/71 (25%)	56/71 (78%)

Conclusions: Although the proportion of HCCs detected pretransplant increased, detection remains a diagnostic challenge. The sensitivity of AFP is low. Most lesions greater than 1 cm can be detected by CT or MRI with comparable sensitivities. To minimize the number of missed tumors, we strongly advocate routine periodic CT or MRI studies in all patients with ESLD who are waiting for liver transplantation.

21,02

RESECTION OF PRIMARY LIVER CANCER FOLLOWING TRANSCATHETER ARTERIAL CHEMOEMBOLIZATION: CLINICOPATHOLOGICAL FEATURES AND POSTOPERATIVE COURSE IN 35 CASES.

Wang YH[1], Liu YX[1], Feng YQ[1], Ji XL[2], Zhao HL[2].

[1]Department of Hepatobiliary Surgery, [2]Department of Pathology, Chinese People's Liberation Army General Hospital. Beijing 100853, P.R.China.

Aims: To study the clinicopathological changes and postoperative course following transcatheter hepatic arterial chemoembolization (TACE) in primary liver cancer (PLC).

Methods: One hundred and eighty-two cases of PLC were resected from 1988 to 1995. 35 cases of them that resected after 1 to 5 times of TACE were evaluated. 11 of the 35 cases were 5cm or less in diameter, 24 cases were larger than 5cm.

Results: Uptake of iodized oil, shrinkage of tumour mass and decrease of AFP level were good clinical features of the tumour after TACE and were related to the times of TACE. Only 7 of the 35 cases after TACE with 100% necrosis were found pathologically. The degree of necrosis was correlated to injured vessels of PLC and was also related to the times of TACE. Post-operative survival rate and disease-free survival rate of the 35 cases in 5 years were 40.5% and 28.9%, respectively.

Conclusions: Single treatment of TACE is not curative to PLC, and it is essential to seize a chance to perform secondary liver resection for primaryly unresectable PLC after 2 to 3 times of TACE.

21,03

RESULTS OF HEPATIC RESECTIONS AND INTERVENTIONAL RADIOLOGICAL PROCEDURES IN PATIENTS WITH ADVANCED HEPATOCELLULAR CARCINOMA (HCC).

D.Granov, P. Tarazov, A. Pivovarov, V. Polysalov, A. Polykarpov.
Research Institute of Roentgenology and Radiation Therapy. St.Peterrsburg, Russia.

Aim: To evaluate the effectiveness of hepatic resections and interventional radiological procedures in pts with advanced HCC.

Methods: Between 1986-1997 we treated 101 pts with HCC. The advanced stage of the disease was diagnosed in 99 cases: the tumor size more then 5 cm. in diameter was in all cases, daughter nodules-89 pts., tumor trombi in segmental or lobular portal branches-73 pts. The underlying liver cirrhosis Child-Pugh «B» or «C» was in 24 pts. Major hepatic resections were performed in 21 pts., interventional radiological treatment in 78 pts.: hepatic artery infusion(HAI), hepatic artery chemoembolization(HACE), HACE in combination with portal vein chemoembolization(PVCE).

Results: At present, 14 pts. died in 7- 55 (32,5±8,6)mo. after hepatic resections. The other 7 pts. alive 10 - 142 mo. In group with unresectable tumors the mean survival among pts. who died was 15,1±5,3 mo. The best results were observed after repeated courses of combined HACE and PVCE(24,2±5,9 mo.) vs HACE(16,6±6,5 mo.) and HAI(7,5± 3,5 mo.,P<0,01). All pts. with advanced cirrhosis died between 3-6 mo. independently of a kind of interventional treatment.

Conclusion: The treatment results of patients with advanced HCC are still unsatisfied. Hepatic resection significantly prolongs survival but is possible in limited amount of patients. Combined HACE and PVCE is the best palliation among other interventional radiological procedures in unresectable cases. Underlying advanced cirrhosis seriously decreases survival independently of treatment method.

KARGER
Fax +41 61 306 12 34
E-Mail karger@karger.ch
www.karger.com

21,04

THE TREATMENT OF THE HEPATO CELLULAR CARCINOMA: PRELIMINARY RESULTS OF A MULTIMODAL THERAPEUTIC PROTOCOL

Berloco P., Borzomati D., Altomare V., Alloni R., Caricato M., Arullani A., Tomini, G., D'Aprile M., Cortesini R.
Dept. of Surgery and Oncology, Campus Bio-Medico Rome,
II. Dept. of Surgery, University La Sapienya, Rome

Alternative „mini-invasive" treatments for patients affected by Hepato-Cellular Carcinoma (HCC) have been well experimented.
Nevertheless Surgical Excision (SE) still maintains an important role, while Liver Transplant (LT) is indicated in selected cases. The presence of an overlapping is present and comparative studies are still not available. In collaboration with a Transplant Centre we attempted a multimodal therapeutical protocol that included Alcohol-Injection (AI) or Radiofrequency Thermo-Ablation (RTA), SE and LT. According to number and location of the lesions and the hepatic function patients were assigned to one of the following therapeutical options:
Group 1: monolat. lesion Child A patients (or without cirrhosis): - SE
Group 2: multiple-bilateral lesions Child A-B-C patients:
- AI/RTA
Group 3: single monolateral lesions Child B patients - LT
At our Department 22 patients affected by HCC were observed from November 1995 through December 1998. Twelve (54.5%) (Gr. 1) underwent SE (1 explorative laparotomy, 2 right- and 1 left-lobe hepatectomy, 3 segmentectomies and 5 wedge resections), perioperative mortality and major morbidity consisted of 8.3% and 25%. Six (27.3%) (Gr. 2) underwent AI (3 cases) or RTA (3 cases) with no mortality and an overall morbidity of 16.6%. Finally 3 (13.6%) (Gr. 3) patients underwent LT (no morbidity or mortality were recorded in this group of patients). At now 1 patient is waiting to undergo RTA. After a mean follow-up of 12.3 months (1-27 months) 2 (10.5%) patients died for unrelated causes, no patients died for the disease and 14 (73.7%) are alive and free of disease. A 15.8% overall disease recurrence eate was recorded (Group 1: 10.5%, Group 2:5.3%, Group 3: 0 %). The development of multiple therapeutical options for the treatment of HCC patients still involves clinical doubts due to an overlapping of these different kinds of treatment. Patients affected by HCC can be properly divided into different groups according to patient's and tumour's features (each group possibly requiring a different kind of treatment). In our Centre we therefore attempted a multimodal therapeutical protocol to offer patients the most safe and effective therapy in order to reduce mortality and morbidity burt also to possibly perform a radical treatment. It is however evident that comparative studies are urgently warranted to clarify indications, advantages and limits of these different therapeutic options for patients affected by HCC.

21,05

RADIOFREQUENCY ABLATION SYSTEM (RFAS) IN THE PERCUTANEOUS AND INTRAOPERATIVE TREATMENT OF HEPATIC PRIMITIVE AND METHASTATIC MALIGNANCIES.

Cillo U. - Tedeschi U. - Zanus G. - Boccagni P. - Brolese A. -Bonariol L. - Urbani L. - Bassanello M. - Montin U. - Gringeri E. - Veroux M. - D'Amico D.F.
DEPARTMENT OF GASTROENTEROLOGICAL AND SURGICAL SCIENCES - UNIVERSITY OF PADOVA (ITALY).

Introduction. Treatment of hepatic nodular malignancies still represents a clinical problem in many istances due to the peculiar morpho-functional carachteristics of the liver. The Radiofrequency Ablation System (RFAS) is a relatively new therapeutic approach of such nodular either primitive or methastatic lesions.
Patients and Methods. Form 1989 until the present time 377 HCC patients (on cirrhosis) were treated at our center. Seventy patients underwent to surgical resection, 20 to OLTx, 51 to non surgical, non ablative treatment (TACE, TACI), 218 underwent to repeated alcol injections cycles and 19 were treated by RFAS. Among the patients observed for hepatic methastases (Colorectal ca., renal ca., surrenal ca.), 19 out of 214 were treated by RFAS. A R.I.T.A. RFAS was adopted in all cases with a 16 Gauge probe drived percutaneously or intraoperatively under U.S. guidance. Single 12 minutes cycles were used in the majority of the cases. Results were evaluated by CAT scan 15 days after the procedure and in selected cases by FNAB of suspected neoplastic residuals. In 3 cases we adopted i.o. stop flow techniques to enlarge the ablation diameter.
Results. A radical ablation was obtained after treatment of nodules <3 cm. In 4 patients a palliative approach of nodules > 3cm requested multiple RFAS applications (max 3) with 7-15 days intervals.
In 1 case (2.6%) we observed a post-procedure bleeding resolved with conservative treatement. Seven patients (18.4%) experienced fever. No procedure related mortality occurred.
Conclusions. Although it is too early to draw conclusions on long term results of RFAS in the treatment of hepatic malignancies, in our experience this procedure showed a high dimension dependent ablative efficacy (< 3- 3,5 cm), a significant flexibility (percuteneous or intraoperative approach) and a low prevalence of procedure related morbidity. If compared with the traditional alcol injection approach, this therapeutic tool is efficient also in the treatment of hepatic sencondaries and its efficacy is optimal also in a one shot pattern. The i.o. stop flow technique and the introduction of new probes will significanly expand the field of applications of this therapeutic approach.

21,06

COMPARISON OF THE UICC TNM AND IZUMI STAGING SYSTEM AS PREDICTORS OF OUTCOME IN 52 CIRRHOTIC PATIENTS UNDERGOING HEPATIC RESECTION FOR HEPATOCELLULAR CARCINOMA

Chiappa, A.C., Zbar, A.*, Beertani, E., Bielle F., Crotti, C., and Staudacher C.
Department of Emeergency Surgery-Surgical Oncology, University of Milan-ITALY-S. Raffaele Scientific Institute, *Imperial Medical College-Hammersmith Hospital-London- UK

Aims: The clinical value of UICC TNM classification and TNM modified (Izumi) regarding prognosis after liver resection for hepatocellular carcinoma (HCC) was evaluated.
Methods: Between January 1993 and January 1998, overall specific survival and disease-free survival (DFS) were evaluated in 52 cirrhotic patients (39 M, 13 F, mean age: 65 years, range 43-81 years) undergoing hepatic resection for supervening HCC.
Results: The 1-year, 3-year, and 4-year overall specific survival rates in patients who underwent hepatic resection were 89%, 53%, and 53% respectively. In multivariate analysis, vascular invasion predicted long-term outcome. The difference between stage 1 and 2 or stage 3 using UICC TNM classification was not significant for prognosis. A modification of the UICC TNM staging system (as used by Izumi et al.) incorporating microvascular invasion as an independent prognostic variable shows the value of stage as a predictor of outcome.
Conclusions: An uniform tumour classification of HCC is advocated. Our results show that the UICC TNM classification for HCC is inadequate and may even on occasion lead to unnecessary resection. The modified staging system of Izumi is superior in determining outcome for cirrhotic patients with supervening HCC undergoing resection.

21,07

CONSEQUENCES OF LONG CONTINUOUS NORMOTHERMIC LIVER ISCHEMIA DURING HEPATIC RESECTIONS

Cerwenka H., El-Shabrawi A., Bacher H., Werkgartner G., Höss G., Mischinger HJ. Department of General Surgery, Karl-Franzens University, Auenbruggerplatz 29, A-8036 Graz, Austria

Aims: In the literature normothermic liver ischemia lasting up to 45 or 60 minutes is described as safe. For extended liver resections we use continuous ischemic periods of more than 60 and 90 minutes. The aim of this study was to evaluate the impact of the duration of ischemia on the postoperative course.
Patients and Methods: This prospective study comprised 66 patients undergoing major liver resections: Duration of ischemia was 30 to 60 minutes in 21 patients (group I), 60 to 90 minutes in 20 patients (group II) and more than 90 minutes in 15 patients (group III). Significant postoperative liver failure was defined as bilirubin above 5 mg/dl for more than 2 weeks or bilirubin above 15 mg/dl and hypalbuminemia, coagulopathy, elevated ammonia and encephalopathy. For liver cell protection tocopherol, ascorbate and cortisol were administered intraoperatively.
Results: The postoperative values of the transaminases were significantly higher in group III (e.g. AST: mean 1086 U/l on the first and 328 on the third postoperative day) than in group II (318 and 125, respectively) and in group I (238 and 114). Prothrombin time also showed good correlation to the duration of ischemia (group III: 47 and 57%, respectively; group II: 56 and 58%, group I: 63 and 70%). The impact on total bilirubin was a bit more delayed but on the fifth postoperative day the values also reflected the differences in the ischemic periods very well (mean: group III: 4.3 mg/dl; group II: 2.9; group I: 1.6). Postoperative liver failure and prolonged hospital stay were significantly more frequent in group III.
Conclusion: In patients who had a long period (more than 90 minutes) of continuous nomothermic liver ischemia postoperative liver failure combined with higher morbidity and prolonged hospital stay was seen more frequently.

21.08

IMPACT OF NORMOTHERMIC ISCHEMIA ON POSTOPERATIVE PATTERNS AFTER LIVER RESECTION.

Nuzzo G, Giovannini I, Giuliante F, Boldrini G, Chiarla C, Vellone M. Dept of Surgery (Chirurgia Geriatrica) Catholic University, Rome, Italy

Aims: Postoperative (p.o.) data from 75 hepatectomies were analyzed to assess the distribution of changes induced by normothermic ischemia (NI). *Methods:* Hepatectomies ranged from minor to superextended resections. NI (continuous or intermittent pedicle clamping, with 9 total vascular exclusions) ranged from 5 to 110 min (mean ± sd = 44 ± 25), or from 5 to 85 min (31 ± 27) in cirrhotic patients. Analyzed variables included duration of NI (DISC), of surgery (DSURG, quantifying magnitude and complexity of the operation) and of p.o. hospital stay (DPOS), plasma variables such as ALT, AST, LDH, cholesterol (CHOL), triglycerides (TRIG), phosphate (PHOS), alkaline phosphatase, gamma-GT, bilirubin, cholinesterase, albumin, amilase, fibrinogen, hematocrit and blood cell counts, and prothrombin time. *Results:* Regression analysis evidenced direct relationships between DISC and increases of ALT, AST or LDH, and decreases in CHOL, TRIG, TRIG/CHOL ratio and PHOS in p.o. day 1-3 (r^2= 0.3 to 0.5, p<0.001). The r^2 associated with DISC fell to 0.1 only, when DSURG was included as a simultaneous independent variable (except for TRIG/CHOL and PHOS). Measurements at p.o. day 7 were unrelated to DISC or DSURG. Morbidity (transient liver insufficiency) increased with DISC (p<0.05), however DPOS was mostly related to DSURG. *Conclusions:* No specific or persistent alteration quantifying the consequences of DISC, or the link with morbidity, was identified. NI in our patients was a safe technique, however more study is needed to provide exact quantitative figures on tolerance to NI in normal and diseased liver.

21.09

SAFE TOLERANCE OF THE CIRRHOTIC LIVER TO CONSECUTIVE INFLOW OCCLUSION FOR UP TO 40 MINUTES

Kim YI, Hwang YJ, Kim JW, Yun YK
Department of Surgery, Kyungpook National University Hospital, Taegu, Korea

Aims: Hepatic inflow occlusion(HIO) is useful for reducing blood loss during liver resection. However, ischemic liver injury caused by this procedure is a serious dilemma particularly in patients with cirrhotic liver. The aim of this report was to clarify a safe limit for normothermic consecutive HIO during hepatectomy on the human cirrhotic liver.
Methods: Between 1987 and 1998, 47 hepatectomies with continuous HIO for longer than 30 minutes (7 resections more than lobectomy, 8 segmentectomies, 2 nonanatomical resections, 11 subsegmentectomies and 19 partial resections) were employed on adult patients (female/male=7/40) with liver cirrhosis (all hepatocellular carcinoma except one). The Child's classification was A in 26 patients, B in 19 and C in 2. Those were divided into 4 groups by the duration of consecutive HIO: group1 (30min≦ HIO≦ 40min, n=18), group 2 (40<HIO≦ 50, n=12) , group 3 (50<HIO≦ 60, n=14) and group 4 (60<HIO, n=3). The liver and coagulation tests, operative blood loss and postoperative complications were analyzed.
Results: The preoperative blood test included ALT(65± 36U/L, mean± SD), total bilirubin (1.0± 0.4 mg%), ICG R_{15} (16.7± 8%) and prothrombin time(101± 30%). All patients tolerated the procedure except one death in group 4 (hospital mortality, 2.1%). Operative bleeding was satisfactorily controlled by this technique with blood loss of 835± 748 mℓ. However, the postoperative peak values for ALT were substantially elevated as the inflow occlusion was extended (237± 169 in group 1, 526± 626 in group 2, 822± 533 in group 3, and 685± 251 in group 4 ; p<0.02, group 1 vs 3 and 4). The peak ALT higher than 1000U/L was occasionally found when HIO was prolonged >40min (2/12 in group 2 and 5/17 in groups 3 and 4). No significant differences were found among the groups in terms of other liver function tests.
Conclusion: Hepatectomy under the condition of consecutive inflow occlusion can be safely performed even in the cirrhotic liver when the patients are selected and the occlusion is released within 40 min.

21.10

SURGICAL MANAGEMENT OF CAVERNOUS HEMANGIOMA OF THE LIVER. OUR FOUR YEARS EXPERIENCE.

Białek P, Biejat Z, Polański J.A.:
3rd Department of Surgery, 2nd Faculty of Medicine Warsaw Medical School, Stępińska 19/25, Warsaw. POLAND

AIMS

Cavernous hemangioma is the most common benign tumor of the liver. We present our last experience in surgical management of this lesion.

METHODS

There were fifteen patients (12 women and 3 men, middle age 46) with cavernous hemangioma of the liver who were surgically treated in our Department from 1995 to 1998. A descriptive study is made of the cases, their treatment and postoperative course.

RESULTS

The surgical indications included uncertain diagnosis and symptomatic giant /more than 5 cm/ liver tumor. All patients received abdominal sonography, computed tomography (CT) and scintigraphy, in which all displayed the hepatic lesions. The tumors were 3.5-15 cm in diameter and the median was 6.7 cm. No biopsy was performed preoperatively. Three hemihepatectomies, nine bisegmentectomies, two segmentectomies and one 2,3,6,7 segments resection were performed. There was no mortality. Surgical complications was limited to one right hepatic duct injury which was repaired on T-drain during the same operation. All patients were dissmissed after 9-20 days (average 12 days) after surgery without symptoms.

CONCLUSIONS

Liver resection is the only radical treatment for liver hemangioma, but there is still no consensus on indications for surgical procedures. We suggest liver resection in giant /more 5 cm/, symptomatic tumors or when imaging studies are not conclusive.

Dig Surg 1999; 16 (suppl 1): 68-70

Liver Transplantation II.

22.01

HEMODYNAMIC AND BLOOD VOLUME MONITORING DURING ORTHOTOPIC LIVER TRANSPLANTATION

Fazekas J., Gondos T., Tóth T., Tóth M., Forró M., Mándli T., Csaba O., Horovitz P
Semmelweis Medical University Transplantation and Surgical Department, Budapest, Hungary

Aims: Evaluation of standard hemodynamic and blood volume monitoring in pts undergone orthotopic liver transplantation (OLTx) from the point of view of postoperative complications.
Methods: 59 consecutive pts were studied with conventional pulmonary and systemic hemodynamic monitoring consisted of Swan-Ganz catheterization to asses cardiac output (CO); filling pressures (CVP, PWCP); systemic and pulmonary arterial pressures and resistance (MAP, PAP, SVR, PVR); cardiac work indexes (LVSWI, RVSWI); and oxygenation parameters (DO2I, VO2I, O2ER, Qs/Qt). At the last few pts addition to the conventional hemodynamic monitoring a blood volume-monitoring technique with fiberoptic catheter for thermo-dye dilution (COLD System, Pulsion Medizintechnik) was apply to asses the extravascular lung water (EVLW); the intrathoracic and global end-diastolic blood volume (ITBV,GEDV). Measurements were obtained after induction of anesthesia (AS), during hepatectomy (H1-H2), in the anhepatic phase (AP) and in the postreperfusion phase (PRP1-PRP2). All pts received the same anesthetic technique. Patients have been classified into two groups according to the postoperative complications. **Group 1**: good graft function, without any complications, 37 cases. **Group 2**: poor graft function with major postoperative complications, 22 cases.
Results: Significant differences were found between Group 1 and 2 only at DO2I-VO2I [ml/min/kg] in the phases AS, H1; PCWP [mmHg] in the phases AS, H2. (DO2 at AS: 520±207 vs 555±166, p<0.05; at H1 660±294 vs 584±190, p<0.05; VO2I at AS: 94±55 vs 80±30, p<0.05; at H1 93±36 vs 74±21, p<0.05; PCWP at AS: 16±5 vs 12±3 p<0.05; at H2: 16±6 vs 14±5). Using volume-monitoring technique every patient belonged in Group 1. We found good correlation between the filling pressures (CVP-PCWP, r=0,77); the volumetric preload parameters (ITBV-GEDV, r=0,63); but we couldn't find any correlation between the filling pressure and the preload parameters (r=0.02).
Conclusion: The volumetric parameters showed the changes of intravascular volumes in the cases where the conventional parameters didn't. That's why the COLD system is seemed to be a very valuable technique in the monitoring of the perioperative phase of OLTX.

22.02

HEMODYNAMIC EFFECTS OF INTRAPORTAL PROSTAGLANDIN E1 INFUSION AFTER LIVER REVASCULARIZATION.

Hidalgo E, *Mora A, Murio E, Lázaro JL, Charco R, Bilbao I, *Cortes C and Margarit C.
Liver Transplant Unit. Department of Anesthesiology*. Hospital Vall Hebron. Barcelona.

Intravenous infusion of Prostaglandin E1 (PGE1) is used to treat preservation injury in liver transplantation (LT). Because PGE1 produces systemic vasodilatation , IV administration is delayed until hemodynamic stability is reached and full doses can only be given hours after graft revascularization, when ischemic-reperfusion injury is already stablished. Our purpose was to study the hemodynamic effects of PG1 administered through portal vein at time of reperfusion until 90 min in order to evaluate the tolerance to this strategy.
Material and Methods:25 adult patients undergoing LT entered the study, and were randomized to recieve placebo (n=13) or PGE1 (n=12) at 0.6µgr / Kg /h, during the first 90 minutes after graft reperfusion, through a catheter placed in portal vein. The piggyback technique was used systematically, portal and arterial anastomoses were performed before graft reperfusion in all cases. Mean arterial presure (MAP), CVP, Cardiac Index, Systemic Vascular Resistance Index were recorded (Swan-Ganz) during reperfusion, and at 5, 30, 60 and 90 min. Mean values and SD were compared by T-Student test.
Results: It was no need to stop or slow down the infusion in any case. The PGE1 group showed a lower MAP at 90 min (p< 0.02)as well as a higher CI (p< 0.04), without clinical relevance. Additionally, SVRI showed a tend to be lower in this group without statistical significance.

		Reperfusion	5 min.	30 min.	60 min.	90 min.
Cardiac Index	PGE1	4.7±1.5L/m/m2	4.9±1.2	5.7±1.9	5.0±1.7	5.2±1.6
	Placebo	3.2±1.5L/m/m2	3.9±1.5	4.4±0.8	4.6±1.2	4.3±0.9
MAP	PGE1	54±20mmHg	62±18	65±12	62±11	63±8
	Placebo	48±18mmHg	57±15	68±17	62±13	67±17
				P<.05		P<.05

Conclusion : High dose intraportal PGE1 infusion administered by portal vein since reperfusion is well tolerated and offers the opportunity to evaluate the effects of early administration of PG1 on ischemia-reperfusion injury.

22.03

PATHOPHYSIOLOGIC RESPONSE AFTER LIVER TRANSPLANTATION.

Chiarla C., Giovannini I., Boldrini G., Castagneto M.
CNR Center for the Study of Pathophysiology of Shock, Catholic University, Rome, Italy

Aims: Purpose of our work was characterization of metabolic and cardiorespiratory patterns after liver transplantation (LTx). *Methods:* Onehundred-thirty integrated measurements from 35 LTx patients (pts) were analyzed, and data compared to those from a reference group of pts after major surgical procedures (GS). Each measurement provided an extensive assessment of metabolic, hemodynamic and metabolic patterns, based on more than 60 simultaneously obtained variables. Although complications occurred, all LTx pts survived the study period of 20 days. *Results:* Compared to GS, LTx pts had higher cardiac index and stroke volume, with lower O_2 extraction (p<0.001 for all), without significant differences in peripheral resistance (even in pts with previous liver cirrhosis). Hyperdynamism was associated with higher wasted ventilation and pulmonary venous admixture (p<0.001). Metabolic rate was also higher in LTx pts (p<0.001); however, these were normo- to hypometabolic in p.o. day 1-4, then tended to develop hypermetabolism, with a peak in the actual/theoretical energy expenditure on the 11th p.o. day. Within these patterns, peculiar changes predictive of different evolutive courses (i.e., recovery, development of sepsis) were also identified. *Conclusions:* The response to LTx is characterized by cardiovascular hyperdynamism without decreases in peripheral resistance, with pulmonary maldistribution of the increased blood flow, and with a biphasic evolution of energy expenditure. These findings may be used to optimize cardiorespiratory and metabolic monitoring and support in LTx.

KARGER
Fax +41 61 306 12 34
E-Mail karger@karger.ch
www.karger.com

22.04

EARLY AND LATE COMPLICATIONS OF ROUX-EN-Y CHOLEDOCHOJEJUNOSTOMY (CDJ) AS TREATMENT OF BILIARY COMPLICATIONS FOLLOWING ORTHOTOPIC LIVER TRANSPLANTATION (OLT).

R.Rai, BR.Davidson, A.Nandy, N.Doctor, L.Horgan, A.Burroughs, K.Rolles.

Hepatobiliary and Liver Transplantation Unit, The Royal Free and University College Medical School, Pond Street, London NW3 2QG.

AIMS: To study the early and long-term outcome of Roux-en-Y choledochojejunostomy (CDJ) for treatment of biliary complications after orthotopic liver transplantation.

METHODS: We reviewed our experience of Roux-en-Y choledochojejunostomy (CDJ) to treat biliary complications after OLT. From October 1988 to January 1998, 46 patients under went CDJ for biliary complications following OLT. There were 32 males and 14 females with age range of 22 to 65 years (median 60). The original biliary reconstruction at the time of OLT was duct to duct (DD) in 41 patients, primary CDJ in 3 and gall bladder conduit in 2. No T-tube was used.

RESULTS: The indication for CDJ was a biliary leak (23 patients), stricture (20), biliary stones (2) and biliary sludge (1). Two patients (4.3%) had associated hepatic artery thrombosis. The bile leaks were diagnosed at a median period of 29 (2 to 65) days post OLT and stricture at median period of 2 years (33 days to 6.5 years). Twenty-five (54%) patients had an endoscopic and/ or radiological therapeutic intervention before CDJ. Median follow up was 5 years (range 1 month to 9 years). Early complications occurred in 12 patients (26%) and there were 3 peri-operative deaths (6%), only one of which was directly related to surgery. Late complications, mainly anastomotic strictures, occurred in 10 patients (22%).

CONCLUSIONS: The procedure related mortality for surgical revision of biliary complications after OLT is low but early and late complications are common. Surgery should be reserved for patients failing non-operative intervention.

22.05

BILIARY COMPLICATIONS IN WHOLE AND REDUCED SIZE LIVER GRAFTS

Maggi U, Rossi G, Reggiani P, Melada E, Latham L, Caccamo L, Gatti S, Paone G, Fassati LR
Centro Trapianti Fegato-Ospedale Maggiore IRCCS Policlinico, Milano-ITALY

Aims To evaluate the rate of biliary complications in adult and pediatric patients (pts), in whole and reduced size liver grafts, aftter the introduction of split liver techniques.
Methods From April 1994 through November 1998, 115 orthotopic liver transplantations (OLT) were performed in adults (mean age 44±10 years), 74 in pediatrics (mean age 5±5 years). In adults, 109 were whole size grafts (WG), 6 reduced size grafts (RG), that is right grafts retrieved with split liver techniques (in situ in 5 cases, ex situ in one). In pediatrics, 49 were WG, 25 RG (11 left split livers –4 in situ, 7 ex situ-, 10 partial and 4 reduced grafts). In WG a cholecoho-choledocho (CC) anastomosis was performed in 72% of adults and in 22% of pediatrics, whereas in RG an hepaticojejunal (EJ) anastomosis was performed in 33% of adults and in 100% of pediatrics.
Mean follow-up from transplantation was 21±18 months in adults, 25±17 in pediatrics. The rate of biliary complications and actuarial survival were evaluated.
Results The global rate of biliary complications was 21% in adults and 14 % in pediatrics. Respectively in adults and pediatrics, WG had complications in 20% and 6% of grafts; RG in 50% and 32%. In pediatric pts, split grafts had biliary complications in 27% of cases, whereas non-split grafts, in 35%.
Considering only WG, in adults an higher rate of complications was present in CC than in EJ (22 vs 17%); lower rates but with similar distribution were found in pediatrics (9% vs 5%). One and 5 years actuarial survival rates were 76% and 73% in adults, whereas 83% in pediatrics.
Conclusion Biliary complications are still a problem in liver transplantation, though the improvement in patient and graft survival. In our 4-years review, the rate of these complications is still high, more in adults than in children. In WG, both in adults and in pediatrics, CC anastomosis had always more problems than EJ; in RG biliary complications had obviously a higher rate than in WG; though the limited number of grafts, right grafts from split livers in adults had the highest rate of biliary complications, whereas left grafts from split livers in children had lower rates. So in split livers, more attention is suitable for right grafts, even for biliary complications.

22.06

. IN SITU SPLIT LIVER (in situ SLT): RIGHT GRAFT POSTOPERATIVE OUTCOME

E.Andorno, A.Antonucci, G.Paraluppi, R.Mondello, R.Valente, A.Genzone, F.Panaro, N.Morelli, G.Dardano, F.Ermili, M.Pittaluga, C.Bottino, L.Saltalamacchia P.Grondona and U.Valente.
Inst.: Department of Transplantation, S.Martino Hospital, Genoa (I).

Purpose - Although the cadaveric donor pool is raising as result of specific donation policy adopted in our region, still liver supply doesn't cover the needs of paediatric and adult patients waiting for OLT. A split liver transplantation program was started at our institution to improve paediatric organ procurement without affecting adult donor pool.
Patients and Methods - From July 1997 to October 1998 21 in situ splitting procedures were performed during multiorgan procurement, following the original X.Rogiers' technique. 20 right split grafts were implanted on 20 adults using Piggy Back technique in 19 cases and side to side cavocavostomy in 1. Right hepatic artery was always given to the right graft while the caeliac trunk was given to the left. RESULTS - Splitting procedure feasibility rate was 100% and obtained 40 grafts for liver transplantation. Mean splitting time was 130min, mean blood loss during splitting was 51.25ml, mean cold ischemia time was 470min, mean donor's age was 31.5yrs. Never the splitting procedure negatively affected multiorgan procurement. 40 in situ SLT were performed; 21 right split grafts were transplanted at our institution (19 SLT in adults, 1 SLT + kidney in a child simultaneously) and 1 right graft was shipped to another institution. The 19 left grafts were shipped to other Italian and foreign centres and implanted in 18 cases on paediatric recipients whilw in 1 on an adult, for auxiliary transplantation.Survival rate of adults transplanted at our institution is 70% (UNOS 3 0%, UNOS 2 70%, UNOS 1 88,9%).
Conclusion - In situ SLT is a feasible procedure and together with a cooperation policy between Italian and foreign centres allows to cover the needs of paediatrics patients waiting for OLT, without reducing adult donor pool.

22.07

IN SITU SPLIT-LIVER WITH MIDDLE HEPATIC VEIN ANOMALY

E.ANDORNO, A.Antonucci, G.Paraluppi, R.Mondello, R.Valente, A.Genzone, F.Panaro, N.Morelli, G.Dardano, F.Ermili, L.Saltalamacchia, M.Pittaluga, C.Bottino, P.Grondona, I.Fontana and U.Valente.

Inst.: Dept. of Transplantation, S.Martino Hospital, Genoa (I).

Purpose - We describe the in situ liver splitting, performed on a cadaveric donor with an hepatic vein anomaly, consisting in intraparenchymal confluence of the middle hepatic vein (MHV) with segment 3 vein (V3) of left hepatic vein (LHV). Two split grafts were obtained (S2+S3) and (S1+S4+S5+S6+S7+S8).

Materials and Methods - Donor: 33 year old man, 1.85m, 75 Kg, dead for head trauma. Splitting: liver splitting was performed during multiorgan procurement (heart, whole-pancreas, kidneys), following X.Rogiers' original technique. During extraparenchymal hepatic vein dissection we noticed the absence of the common trunk (LHV+MHV) and the caval ending of the LHV. After dissection of hilar plate and parenchymal transection, we observed that MHV (diameter 1,5 cm) met V3 vein. In order to obtain venous drainage of both grafts, we divided MHV at its ending in V3. Left graft drainage was given by LHV after V3 reconstruction at MHV end orifice. Back table procedure (right graft): caval drainage of MHV was obtained using donor's iliac venous graft to bridge the gap between MHV and the caval ending orifice of LHV. Recipient: Left graft (weight 280gr.) was shipped to a foreign transplantation centre and was implanted on a paediatric recipient following segmental liver transplantation technique. Right graft (weight 1100gr.) was implanted on a 59 year old man affected by HCC on HCV related cirrhosis, using side to side cavacavostomy.

Results - Functional recovery of both grafts was immediate with early estubation of both recipients. Adult recipient liver function tests: ALT peak level 820 UI/dl, lactacidaemia 3.1 mmol/dl, PT 45% on 24th hour. Postoperative US allowed determination of MHV patency. Adult patient was discharged from hospital on Day 24.

Conclusion - MHV division during in situ liver splitting procedure and its reconstruction using donor iliac venous graft, permitted to obtain two well functioning split grafts, despite hepatic vein anomaly.

22.08

FIRST REPORT OF CAVOPORTAL HEMITRANSPOSITION IN PEDIATRIC REDUCED SIZE LIVER TRANSPLANTATION

Hanack U.,Lorf Th.Talaulicar R.,Canelo R.,Schiffman J-H.,Ringe B.

Klinik für Transplantationschirurgie,Klinik für Kinderheilkunde der Georg-August-Universität Göttingen

Aims: Recipient portal vein thrombosis is currently not considered as contraindication for liver transplantation. Even in cases of diffuse thrombosis of the portal venous system cavoportal hemitransposition was successful used in adult patients (Tzakis et al. Transplantation 1998). We describe a reduced size liver transplantation in a child with splanchnic vein thrombosis necessitating cavoportal transposition.
Methods: A female 1 $^{9/12}$ year old child suffering from hepatoblastoma showed partial response to systemic chemotherapy (starting with itosfamid, cisplatin, adriamycin) and was evaluated to reduced size liver transplantation. In backtable preparation the graft was cut down to the left lateral segment (segments II and III) yielding 500 g. Hepatectomy was performed including the retrohepatic portion of the inferior vena cava (IVC). During the preparation it became obvious that the hole portal vein system (including splenic, superior mesenteric and inferior mesenteric vein) was occluded. Thrombectomy failed and the decision for cavoportal hemitransposition was made. Left hepatic vein from the reduced graft was anastomosed end-to-end with the superior hepatic IVC. The infrahepatic IVC was anastomosed end-to-end with the portal vein of the graft. The stump of the recipient portal vein was sutured. Arterial and bile duct anastomoses were conducted in end-to-end standard technique.
Results: The postoperative course showed satisfactory liver function, mild (400 ml/day) ascites, no signs of encephalopathy or gastrointestinal bleeding.
Conclusions: We describe for the first time the cavoportal hemitransposition performed in association with reduced size liver transplantation and conclude that this technique can safely carry out in the presense of diffuse splanchnic vein thrombosis in pediatric recipients.

22.09

SAFE USAGE FOR HEPATIC TRANSPLANT OF GRAFT LIVERS PROCURED FROM OLD DONORS (FROM 70 TO 87 YEARS OLD).

Cescon M, Mazziotti, A, Grazi GL, Ercolani G, Quintini C, Montalti R, Cavallari A
Dept of Surgery and Transplantation, Sant'Orsola Hospital, University of Bologna, Bologna, Italy

The limiting age for accepting organs for orthotopic liver transplantation (OLT) has been continuously extended over the past years. We report herein our experience with the usage of hepatic grafts procured from very aged donors.
Methods: A retrospective, case-control study was carried out to assess the outcome of 17 OLTs (Group A) performed with livers procured from donor older then 70 years (mean age 73.8 ± 4.1; range 70-87) in the period '96 - '98; the outcome of these operations were matched with 17 OLTs (Group B) performed with organs obtained from donors younger then 40 years (mean age 24.8 ± 8.4; range 13-40) which were chronologically performed thereafter. The two groups were comparable for gender, mean age, indication for OLT and technique of procedures. The 1-year actuarial survival rate for these 34 transplanted pt. was 90%. The following variables were crosstabulated according to donor age, cold ischemia time, i.o. blood and plasma replacement, 30-day mortality, incidence of primary graft dysfunction, incidence of acute rejection, incidence of arterial complications, long term survival. Furthermore, the postoperative GOT, GPT, total bilirubine, alkaline phosphatases, γ-GT, prothrombin activity, aPTT were collected and compared for the first 14 postoperative days. Liver biopsy was obtained in 9/17 donors older than 70 years, revealing less than 10% of steatosis in all but one of them.
Results: There were 3 (8.8%) postoperative deaths; 1 in Gr. A and 2 in Gr. B (p = NS). The only 2 arterial problems were observed in Gr. A livers (p = NS): one arterial thrombosis was treated by thrombectomy, while the haemoperitoneum secondary to the rupture of an atherosclerotic artery was the direct cause of death in the second. Only one patient, in Gr. A, required retransplantation (p = NS). There were no other differences in the considered variables, except for total bilirubin at day 8, prothrombin activity at day 4, aPTT at days 6 and 13 and albumin at day 5. The 1-year actuarial survival rates were 86.2% and 93.5% for Gr. A and Gr. B respectively (p = NS).
Conclusions:: The use of liver grafts procured from aged donors is to be considered safe. Greater care must be placed to pathological vascular conditions related with advanced stage atherosclerosis, as revealed by calcified plaques on the hepatic artery, which may be the cause of severe postoperative complications.

22.10

ANATOMIC VARIATIONS OF THE HEPATIC ARTERY: CLASSIFICATION AND THEIR SIGNIFICANCE IN LIVER TRANSPLANTATION.

Felekouras ES[1, 2], Tsamandas AC[1], Blesios G[1,] Pierrakakis S[2,] Álexiou D[3], Setakis N[2], Salakou S[1], Tepetes K[1], Karavias D[1], Papalampros E[3] Bastounis E[3]
T.Å. Starzl Transplantation Institute[1], University of Pittsburgh Medical Center, Pittsburgh, PA, USA, Department of Surgery, Thriasion General Hospital, Athens, 1st Department of Surgery, University of Athens Medical School[3].

Aims: Objective of the study was to report our experience in liver transplantation, using allografts with anatomic variations of hepatic artery
Methods: During a 3-year period (from 1993-1995) we performed 167 multiple organ recoveries, from cadaveric donors in Pittsburgh Transplant Institute. All liver grafts were systematically prepared for implantation in a back table procedure. During the dissection of the hepatic artery, all hepatic artery variations were listed according to a schema we developed.
Results: The right hepatic artery was coming from: the SMA in 11, 37%, the AA in 1, 79%, the CHA in 1, 19%, the ÑÇÁ in 85,65% (normal position). The left hepatic artery was coming from the LGA in 14,97%, the ÁÁ in 2,39% and in 82,6% from the ÑÇÁ (normal position).
Conclusions: Meticulous dissection and preparation of the hepatic artery helps the prevention of its trauma and subsequently successful Liver Transplantation. Injury of the hepatic artery leads to the hepatic artery thrombosis and the patient to death or retransplantation.

Dig Surg 1999; 16: 71-73

Liver tumor IV.

23.01

EXTENSIVE SURGERY FOR HILAR CHOLANGIOCARCINOMA: EARLY RESULTS

J P A Lodge, B J Ammori, G V Miller, K R Prasad, S G Pollard
Departments of Hepatobiliary Surgery, St. James's University Hospital, Beckett Street, Leeds LS9 7TF, UK

AIMS: Local resection for hilar cholangiocarcinoma failed to improve its dismal prognosis. More recent reports, however, demonstrated improvement in survival and quality of life following aggressive resection. This paper describes our early results of extensive surgery for hilar cholangiocarcinoma. **METHODS:** Between January 1991 and July 1998, 36 patients (23 males) underwent laparotomy for radiologically operable hilar cholangiocarcinoma. Twenty nine patients underwent resection (local resection 2, major liver resection 19, orthotopic liver transplantation 8) and radical lymphadenectomy. Of the seven unresectable cases, two underwent surgical biliary bypass.
RESULTS: The resection rate was 80.6%. Hospital mortality was 9.5% for resection alone and 13.8% when liver transplantation was considered. Postoperative morbidity developed in 19 of 36 patients (52.8%). The Kaplan-Meier 1- and 3-year actuarial survival for resection alone, transplantation and 'no resection' was 61% and 37.4%, 62.5% and 31.3%, and 21.4% and 0% respectively. The mean (median) cumulative survival time (including postoperative deaths) for the above three treatment modalities was 21.5 (16.7), 22.3 (18.2) and 7.9 (3.8) months respectively. Resection and transplantation significantly prolonged survival over 'no resection' (p=0.0257).
CONCLUSIONS: Aggressive resection and liver transplantation improved survival of patients with hilar cholangiocarcinoma. This was achieved with acceptable morbidity and mortality rates.

23.02

SURGICAL TREATMENT OF HEPATOCELLULAR CARCINOMA

Geissler F.*, Witzigmann H.*, Uhlmann D.*, Tannapfel A.**, Hanss I.*
*Dep. of Surgery II., **Institute of Pathology, University of Leipzig, German

The prognosis of patients with multiple hepatocellular carcinoma (HCC) remains disappointing. Hepatic resection and liver transplantation (OLT) offer the only chance for cure.

Methods: Between 4/94 and 12/98 102 patients, mean age 61 (19-82), with HCC were admitted to our department. Male/female ratio was 74:28 = 2,6:1,65 patients received no therapy or palliativ treatments. Hepatic resection was performed in 37 and OLT in 11 patients. Each carcinoma was re-evaluated in terms of staging and grading. Furthermore p53, apoptosis and proliverative activity was measured.

Results: The 30-day (operative) mortality rate for resection was 10,8%. Curative resection (RO) was possible in 25/37 patients. The cumulative survival rate in the RO-resection group was 42% at 3 years. In the OLT group 3/11 patients died in the early postoperative period because of complications. At present 8/11 patients are alive with a mean follow up 585 days. Only one patient acquired lung and bone metastases 7 months after OLT. The status of p53, apoptosis and proliferation did not influence the outcome significantly.

Conclusions: Surgical resection is the preferred treatment for HCC in patients without cirrhosis. Patients with advanced cirrhosis and HCC are candidates for transplantation. Accurate patient selection are important for both procedures. To improve surgical results, multimodality treatment protocols are necessary.

23.03

HEPATOCELLULAR CARCINOMA IN CIRRHOTIC PATIENTS. OUR EXPERIENCE WITH ECHO-GUIDED RADIOFREQUENCY PERCUTANEOUS ABLATION

Puleo S, Azzarello G, Astuto M, Lombardo R, Di Carlo I.

First Surgical Clinic, University of Catania, Catania, Italy

Hepatic resection and orthotopic liver transplantation are the most effective therapy for hepatocellular carcinoma (HCC) in cirrhotic patients. In patients not suitable for surgery, many alternative procedures are today utilized.
Aim of this study is to verify the therapeutical effectiveness of radiofrequency interstitial thermal ablation (RITA).
Materials and methods.
From January 1995 to December 1998, 78 cirrhotic patients affected by HCC were observed in our Institution. Seven (8,9%) of them have been submitted to RITA, in the last year. All the patients were males and aged from 60 to 76 years (mean age 68,4). Four patients (57,1%) were classified as Child B and 3 (32,9%) as Child A, all had a single nodule variable from 2 to 5 cm in size, diagnosed by US, echo-color-doppler and CT scan. The indications for RITA were : general contraindications to surgery (3 cases), not given consensus for surgery (4 cases).Percutaneous "one-shot" RITA was performed under general anesthesia.
Results.
In all patients thermal injuries were usually applied for 25 min. No intra or post-operative complications were observed, and the patients were discharged after 24-48 hours. The effectiveness of treatment was assesed at 20 days, 3, 6 and 9 months with CT scan. Complete disappearance of the lesion was achieved in in 3 patients (42,8%) in the remaining patients partial response was obteined.
Conclusion.
RITA seem to be a safe and effective alternative treatment in patients affected by HCC. Further investigations and major number of patients should be rquested for controlled trials in order to define the therapeutic role of this method.

23.04

INCREASED SURVIVAL AFTER LIVER RESECTION FOR HCC IN CIRRHOSIS GIVES THE PROCEDURE ADDITIONAL EFFICACY.

Grazi GL, Mazziotti A, Ercolani G, Pierangeli F, Montalti R, Del Gaudio M, Cavallari A
Dept of Surgery and Transplantation, Sant'Orsola Hospital, University of Bologna, Bologna, Italy

After the performance of liver resection (LR) for the treatment of cirrhotics with hepatocellular carcinoma (HCC) during the '80s, different non operative procedures have been proposed for these same patients, but all of them had to face with surgery in term of effectiveness. During the past years resective surgery had further developed and refined; we have reviewed our more recent results and compared them with previous data.

Methods: A retrospective study was performed with all 258 LRs performed for HCC on cirrhosis from 1983 to 1998. There were 211 (81.8%) man and 47 (18.2%) female. Mean age was 61.6 ± 7.8 years (range 22 - 80). Nine pts. received palliative procedures for symptoms and thus were excluded from survival analysis. 30-day mortality rate for the entire series was 5.0% (13 pts.); the 3- and 5-year actuarial survivals were 63.4% and 41.3%; the 3- and 5-year recurrence rates were 35.9% and 55.8%. The year 1992 was arbitrarily chosen as a cut-off for categorising patients: Group A < 1992 (107 pts., 41.5%), Group B ≥ 1992 (151 pts., 58.5%). During this latter period surgery radically changed in our Department, in particular for the operative technique, with a more meticulous and bloodless parenchyma mapping and division.

Results: The two groups were similar for major operative selection criteria, even if an higher proportion of Child A pts. underwent surgery more recently: 64.5% (69/107) in Gr. A vs. 87.3% (131/150) in Gr. B ($p < 0.05$). On the other hand, pts. in Gr. B had more advanced diseases (Stage 1-2: 61.0% in Gr. A vs. 45.3% in Gr. B, $p < 0.05$). There was no difference in the extension of the procedures performed, but the need for intraoperative blood transfusions decreased from 68.6% (72/105) of Gr. A to 24.0% (36/150) of Gr. B ($p < 0.0005$). 30-day deaths were also reduced in the second period: 10/107 (9.3%) in Gr. A vs. 3/151 (2.0%) in Gr. B ($p < 0.005$). Postoperative complication rate was similar among the two groups. The 3- and 5-year actuarial survivals were 52.9% and 32.3% respectively for Gr. A; 72.5% and 50.0% for Gr. B ($p < 0.005$).

Conclusions: The experience gained in the more recent years in LRs for cirrhotics with HCC has led to significantly improve operative results and long term outcome, with half of the patients still alive 5 years after surgery. LR is an extremely effective therapeutical option for well compensated cirrhotic with limited disease.

23.05

RESULTS OF OPERATIONS FOR PRIMARY MALIGNANT HEPATIC TUMORS

Tóth P., Takács I., András Cs., Szappanos M., Varga G., Sápy P.*
2nd Department of Surgery, University Medical School of Debrecen
*3rd Department of Internal Medicine, University Medical School of Debrecen
4004, Debrecen, Móricz Zs. krt. 22., Hungary

Aims: Authors evaluate the results of 26 operations performed because of primary malignant hepatic tumors.

Methods: Between the 01.01.1992 and 31.12.1998 14 patients had hepatic resections because of primary malignant tumors. In 12 cases the tumors proved to be inoperable. The average year of the 14 females and 12 males was 63.5 years (43-77). Causes of the surgical interventions were hepatocellular carcinoma (18 cases), cholangiocellular carcinoma (6 cases), primary hepatic carcinoid and cystadenocarcinoma (1-1 cases). Resections were performed by CUSA ultrasonic aspirator equipment. The procedure of total vascular exclusion was not used during the operations. Tumors were removed with a safety edge of 1cm. Six segment resections (one segment resection in 1 case, two segments resection in 4 cases, three segments resection in 1 case), 5 hemihepatectomies and 3 extended hepatectomies were executed. The average size of the removed tumor was 12.9 (7-26) cm. The average volume of blood transfused was 600 (0-1800)ml during the operations. After the surgery 4 from the patients who underwent resections and 6 patients with inoperable tumors received adjuvant cytostatical treatment.

Results: There were no casualties in the early postoperative period. We observed transitional elevation of liver enzymes in 3 patients, emergence of hypertonic crisis in 2 patients and the complication of bile flow, that needed permanent drainage, in 1 patient. There was no any surgical reintervention. Local recurrence of the tumor was not detected, so far. The average one year survival rate of the patients who had resection was 72 %. Patients with inoperable tumor have an average one year survival rate of 60%.

Conclusions: The inoperability of the primary malignant hepatic tumors is often observed in the period of their first detection. The risk of these operations is high mostly because of severe concomitant diseases. By increasing the number of cases of resections we can hope better survival data. The adjuvant and neoadjuvant chemotherapy is useful treatment that makes the patients suitable for the surgery and improves the survival parameters.

23.06

EARLY SURGICAL RESULTS OF LIVER RESECTIONS

Takács I., Tóth P., András Cs., Vágvölgyi A., Halász L., Sápy P.*

2nd Department of Surgery, University Medical School of Debrecen
*3rd Department of Internal Medicine, University Medical School of Debrecen
4004, Debrecen, Móricz Zs. krt. 22., Hungary

Aims: Authors evaluate the results of 69 liver resections performed because of metastatic tumors in the liver.

Methods: Between the 01.01.1992 and 31.12.1998 69 patients were operated for metastatic hepatic tumors. Resections of the liver were performed in 49 cases because of metastases of colorectal tumors, tumors of pancreas and of the papilla of Vater (in 9 cases), tumors of the stomach (in 3 cases), tumors of the breast (in 5 cases), tumor of lung, testis, carcinoid of the small intestine (in 1-1 case). Male/female ratio was: 38:31. The average year of the patients was 57.1 years (19-85). Simutaneously with the hepatic resection we performed resection of the colon in 16 cases. In 33 cases resections of the liver were executed 7(1-16) months after the resection of the colon. In 8 of the 33 cases the liver metastases were known in the period of the primary surgical intervention. Simultaneous resections of the pancreas were performed in 8 cases, simultaneous gastric resections were performed in all of the 3 cases, 24 atypical hepatic resections, 36 segment resections (one segment resection in 16 cases, two segments resection in 14 cases, three segments resection in 6 cases), 5 hemihepatectomies and 4 lobectomies were executed. After the surgery 31 patients received adjuvant cytostatical treatment

Results: There were no casualties in the early postoperative period. We observed fever (4 patients), transitional elevation of liver enzymes (9 patients), pleuropneumonia (2 cases), TIA (1 patient). There was no any surgical complication. Three patients had local recurrent tumor, lately. The one year average survival rate was 64 %.

Conclusions: In cases of elective surgical procedures the resection of the tumor of colon (or other abdominal organ) simultaneously with the resection of hepatic metastases is the choice of treatment when the oncological and the general state of the patients makes the surgical intervention possible. The adjuvant chemotherapy is useful treatment to improve the survival parameters.

23.07

HEPATIC RESECTION FOR CANCER IN THE ELDERLY.

Chiappa A, Zbar AP, Biella F, Bertani E, Crotti C, and Staudacher C.*
Dept. of Emergency Surgery-University of Milan-ITALY
S. Raffaele Scientific Institute
**Imperial Medical College-Hammersmith Hospital-London-UK*

Aims. This report analyzes liver resection in 46 patients with primary and metastatic liver cancer aged 65 years or older.

Methods. Between December 1992 and January 1998, 46 patients aged over 65 years (28 M, 18 F; mean age 70; range: 65-82 years) underwent liver resection. The type of hepatectomy was classified according to Coinaud. The American Society of Anesthesiologists (ASA) Physical status scores were preoperatively evaluated. Data were compared using Fisher's exact two-tailed test, X^2 test and Student's *t* test.

Results. Hepatic resections were performed for metastases (n=22;48%) and hepatocellular carcinoma (HCC) complicating cirrhosis (n=24;52%). Major hepatectomies were performed in 15 patients (33%), with 2 deaths (1 from hepatic failure and 1 from non hepatic causes). Non-anatomical hepatic resections were performed in 31 patients (67%), with 2 deaths from hepatic failure. Of the 46 malignancies, 24% were multiple. The median size of the tumors was 4,5±4 cm (range: 1-15 cm). Mean operative blood loss was 800±790 ml (range: 100-4500 ml). Mean post-operative hospital stay was 13±7 days. The overall mortality rate was 9% (n=4) The overall complication rate was 15%. The 1, 3, and 4-years specific survival rates were 87%, 51%, and 47%, respectively. By multivariate analysis only preoperative jaundice (bilirubin level ≥2mg/dl) ($p<0.001$) and intraoperative blood transfusions ($p<0.05$) predicted major complications. Preoperative ASA grading did not influence complications or mortality (p=0.22).

Conclusions. Five previous studies have specifically examined outcome following liver resection in the elderly, however results were generally poor with operative mortality rates being 19% - 40%. This study demonstrates that major and minor hepatic resections can be performed safely in elderly patients with acceptable morbidity and mortality, and that chronological age alone should not be considered a contraindication to liver resection.

23.08

LIVER TUBERCULOSIS (SELECTIVE DAMAGE)

Severtsev A., Mironov N., Nikolaenko E., Laptev V., Gribunov Yu., Merzljakova E., Ivanova E., Nazarenko V., Zemskova Z., Sedova L., Tupikova E.
MED CENTRE FOR RUSSIAN GOVERNMENT (Moscow; Russia): ① United Hospital & Policlinics ("Volynsky" Hospital), ② Postgraduate & Research Centre (Dept. of Surgery), ③ Central Clinical Hospital; ALL – RUSSIAN RESEARCH INSTITUTE OF TUBERCULOSIS (Moscow, Russia)

We report a surgical case of selective tuberculosis of liver with the absence of any additional tuberculosis sites in other organs.
A 72-year-old-man with the diagnosed multiple (8 nodules; diameter is up to 1 cm) round tumors of the right lobe was admitted to our department. These tumors were diagnosed accidentally by US-examination. He hadn't any signs or symptoms of liver or any other organ disease. All lab tests were normal. He was taking no any liver damaged drugs. His HAV, HBV, HCV, HDV, HGV, TTV tests were negative, and CEA and α-FP levels were not elevated. During CT scan, MRI and scintigraphy repeated in 3 different diagnostic centers the presence of nodules in liver was not confirmed, but repeated US examinations (including Doppler) in all these diagnostic centers (3) showed the presence of nodules. US exam of liver after food intake demonstrated disappearance of these nodules, and they occurred again on the next day. The bone scintigraphy didn't give any pathology. The biopsy of liver nodules under US-scan was not informative.
The patient was treated surgically with the suspicion of HCC or metastases of unknown origin. Intraoperative specimen showed the liver tuberculosis. At the same time intraabdominal investigation of all-abdominal organs and lymph nodes didn't give any pathologic sites. Additional postoperative investigations of lungs, lymph nodes, bones, kidneys, brain rejected TBC pathology in these organs.
In the post-operative period patient had a specific chemotherapy (1/2 of conventional doses of anti – tuberculosis drugs). Long term results (3 months) showed good conditions of patient
According to the data from the All-Russian Research Institute of Tuberculosis (Moscow, Russia) the sole case of selective tuberculosis of the liver was registered in Russia in 1920.

23.09

QUALITY OF LIFE IN PATIENTS WITH OBSERVED AND RESECTED FOCAL NODULAR HYPERPLASIA

Mössinger M, Fronhoff K, Nadalin S, Tusch G, Raab R, Weimann A
Klinik für Abdominal- und Transplantationschirurgie,
Medizinische Hochschule Hannover, Germany

Aims: Focal nodular hyperplasia (FNH) is a benign liver tumor entity with a predominance in young women. Diagnosis is often an incidental finding. An association with contraceptive steroids has been discussed. Agreement exists that surgery should be only performed in case of symptoms and tumor growth. Frequently, there is onset of symptoms at time of diagnosis which makes the indication for surgery difficult in individual cases. It is recommended that women with observed tumors should withhold from contraceptive steroids and pregnancy. In comparison to surgery no data are available with regard to long term observation and quality of life.
Patients and Methods: Between 1978 and 1996 119 patients (109 women, 10 men; mean age 36.4±9.0 yrs) underwent surgery for FNH. During the same period 89 patients (82 women, 7 men; mean age 34.7±10.4 yrs) were observed for FNH. Median tumor size in surgically treated patients was 7.0 (1.0-20.0) cm and in observed patients 6.7 (1.2-13.8) cm. Seventy-two patients after surgery (92.3%) and 66 of the observed group (74.2%) underwent follow-up after 34.7 (0.4-83.6) and 90.3 (4.9-197.7) months respectively. Diagnostic imaging used sonography if necessary added by contrast enhanced computerized tomography. A change in tumor size of 2cm was considered significant. Quality of life was assessed with the Gastrointestinal Quality of Life Index (GILQI) according to Eypasch et al.
Results: GILQI scores were without significant difference: surgery 113.4±17.8; observation 119.2±18.6. At the time of follow-up tumor size was constant in 42 of the observed patients (63.6%). Significant decrease was found in 22 patients (33.4%) while no increase could be observed. In two patients (3.0%) reliable comparison was not possible. 5 patients who were primarily observed had been operated before: 3 of them due to increase of tumor size. 15 of the patients had an observation period for more than 10 years. During observation 11 women had 14 pregnancies. All pregnancies were uneventful: 9 spontaneous, 4 cesarian , and 1 forceps delivery. Five women continued intake of contraceptive steroids with an increase of tumor size in none of them.
Conclusions: Observation of FNH can be also justified with regard to quality of life. During long-term observation significant increase of tumor size is uncommon. Withdrawal from pregnancy and hormon medication is not supported by these results.

Dig Surg 1999; 16 (suppl 1): 74-76

Liver tumor V.

24,01

RISK FACTORS IN LIVER SURGERY - A NEW SCORE

Lamesch P, Tanev I, Geißler I, Hauss J
Klinik für Abdominal-, Transplantations- und Gefäßchirurgie
University of Leipzig, Liebigstr. 20a, 04103 Leipzig, Germany

Introduction:
Preoperative risk scores before liver resection are currently under investigation and controversely discussed. Individual laboratory tests (LT) and liver function tests (LFT) are misleading as they represent the result of a *single* metabolic pathway only. The aim of the present study was to analyse the value of an empiric score on the basis of routine parameters and liver function tests.

Patients and Methods:
51 patients with primary liver tumors scheduled for an elective liver resection were included in this study. Preoperative LT ASAT, ALAT, GLDH, PTT, bilirubine, AT III, NH_3 and the LFT MEGX (lidocaine-test) and ABT (Amino-pyrine-breath-test).Each paremeter got 1-4 points on the basis of the severity of pathologic changes. Total score: Σ points / Σ parameter. The postoperative complications were analysed retrospectively.

Results

(χ^2: p=0.00023

Score Patients (n)	3	4	5	6	7	8	9
no comp.	1	9	6	0	0	0	0
mild comp.	0	0	4	0	1	0	0
severe comp.	0	0	2	7	3	0	2

Conclusion:
The rationale of this score was to include a large number of routine LT and LFTs. Although preliminary, these highly significant results demonstrate, that patients withr severe postoperative complications had more than 6 points, patients with less than 6 points only mild complications. None of the patients with 3 or 4 points had any complication. The definite value of this score needs to be evaluated on the bases of larger studies.

24,02

DOES SMALL HCC CORRESPOND TO EARLY TUMOR STAGE ?

Weimann A, Hoberg S, Lang H, Schlitt HJ, Tusch G, Raab R, Klempnauer J
Klinik für Abdominal- und Transplantationschirurgie,
Medizinische Hochschule Hannover, Germany

Aims: Agreement exists that liver transplantation for hepatic malignancy should be abandoned in advanced tumor stage. An ongoing discussion is addressing the issue of whether transplantation might successfully cure the underlying disease in patients with small resectable hepatocellular carcinoma (HCC) with cirrhosis. While small HCC can be defined as one or two tumor nodules $\leq$ 5cm, the Union Internationale Contre le Cancer (UICC) classification for stage II also includes larger solitary tumors without microvascular invasion. For selection of appropriate candidates for liver transplantation criteria have to be related to preoperative diagnostic imaging which is limited to the detection of tumor number and size. A retrospective analysis was performed in order to investigate whether the definition of small HCC really corresponds to early tumor stage.
Patients and Methods: Between 1971 and 1996 374 patients underwent surgical treatment for HCC. Forty-three (11.5%) could be classified as small according to the definition of Tang. Twenty-nine of these patients underwent resection and 14 liver transplantion. Additionally, histological examination of the resection and hepatectomy specimen discovered 86 patients (23.0%) with UICC stage I and II tumors, 64 after resection and 22 after liver transplantation. Survival of patients with small HCC and those with stage I and II tumors was compared. Statistical analysis: logrank and Wilcoxon test; $p<0.05$.
Results: Univariate analysis of 374 patients revealed UICC tumor stage and tumor size > and $\leq$5cm prognostic factors. 35 of 43 patients (81.4%) with small HCC had UICC stage I and II tumors while only 8 (18.6%) showed advanced tumors in stage III and IV due to lymph node metastases and macrovascular invasion. The 1-, 3-, 5- and 10yr survival rates after liver resection for small HCC were 86, 59, 43 and 43% resp., after liver transplantation 83, 83, 83 and 0% resp. No significant difference in survival could be observed with regard to the patients with UICC stage I and II tumors: resection group 76, 60, 49 and 40% and transplantation group 73, 58, 50 and 34%.
Conclusion: The definition of small HCC fulfills prognostic value with regard to early tumor stage. Therefore, it is helpful for decision making about appropriate surgical treatment in HCC.

24,03

PREOPERATIVE SEGMENTAL LIVER MASS EVALUATION

O.Tsiroulnikova, A.Filin, A.Semenkov and S.Gautier
National Research Centre of Surgery, Moscow, Russia.

The sufficiency of liver fragments' mass is very important for successful split or living related liver grafting. Since the routine CT-scan obtains adequate calculation only for left lateral segment and for the whole liver, it cannot be used successfully for estimate of lobes or segments. Some formulas created for mathematical prediction of liver lobes' mass or volume also cannot estimate liver segments. The study performed on 54 cadaveric livers to evaluate mass percent ratio of each C.Couinaud segment showed the following correlation: I – 1.6 ± 0.2%, II – 11.8 ± 0.7%, III – 10.4 ± 0.5, IV – 22.7 ± 1.3%, V – 15.1 ± 0.6%, VI – 12.3 ± 0.5%, VII – 14.1 ± 0.4%, VIII – 12.0 ± 0.4%. The revealed percentage (N) can be combined with any formula or other method of total liver mass calculation:

$$M_{segm} = \frac{M_{liver} \times N\,(\%)}{100}$$

The method was called segmental liver mass evaluation (SLME). The described method was practically utilized to make a choice between the left lateral segment and the total left or right lobe for living related liver transplantation in 8 children of 14 to 43 kg. body weight and to predict the mass of hepatic remnant after 32 extended hepatectomies. Using SLME we have withdrawn CT for liver volume measurements since 1996. SLME appears to be correct for split- as well as for reduced sized liver grafts mass. In the same time it can avoid X-ray radiation during the traditional CT which is not indifferent for the health of living donor.

KARGER
Fax +41 61 306 12 34
E-Mail karger@karger.ch
www.karger.com

24,04

SURGICAL CLASSIFICATION OF LIVER TUMOURS

S.Gautier, O.Tsiroulnikova
National Research Centre of Surgery, Moscow, Russia.

The universal utilization of any available contemporary classification of hepatic focal lesions is limited by numerous variants of hepatic anatomy, tumour size, localization and morphological type. The observation of 143 patients with different large hepatic focal lesions had demonstrated that success of curative liver resection depended on the opportunity to keep some tumour free part of the liver (not less then 2 C.Couinaud segments) to carry out the liver function after surgery. As a result of 64 curative extended anatomical liver resections a new variant of liver tumour classification had been created. According to anatomical resection's principles it supposes to present the size of hepatic focal lesions by number of C.Couinaud segments involved using the main TNM symbols combined with letters and figures as indexes to show other intrahepatic and/or extrahepatic structures affected if any. Letter indexes are corresponding to the wide-spread English medical terms and not to be repeated. T – tumour or some other hepatic focal lesion is followed with Roman figures to show the liver segments it spreads over. In the case of one big tumour and some satellites the Roman figures are being summed up (+). TC – tumour in cirrhotic liver. TR – tumour recurrence after previous resection. V – hepatic veins or caval vein involvement or/and portal thrombosis. D – bile ducts' lesion with jaundice. O – other organs involvement: O_a – adrenal, O_c – colon, O_d – diaphragm, O_k – right kidney, O_s – stomach, O_w – abdominal wall. N – lymphatic nodes' involvement: N_1 – celiac artery group, N_2 – paraaortal group, N_3 – mediastinal group. M – metastasis: M_b – bones, M_e – encephalon, M_l – lungs, M_p – peritoneal dissemination. For example: HCC $TCR_{II-III+I}$ V $N_{1,2}$ M_l means recurrent hepatocellular carcinoma of cirrhotic liver with the II and III C.Couinaud segments involved, with satellite in the caudate lobe and portal thrombosis, with metastasis into lymphatic nodes of 1 and 2 groups and lungs. The classification is supposed to be convenient to present malignant as well as benign liver tumours and other focal lesions of the organ and may be developed by some extra letter symbols if necessary.

24,05

GENERAL ANAESTHESIA FOR PATIENTS WITH LIVER DISEASES: INTRAVENOUS OR INHALATED ANAESTHESIA ?

Darvas K., Tarjányi M.,Pinkola K., Molnár Zs., Kupcsulik P., Flautner L.
1st Department of Surgery, Semmelweis Medical University, Budapest, Hungary

Patients with liver diseases are in the high risk anaesthesiology category. Changes in circulation, the intrapulmonal shunt fraction and the altered dug metabolism must be considered when the anaesthetic method is chosen.
In our study 102 patients with liver disorders undergoing abdominal surgery were investigated in 4 groups. The applied volatile anaesthetics were isofurane (n=30) or sevoflurane (n=12) in 0,5-1,0 % inhaled fraction. The intravenous drugs were diazepam (n=30; 0,1 mg/kg) and propofol (n=30; 1 mg/kg). Atracurium (0,2 mg/kg) was given as a muscle relaxant. Mean arterial pressure (MAP), pulse rate (P), O_2 saturation and end tidal CO_2 pressure ($etCO_2$) were continuously monitorised. The acid-base state, blood gases, serum electrolytes (Na, K), glucose and liver tests (prothrombine, alcalic phosphatase (ALP), γ-glutamil-transpeptidase (γGT) and total bilirubine) were recorded. The statistical analysis was performed by Student's t-test. Statistical significance was judged by p value less than 0,05.
In isoflurane and sevoflurane groups MAP decreased during the surgery (95-90 mmHg). There was no significant pulse rate difference between the inhalation and the intravenous groups (86-89 /min). Acid-base and blood gas values were in normal ranges in all groups and there were no significant differences. The blood glucose increased in both intravenous but not in the volatile group (4,3-5,5 mmol/L). The changes in liver function during the first 7 postoperative days: prothrombine (60-68%), ALP (380-290 U/L), γGT (52-48 U/L), bilirubine (68-59 μmol/L).
In liver diseases, the intravenous diazepam or propofol anaesthesia as well as inhaled isoflurane or sevoflurane anaesthesia are convenient. In case of patients with hyperdynamic circulatory state or impaired glucose tolerance, volatile anaesthesia is preferable. The rapid onset and quick elimination of sevoflurane make it useful at short surgical procedures. Because the renal biotransformation of sevoflurane can produce anorganic fluoride metabolites, we avoided to use the drug in case of hepatorenal dysfunction.
The changes of liver function during and after propofol, diazepam, isoflurane and sevoflurane anaesthesia depend on the types of liver disorders and the performed operations.

24,06

p53 MUTATION IN CHOLANGIOCARCINOMA IS ASSOCCIATED WITH WORSE PROGNOSIS AFTER SURGICAL RESECTION

Havlik R[1], Jiao LR[1], Sbisa E[2], Tullo A[2], Saccone C[3], Honda K[1], Ragai RR[1], Habib NA[1]

[1]Liver Surgery Section, Imperial College School of Medicine, Hammersmith Hospital, London, UK
[2]Centro di Studio sui Mitocondri e Metabolismo Energetico, Bari, Italy
[3]Dept. of Biochemistry and Molecular Biology, University of Bari, Italy

Aims: Mutations of the tumour-suppressor gene *p53* is the most common genetic defect seen in human cancers. Furthermore, the presence of *p53* mutation has been shown to be a poor prognostic indicator after resection for hepatocellular carcinoma when looked at independently from other clinicopathological factors. Its presence and significance in cholangiocarcinoma has not been fully established.

Methods: We reviewed 18 patients undergoing surgical resection for cholangiocarcinoma at The Hammersmith Hospital. DNA samples extracted from tumour and corresponding non-tumour tissue were analysed using denaturing gradient gel electrophoresis, single-strand conformation polymorphism and DNA direct sequencing to detect point mutation(s) in *p53* gene. Patient survival was analysed by the Kaplan-Meier method. Prognostic factors were calculated by both univariate and multivariate analysis using Cox proportional hazards regression model.

Results: Five out of 18 patients had *p53* mutation. Mutations were observed in exon 5 (3 times) and exon 6 (2 times). Survival analysis of these patients after surgery showed the median survival of patients with wild-type *p53* to be 23 months. In the group with *p53* mutations the median survival was 11 months. The difference is statistically significant ($p=0.045$). Statistical analysis also identified positive lymphnodes, arterial invasion, late tumour stage and positive tumour margins as carrying the worse prognosis. Tumour dimention, type of procedure and tumour differentiation were not significant prognostic indicators.

Conclusion: *p53* mutation occurs in cholangicarcinoma and is a poor prognostic indicator for survival after liver resection.

24,07

LARGE HEPATIC HEMANGIOMAS: TO TREAT OR NOT TO TREAT?

Bonzomati Domenico
Dep. of Surgery, Campus Bio-Medico, Rome

The indication of surgical treatment of hepatic hemangiomas include the presence of symptoms or the occurrence of complications. An analysis of the literature shows that the dimension of the lesion is rarely considered an indication to surgery. Nevertheless in presence of an hepatic hemangioma of exceptional dimension, surgical treatment must be considered for the increased risk of rupture and of complication. We describe the case of a 31 years old woman, referred us for the presence of diffuse abdominal pain and dysuria. The patient underwent diagnostic instrumental examination. An abdominal US showed the presence of a 42 cm right lobe hepatic hemangioma determinig huge compression on the bladder and displacement of right branch of the hepatic artery, and of the right renal artery. The patient underwent a right-lobe hepatectomy with partial inflow occlusion by Pringle Manouvre. Intra-operative blood loss consisted of 200 ml. Major and minor morbidity were absent and the patient was discharged at VI post-operative days. Following radiological examinations executed after 12 and 24 months did not show the presence disease's recurrence. The present case, shows that a so large hepatic lesion (10 times larger thabn minimal dimension used to consider en hemangioma as „giant") can determine only scarce and often aspecific symptoms. If performed in centres highly skilled in hepatic sdurgery, the romoval of the lesion (compulsory for the high risk of complicances like rupture, coagulopathy and post hepatic hypertension) is a therapeutical option without mortality and morbidity.

24.08

HEPATIC CAVERNOUS HAEMANGIOMAS -DIAGNOSTIC TOOLS AND CHOICE OF SURGICAL PROCEDURES

João Raposo; Henrique V.Dias; Jorge L.Correia, M J Queirós Medeiros.
Pulido Valente Hospital - Faculty of Medical Sciences - Lisbon - Portugal

INTRODUCTION – Hepatic haemangiomas are the most frequent benign hepatic mesenchymal tumour. We exclude the incidental small capillary haemangiomas, because we only concern about the large cavernous haemangiomas.

PATIENTS and METHODS – We have analysed a series of 15 patients operated on due to huge cavernous haemangiomas. All of them were symptomatic (spontaneous rupture - 1 case) and had more than 10 cm Ø.
All patients had clinical, laboratory , US, contrast CAT scan evaluations, and selective hepatic angiography and in some M.R.I. and scintigraphy. We have analysed the surgical procedures: haemangiomectomy - 11 cases; hepatic segmentectomy - 2 cases; right hepatectomy - 1 case; left lobectomy - 1 case . In this series there were neither complications nor mortality.

CONCLUSION – We only operated on huge and symptomatic lesions. In our series CAT contrast scan have been the best diagnostic tool. Preoperative angiography is important to define the hepatic and lesional vascular map in order to localise the nutritive vessels. The procedure of choice was haemangiomectomy, as in all of them it was possible to deal a well defined plane between the lesion and the hepatic parenchyma. Elective ligation of nutritive blood vessels makes the haemangiomectomy easier to carry out. We only perform hepatic resection for some anatomic locations and when there are diagnostic problems.
We consider haemangiomectomy a safe and reliable operation.

Dig Surg 1999; 16 (suppl 1): 77-78

HPB Egypt

25,01

PARTIAL AUXILIARY LIVER TRANSPLANTATION IN DOGS

Ahmed A. Maharan, Gamal A. Ahmed, Bahjat A. Thabit, Mohamed M. El Shafie, Hassan B. El-Badawy, Mustafa A. Hassanien and Golnar M. Fathy*
Department of Surgery and Anaesthesia
*Faculty of Medicine Assiut University

This work included 30 healthy mongrel dogs weighting between 10-25 kgs (mean 17.5 kgs). The dogs were divided into 2 main groups.
I. The first group was subjected to partial auxiliary autotransplantation. The immunological factors were behind this choice. The left lobe of liver in 5 dogs was dissected and transplanted in the right flank or pelvic regions of the same animals. The outcome of these animals was not encourging. This enforced us tho change the procedure to be homotransplantation in the second group.
II. In the second group heterotopic transplantation was studied in 25 cases as follows:

1 - Subgroup II-A: was subjected to partial auxiliary transplantation without porto-caval shunt in 10 cases.

2 - Subgroup II-B: was subjected to partial auxiliary transplantation and porto-caval shunt in the same sitting (10 cases) in order to minimize the effect of functional competition which is usually developed between the host liveer and the graft.

3 - In subgroup II-C: we started firstly by porto-caval shunt and after 3 weeks we transplanted the graft.

We can concluded that:
1. Auxiliary transplantation will be simple, safer and may be more convenient in all diseases which do not require hepatectomy.
2. Portal blood represents an absolute factor for functioning of the graft.
3. Auxiliary transplantation is more suitable as we leave the host liver in its place.
4. The auxiliary grafts from a living related donor will be more convenient after further confirmatory and complementary studies on animals.

25,02

PRIMARY CARCINOMA OF THE GALLBLADDER EXPERIENCE OF 18 CASES IN ASSIUT UNIVERSITY HOSPITALS

Mohammed M. El Shafie
Department of General Surgery, Faculty of Medicine, Assiut University

Carcinoma of gallbladder is not a rare entity. This study presents 18 cases (15 remales and 3 males) of histologically proven primary carcinoma of the gallbladder among 866 patients operated in the General Surgery Department of Assiut University Hospital for different biliary troubles during the last 4 years. In only five cases the diagnosis of gallbladder tumour was suggested preoperatively by the help of CT scan and abdominal sonography. In 83.3% of cases (15 out of 18) galistones were associated. Diagnosis wqas confirmed only by laparotomy and histopathological examination. Adenocarcinoma (77%), undifferentiated carcinoma (16%) and squamous cell carcinoma (5%) were the pathological types of the tumours. Areas of spred included liveer bed, portahepatis and caeliac lymph nodes. Distant metastasis included mesenteric lymph nodes, bones and umblicus.

Clinical presentations included pain, fever, vomiting, jaundice, dyspepsia and upper right quadrant mass. Surgical manoeuvers included laparotomy and external billiary drainage, gastrojejunostomy and wedge hepatic resection. lThe mean survival time postoperatively wa 7 months with 2 cases living for 18 and 22 months.

The best hope to improve this dismal lies in earlier cholecystectomy in patients with calcular or benign gallbladder disease.

25,03

SPECTRUM AND MANAGEMENT OF COMPLICATIONS AFTER CHOLECYSTECTOMY

Samy Osman, Mohamed K. El-Ammary
From the General Surgery Department, Sohag Faculty of Medicine, South Valley University, Egypt

Background: Death is an uncommon complication of open or laparoscopic cholecystectomy. The rapid introduc tion of laparoscopic cholecystectomy has been associated with apparently increased incidence of bile ducts injury which has provoked worldwide concern.

Patient and Method: The true incidence and mechanism of post-cholecystectomy complications wheather open or laparoscopic during the last 6 years in our hospital were studied.

Results: Open cholecystectomy was associated with biliary complications as retained stones, leakage of bile, bile duct injury Unusual lte biliary complications were retained gall bladder remnant containing stones and ampullary stenosis consequent to passatge of calculi or operative manipulation. A long cystic duct remnant has been implicated as a cause of postoperativd symptoms. Laparoscopic specifically complications were bile leakage, major bile duct injuries which was the most heralded complication and management are discussed.

Conclusion: Both open and laparoscopic cholecystectomy are highly safe and effective procedures for the treatment of patients with symptomatic gallbladder disease. Toay, adverse outcomes after open cholecystectomy are largely limited to elderly patients with co-morbid conditions and complicated biliary tract disease. Although infequent major biliary complicationsstill occur and have been slightly more common in the initial experience with laparoscopic cholecystectomy.

KARGER
Fax +41 61 306 12 34
E-Mail karger@karger.ch
www.karger.com

25,04

WHIPPLE'S PROCEDURE (PANCREATICODUODENECTOMY), MANSOURA EXPERIENCE

El-Ebidy G., Fathy O., Soltan A., Abd el-Wahab M., El-Hak N., Abu Zid M., Abu El-Enin A.
Gastroenterology Center, Mansoura University, Mansoura, Egypt

Aims: To review the experience of Gastroenterology Surgical Center in Mansoura University as regards outcomes of Whipple procedure of pancreaticodudenectomy.
Methods: Between January 1990 and August 1998, 95 consecutive patients of pancreatic head and periampullary carcinoma underwent pancreaticoduodenectomy. Main presention was obstructive jaundice in 85 patients (89%)). Mean serum bilirubin was 5.5±2 mg%. Preoperative ERCP was done in 69 patients (72.6%) as a diagnostic toal and for decompression of the obstructed biliary system as well. Preoperative abdominal CT scan revealed a resectable mass in 60 patients (63%) with vascular encasement in 9 cases. Pancreatico-duodenectomy was done using Whipple procedure with preserving in 5 cases. Pancreaticofejunostomy was done in 49 cases (51.5%) and pancreaticogastrostomy in 46 cases (48.5%).
Results: From total of 95 patients we had 61 males and 43 females with mean age of 58±11 years. The number of resections per year increased from 5 cases in 1990 to 40 resections in 1998. Histopathology revealed pancreatic head carcinoma in 62 cases (65%), ampullary carcinoma in 17 cases (18%), cholangio carcinoma of the distal third of conunon bile duct in 12 patients (13%) and duodenal tumor in 4 patients (4%). The median intraoperative blood loss was 1000cc, median units of blood transfusion was 2 and the median operativer time was 5 hours. Hospital mortality occured in 6 patients (6.3%) mostly due to pancreatic fistula. Hospital staw was 20 ± 8 days. Postoperative complication involved pancreatic fitula in 15 patients (15.8%) being mostly after pancreaticojejunostomy in early years of performance. Pancreatic fistula complicats only one case after pancreatico gastrostomy out of 46 cases (2%). All cases managed consevatively except 2 cases where total pancreatectomy was needed to control the fistula. Reoperation for bleeding pancreaticogastostomy or gastojejunostomy was done in 5 cases. Intraperiotoneal collection in the lesser sac occure in 8 cases treated with ultrasonography-guided tube drainage.
Conclusion: Pancreatico-duodenectomy could be performed safely for the malignant disorders of the pancreas and perianpullary region. The rate of complications decreases with pancreaticogastrostomy and with high volume experience.

25,05

MYOELECTRICAL ACTIVITIES OF THE STOMACH BEFORE AND AFTER LAPAROSCOPIC CHOLECYSTECTOMY

Nabil Gad El-Hak, M.D.
Gastroenterology Surgical Center, Mansoura, University
Mansoura, Egypt

The effects of chronic calcular cholecystitis and of laparoscopic cholecystectomy (LC) on gastric myoelectrical activities have not been well documented.
Aim: Was to investigate the pattern of gastric myoelectrical activities in patients having chronic calcular gall bladder disease and to evalute the effect of LC on EEG.
Methods: 46 patients (20 male, 25 female, mean age 41 years) with chronic calcular cholecystitis were included in the study. Gastric myoelectrical activities was measured using surfacce electrogastrography (EGG). The study was performed to all patients before and one year after LC. The EGG recording was made for 0.5 hour in the fasting state and 1.5 hour in the postprandial state. Power spected analysis was applied (1). The peercentage of abnormal waves (outside the range of 2.4-3.7 cycles/min) (2). The amplitudeof the gastric slow waves.
Results: EGG abnormal frequency was detected in 16 patients (34.8%) before LC (preprandial abnormatities in 12 and postprandial in 9 patients). One year following LC the EGG abnormal frequency was detected in 6 patients (13%) (4 had preprandial and 2 postprandial abnormalitics). The EGG peak power decreased after meal in 2 patients (4.4%) before LC compared to 13 patients one year after surgery.
Conclusion: This study suggested that gastric dysrhythmias decrease one year after LC but there is an increas in the percentage of patients with decreased poer peak after meal.

Dig Surg 1999; 16 (suppl 1): 79-82

Video Session

26,01

HEPATO-JEJUNAL ANASTOMOSIS IN LOOP EXCLUDED BY LAPAROSCOPY IN THE TREATMENT OF IATROGENIC LIGATURE OF THE BILE DUCT

Crema,E; Silva,AA; Ferreira,DA;Oliveira C.B.; Martins Jr, A ; Alves, J.R;.
Department of Digestive Surgery – Federal School of Medicine of Triângulo Mineiro, Uberaba – MG, Brazil.

The video shows the authors' experience in the treatment of the iatrogenic ligature of the main bile duct. Using this technique, a bile duct anastomosis (hepato-jejunal) with transmesocolic, excluded jejuno loop was performed. Five accesses were used. 10 mm (2) and 3,5 mm (3).
Case 1: A 30 year-old white female presenting with obstructive jaundice on the 18th postoperative day of laparoscopic cholecystectomy reported reported jaundice from the third postoperative day. US showed dilated intraheptic bile duct without visualization of the choledoch. The transparietohepatic cholangiography (TPHC) showed discreet dilation of the bile duct and contrast stopping by a metallic clip image in the common hepatic duct. Following the identification of the proximal stump of the bile duct and the withdrawal of the two clips iatrogenically placed in the hepatic duct. A termino-lateral hepato-jejunal with two separated stitches of 3.0 Prolene was performed, then section of the jejuno loop and latero-lateral anastomosis with exteriorization of the loop by the access of 10 mm using the linear cutting of 75 mm.
Case 2: A 23 year-old white female with obstructive jaundice on the 16th postoperative day of cholecystectomy with subscostal incision about 10 cm long reported jaundice from the second postoperative day. US showed dilation of the intrahepatic bile duct with inner echogenic region, which obstructed ... with no further acoustic shadow. TPHC showed dilation and contrast stopping at the level of the hepatic junction.Through laparoscopy it was identified ligature of the hepatic duct wiht catgut. After the longitudinal anterior opening of the bile duct, the latero-lateral anastomosis was performed with separated stitches of 3.0 Prolene. The treatment of the jejuno loop was similar to the previously described. The postoperative outcome was satisfactory and the contrasted bile duct, in the 8th postoperative day showed reduction of the lumen and good flow of contrast through the anastomosis with no fistulae. The 6-month follow-up showed no dilation of the bile duct and good drainage to the intestinal loop.
We considered that the described procedure is feasible, technically safe and should bee performed by a skillful team trained in advanced laparoscopic procedures.

26,02

LAPAROSCOPIC MANAGEMENT OF COMMON BILE DUCT CALCULI BY CHOLEDOCHOTOMY IN SELECTIVE PATIENTS.

Karaliotas C., Kouris N., Liosis A., Lanitis S.,Doukas S.,Papaevangelou E.
2nd Surgical Department and Surgical Oncology Unit.
Red Cross Hospital Athens - Greece.

The aim of study is to prove that the laparoscopic management of common bile duct stones by choledochotomy in the era of the laparoscopic cholecystectomy is a very reliable method with many benefits.
Methods: In our department from Jan.1993 to Dec 1998 we operated on 1830 patients with gallbladder stones. 1665 patients (91%) were treated laparoscopically and 165 patients (9%) by conventional open method from which 73 cases (4%) were started with laparoscopic approach and converted to open surgery. Among the total population of these patients we found out 110 cases (6%) with concomitant stones of common bile duct. From the last group we select 17 patients which were treated by laparoscopic choledochotomy. The criteria of this selection were: a) The diameter of common bile duct > 10mm. b) Failure to remove stones preoperatively after a successful endoscopic sphincterotomy, c) Failure of doing a preoperatively endoscopic sphincterotomy. The exploration was done before cholecystectomy and after laparoscopic transcystic cholangiography.Via the choledochotomy we were inserted irrigating catheters, flexible choledochoscope - 12F in diameter-, fogarty catheters for impacted stones and four wire type basket. Immediately after the clearance of common bile duct a thin T-tube was inserted and the choledochotomy was closed with 3-0 or 4-0 absorbable interrupted sutures. Two or three sutures are all that are needed for closure of the cloledochotomy. The operation is completed with cholecystectomy.
Results: We had a full clearance of common bile duct in all 17 cases. The mean postoperative hospitalization was 4 days and the patient returned back in order to remove the T-tube. We had no complication. The follow up is from 5 years to 4 months and all patients are free of symptoms.
Conclusion: We believe that the laparoscopic choledochotomy for common bile duct exploration is a safe and reliable technique in experienced hands and we have to extent the indications in such a manner that it could replace the preoperative endoscopic sphincterotomy in the most cases.

26,03

OPERATIVE TECHNIQUE OF LAPAROSCOPIC PANCREATECTOMY

Ammori BJ, Vezakis A, Davides D, Larvin M, McMahon MJ
Leeds Institute for Minimally Invasive Therapy (LIMIT), Wellcome Wing, The General Infirmary, Great George Street, Leeds LS1 3EX, UK

AIMS: To demonstrate the operative technique of laparoscopic pancreatectomy, and to discuss its limitations and future perspective.
METHODS: Between 1993 and 1998, 9 patients underwent laparoscopic distal pancreatectomy for endocrine tumours (n=4), cystadenoma (n=3), adenocarcinoma (n=1) and chronic pancreatitis (n=1).
RESULTS: Distal pancreatectomy with splenic preservation was performed in 9 patients. The ultrasonic dissectors were utilised and facilitated dissection. The splenic vessels were preserved in one patient. The procedure was converted to open pancreatectomy in two patients. The pancreas was divided with a linear stapler in 8 patients and with the harmonic scalpel in one. Pancreatic fistula developed in two patients in whom the pancreatic stump was not oversewn.
CONCLUSION: Laparoscopic pancreatectomy is a technically demanding procedure, but appears feasible and safe. Oversewing of the divided pancreatic stump may reduce the risk of pancreatic fistula.

KARGER
Fax +41 61 306 12 34
E-Mail karger@karger.ch
www.karger.com

26,04

FIBRIN SEALING IN THE PREVENTION OF PANCREATICO-JEJUNOSTOMY LEAKAGE - experimental study

M. Stoianovic. M. Jeremic, M. Stojiljkovic, Z. Cvetkovic, P. Stojanovic, D. Gmijovic, V. Savic, V. Djordjevic, V. Katic, M. Kostov
Surgical clinic, Clinical
Center Nis, Yugoslavia

Aims: The aim of this study is to affirm the protective effects of fibrin sealing on the pancreatico-jejunostomy (PJA), the highest-risqué anastomosis following pancreas head resection.
Methods: Experimental study has been performed on the mongrel dogs, divided in two groups (20 animals each): Experimental group - performed pancreas resection with end to end "dunking" PJA, protected by temporary occlusion of the pancreatic duct with fibrin sealant /Tissucol /Immuno Ag/. Control group -performed pancreas resection with PJA, without any protective procedure. The animals have been followed 5 months to study: *protective effects* of such procedure on the PJA quantified with the percent of anastomotic leakage, negative effects of such procedure on the *exocrine* pancreas secretion (amylase levels, cholecystokinin or secretin test, patohistology and electron microscopy), negative effects of such procedure on the *endocrine* pancreas function (imunohistochemical and ultrastructural examination of the Langerhans islets).
Results: PJA leakage occurred in 13.33% in control group. No dehiscence registered in experimental group (statistical significance). Biochemical, histological and EM examinations showed slight transitory elevation of amylase levels, with mild subclinical pancreatitis following pancreatic duct occlusion. Fibrin flue plug was dissolved and pancreatic juice output was reestablished into the 12 days postoperatively. Long term follow-up no showed damages of the endocrine and exocrine pancreas.
Conclusions: Pancreatic duct occlusion using fibrin glue is useful method in the prevention of pancreatico-jejunostomy leakage, without negative effects on the exocrine and endocrine pancreas.

26,05

THE DIFFICULT CHOLECYSTECTOMY

Savanis G., Velimezis G., Antoniades J., Patrikakos V., Banter A., Mitropapas G., Perrakis E.

Dept. of Surgery, Western Attica General Hospital, Athens, Greece

In the first ten years of performing the laparoscopic cholecystectomy, several situations that considered contraindications or reasons to be converted to open procedure have been reconsidered. As contraindication have been reported the following situations: previous abdominal operation, acute cholecystitis, empyema, excessive obesity, hepatic cirrhosis and cardiopulmonary disease. From these situations only the last one and the consequent inability to provide general anesthesia still remains a conraindication, unless another kind of anesthesia will be used.
Reasons to convert to open procedure were: acute cholecystitis, empyema, multiple upper ubdominal adhesions, inability to recognize the elements of trigonum cystohepaticum, biliodigestive fistula, cancer of the gallbladder, uncontrollable bleeding, injury of the bile duct, very large cystic duct and hepatic cirrhosis not previously diagnosed.
Most of these situations are no longer reason to convert to open procedure. In this video we demonstrate some borderline situations representing the so called 'difficult cholecystectomy' and how they can be overcome, based on necessary experience.

26,06

POSSIBILITIES OF NEW SURGICAL UNIT – PLASMA FLOWS – IN LIVER SURGERY

Severtsev A., Brekhov E., Mironov N., Ivanova E., Laptev V., Suslov N., Bashilov V., Tupikova E.
MED CENTRE FOR RUSSIAN GOVERNMENT (Moscow; Russia): ① United Hospital & Policlinics ("Volynsky" Hospital), ② Postgraduate & Research Centre

From 1997 liver surgeons got a new unit (plasma flows) to control bleeding on the raw liver surface, but it has some peculiarities.
Main advantages of new method of the final processing of liver tissue at the end of surgery are: A) non –contact method; B) the absence of electro hazard; C) a well – defined and more deep (then other physical methods) spongy layer of damaged liver tissue, which gives a final haemostasis on the raw liver surface; D) the highest temperature (up to 10 000 C°), which could vaporize left tumor cells and some infected and necrotic tissues.
The purpose of this video is a demonstration of new physical method possibilities in different cases of liver surgery.

Case 1: Patient with right lobotomy of the liver (secondary tumor): the use of plasma flows for final control of bleeding on the raw liver surface.
Case 2: Patient with non – resectable tumors of liver: the plasma flows unit was used to vaporize of some visible nodules.
Case 3: Patient with hydatid liver disease: non –complete pericystectomy was done. Plasma flows unit was used for final haemostasis and to destroy of left cystic tissues.
Case 4: Patient with polycystic liver disease: after some conventional maneuvers, plasma flows unit was used for complete destroy of cystic epithelium.

In all cases, all patients were discharged from hospital in good conditions and we did not have any complications connected with the use of new surgical unit.

Conclusion: A plasma flows unit is acceptable equipment for the use in liver surgery.

26,07

VIDEO ASSISTED MODALITY FOR SAFE DECOMPRESSION OF LARGE HEPATIC HYDATID CYSTS

Karaliotas C., Kouris N., Nomikou-Papaevangelou A., Tsiripidis G., Lanitis S., Chatziagelli H., Papaevangelou E.
2nd Surgical Department and Surgical Oncology Unit.
Red Cross Hospital, Athens - Greece

It is widely acceptable that the treatment of choice in liver hepatic cysts is surgical and the kind of procedure depends on the surgeon's experience, the local condition and the magnitude of the cyst. When the hydatid cyst is very large and is located more deeply and centrally into the hepatic parenchyma is obvious that a full pericystectomy is impossible and a kind of hepatectomy seems to be a very large and heavy procedure for a benign disease. So we recommend a new modality of treatment with laparoscopic approach .
Method: From Jan 1994 we developed a new therapeutic protocol for large hepatic hydatid cysts by laparoscopic approach. This method should be contemplated in those cases that are fulfilled the following criteria simultaneously: a) Solitary or double cyst, b) maximum cyst diameter more than 10cm in CT, c) overt projection point of the fibrin capsule in the front upper surface of the liver, d) possible access of the cyst from the front or lateral abdominal wall, e) pre and postoperative regimen with albendazol. These criteria were fulfilled by five patients which operated on laparoscopically, with an initial transabdominal puncture of the cyst via a wide port and decompression of the cyst with extracorporeal suction. After the decompression and partial evacuation of the cyst, scolicidal agent is injected and the cyst wash down for 4-5 minutes. The next step is a fenestration which is created onto the cyst wall and the rest fluids and daughter cysts are removed too easy with the laparoscopic suction under direct vision of the cavity of the cyst. The operation is finished with subsequently drainage of the cavity alone or with omentoplasty if it is possible.
Results: With the above method we had excellent results with one postoperative bile leakage from cyst which was treated by endoscopic sphincterotomy. The remnant cavity was disappeared in three patients after six months and in two was diminished to 3-4 cm.
Conclusion: We believe that the above therapeutic modality is safe, without spillage and contamination for treatment of large hepatic hydatid cysts.

26.08

EXTENDED RIGHT HEPATECTOMY FOR HEPATOCELLULAR CARCINOMA

Ercolani G, Mazziotti A, Grazi GL, Pierangeli F, Cescon M, Cavallari A.
Dept of Surgery and Transplantation, Sant'Orsola Hospital, University of Bologna, Bologna, Italy

Hepatocellular carcinoma (HCC) arising from not cirrhotic liver is often discovered with large size. The video shows a right hepatectomy extended to the segment 4 for a huge symptomatic HCC. Some anatomical variations are individuated: the presence of a trifurcating portal vein, a corresponding trifurcating hepatic duct and the drainage of the right hemiliver in three right hepatic veins. The right posterior and right anterior branches of the portal vein and hepatic artery are dissected and sectioned. Then, the corresponding right posterior and right anterior branches of hepatic duct are interrupted. The superior right, middle right and inferior right hepatic veins are divided. Following the umbilical portion of portal vein, the portal branches for segment 4 are tied and sectioned. This technique allowed performing the extended right hepatectomy without the need for pedicle clamping. No blood transfusion was required.

26.09

HEMANGIECTOMY : THE SURGICAL TREATMENT OF CHOICE IN THE HEPATIC CAVERNOUS HEMANGIOMA

J. Grondona, R. Bracco, A. Michetti and M. Duhalde
Centro Médico Martin Omar of San Isidro and Clinica Pueyrredón of Mar del Plata, Bounes Aires, Argentina

The cavernous hemangioma (CH), the most frequent solid benign tumor of the liver is found in 5%-7% of the autopsy series. Its incidence is higher in woman and in adults. Usually small, asymptomatic and being an unexpected finding at imaging studies. In this video, the operation of two different patients with symptomatic CH complaining pain in the upper right quadrant, is presented. The first one, was a 68 years old male patient, assessed by ultrasonography (US) that showed an hiperechoic mass of 10 cm. in diameter located in segment VII near the trunk of the right hepatic vein. Enhanced computed tomography scan (CT) confirmed the diagnosis of CH. The second case, was a 39 years old female patient. evaluated by US, CT and magnetic resonance imaging (MRI) revealed a mass of 12 cm in diameter located in segments VI and VII with the pattern of the CH. The MRI showed a close relationship between giant CH and the inferior vena cava. In both cases a surgical approach through bilateral subscostal incision and epigastric additional incision was performed. Infra-operative ultrasonography was carried out to visualize portal and hepatic veins and for delimit the CH. The ultrasound dissector is equipped with irrigation and aspiration systems and bas the advantages of fracture the parenchyma preserving the vessels and ducts where the smallest are coagulated by cautery and larger closed with metal clips or ligated with sutures. Therefore the surgical planes the CH and the hepatic parenchyma are easily found with the ultrasound dissector and the selected resections so-called hemangiectomies are carried out safely and with minimal bleeding. Argon beam coagulator and fibrin glues were used for complete the hemostasis and biliostasis. No operative complications were obseerved and the hospital-stay were of 7 and 8 days respectively.
This kind of resection therapy should accomplish complete removal of the lesion while maximizing preservation of the normal hepatic parenchyma.

26.10

IATROGENIC LESION OF THE MAIN BILE DUCT: CHOLANGIO-JEJUNOSTOMY AS DEFINITIVE TREATMENT.

G.B. Doglietto, S. Alfieri, C. Carriero, F. Pacelli.

Department of Digestive Surgery, Catholic University, Rome, Italy.

We report a clinical case of a 56-year-old male patient, referred to our unit for obstructive jaundice due to iatrogenic lesion of the main bile duct occurred during open cholecistectomy. The patient had been already treated by external biliary drainage.

The video shows the surgical treatment performed to repair the bile duct lesion.

Operative technique: *bilateral subcostal incision and adhesiolysis. Dissection of the hepatic hilum vascular and biliary elements. Intra-operative finding of tied and dissected choledocus. The proximal tract of the bile duct was resected up to the confluence after stitches and scar tissue were removed. The operation was completed with an end to side extramucosal cholangio-jejuno-stomy on a Roux-en-Y loop at the hepatic confluence.*

26.11

HEMIHEPATIC VASCULAR EXCLUSION FOR RIGHT SEGMENTECTOMIES IN CIRRHOTIC PATIENTS USING AN EXTRAGLISSONIAN ANTERIOR APPROACH TO THE PORTAL PEDICLE.

Batignani G., Passini S., Tonelli F.
Departement of Physiopathology - Unit of Surgery -
University of Florence
Viale Morgagni 85 - 50134 - Florence - ITALY

Right hepatic segmentectomies for HCC in a cirrhotic liver usually require Pringle manouver, US guided puncture of segmental pedicle with the injection of dye and/or intraglissonian preparation of segmental hepatic artery, portal vein and intraparenchimal clamping of hepatic vein. Extraglissonian isolation and intermittent clamping of the right hepatic portal pedicle for right lobe segmentectomies may present several advantages such as:

1. ischemic liver damage confined to the right lobe;
2. possible isolation "en-bloc" of the segmental pedicle which may also be injected with dye to better visualize segmental boundaries;
3. no need for dissection in the hepatoduodenal ligament;
4. less possibilities of an error in the suture of segmental artery, vein and bile duct compare to intraglissonian approach.

Moreover dissecting out the right hepatic vein(s) at its caval junction a total hepatic exclusion may be used to further reduce bleeding.
This video shows the extraglissonian anterior approach to the right portal pedicle for the resection of segment V, VI, VII and VIII in two patients, the first had segment VI resection while the second one had segment VII and VIII resection with clamping and following preservation of right hepatic vein (hemiliver vascular exclusion).
The technique used for the extraglissonian approach to the right portal pedicle differs from Professor Lounois' technique, because it was mainly accomplished from the anterior aspect of hepatic hilum using a bent clamp. We found that, using this technique, it was actually difficult to dissect out the pedicles of the posterior-superior segments (VII and VIII) whereas it was very easy to dissect the anterior ones (V and VI) but this may depends from our inexperience with this technique.
Results on post-operative liver function were instead remarkably good probably because of the ischemic injury limited to half liver with uneventfull post-operative recovery in both patients.
In conclusion we strongly reccomend to consider this approach in cirrhotic patients who has to be resect for HCC or in patients with metastasis of the right lobe far enough from the right portal pedicle. Furthermore total vascular exclusion of the right lobe may be accomplished reducing even further the blood loss.

26.12

LIVER SURGERY AND "BASKET BALL" METASTASECTOMY BY MEANS OF HIGH PRESSURE WATERJET METHOD.

F. JAKAB

Aim: It is desirable in the field of liver surgery to reduce early and late complication of blood transfusion. Vascular exclusion is generaly accepted as an effective tool of ***bloodless surgery*** Nowadays the new method in liver surgery is the ***waterjet method*** which carries the advantage of bloodless surgery also.

Method: Patients with primary and secondary liver tumors were selected for liver surgery. Earlier liver surgery has been carried out in inflow vascular exclusion. The 20' ischemic time can be repeated after 5' minutes reperfusion according to need. In this study high-pressure waterjet method has been used as a tool for surgery. After mobilisation of the liver the final plan for surgery has been set up. The resection was carried out by high pressure waterjet technique. Vessels and ducts were ligated on both side, that is on the resectional and on the remaining side. Vascular exclusion has not been applied in these interventions.

Results: At the patients included into the study there was no need for blood restoration at all, on the other hand having finished the liver surgery (segmentectomy, multisegmentectomy, ***horisontal liver resection***, basket ball metastasectomy) the resectional surface seemed to be absolutely dry.

Conclusions: The high-pressure handyjet technique does not require vascular exclusion for the bloodless liver surgery. This new procedure is suitable for delicate preparation of maior vascular structures, not mentioning that is can be easily learn and use ("See and use technique")

Dig Surg 1999; 16 (suppl 1): 83-121

P 1

IN VIVO ASSESSMENT OF HEPATIC TISSUE OXYGENATION WITH GRADED HYPOXIA

El-Desoky AA., Seifalian AM, Davidson BR
University Dept. of Surgery and Liver Transplant Unit, Royal Free and University College Medical School, London, U.K.

Aim: Hepatic tissue oxygenation has been identified as an indicator of the severity of ischaemia-reperfusion injury and has prognostic value for survival in liver transplantation. Near infrared spectroscopy (NIRS) could measure tissue oxygenation. It monitors extracellular oxygenation by measuring oxyhaemoglobin (HbO_2) and deoxyhaemoglobin (Hb). Also, it monitors intracellular oxygenation by measuring cytochrome oxidase (Cyt Ox) oxidation. We used NIRS for measuring hepatic tissue oxygenation with graded hypoxia.

Methods: New Zealand white rabbits (n= 9) underwent laparotomy for liver exposure. Heart rate, blood pressure, temperature, arterial blood pH and blood gas partial pressures were monitored during the experiment. NIRS probes were placed on the liver surface to measure continuously hepatic HbO_2, Hb and Cyt Ox changes. Graded hypoxia was achieved by stepwise reduction of fraction of inspired oxygen (FiO_2) from 15 to 4%.

Results: With all hypoxic periods there was an immediate reduction of hepatic HbO_2 with a simultaneous increase of hepatic Hb. Hepatic HbO_2 showed a positive correlation with arterial oxygen pressure (PaO_2) (r= 0.77, p< 0.001). Hepatic Hb showed a negative correlation with PaO_2 (r= -0.75, p< 0.001). Hepatic Cyt Ox started to reduce significantly from FiO_2 of 10% and showed a positive correlation with PaO_2 (r= 0.90, p< 0.001).

Conclusion: NIRS could be used to monitor the hepatic extracellular and intracellular tissue oxygenation. Cyt Ox changes could be used as an index of intracellular tissue oxygenation changes.

P 2

TISSUE ENGINEERING USING HEPATOCYTES UNDER FLOW BIOREACTOR CONDITIONS ON 3-DIMENSIONAL BIODEGRADABLE POLYMER PRIOR TO IMPLANTATION

Pollok JM[1], Török É[1], Ma PX[2], Kaufmann PM[1], Topp S[1], Kluth D[1], Rogiers X[1].
[1]Dept of Surgery, University of Hamburg, Germany;
[2]Dental School, University of Michigan, Ann Arbor, USA.

Aims: The aim of this study was to optimize the culture conditions for hepatocytes on biodegradable polymer in a flow bioreactor with respect to the cell seeding concentration and the flow rate. Our laboratory has investigated heterotopic hepatocyte transplantation on biodegradable polymer matrices as an experimental treatment for liver diseases. One of the limiting factors for clinical application so far has been survival of sufficient cell mass after transplantation. We hypothesize that in vitro conditioning of hepatocytes within polymer matrices prior to implantation may increase hepatocyte survival and function.

Methods: Highly porous poly-L-lactic acid (PLLA) discs were manufactured as to 18 mm diameter by 1 mm thickness and a pore size of 200-400 μm. Hepatocytes were isolated from adult, male Lewis rats (200-300 g) using a two-step collagenase digestion. PLLA discs were seeded with hepatocytes in a concentration of 2.5, 5, 10, 20 and 40 x 10^6 cells per ml. Seeded discs were exposed to recirculated flow of 0, 7, 15, 24, 32, 52 ml/min of supplemented William's Medium E and harvested after six days in flow culture. The number of spheroidal aggregates (SphA) was measured by phasecontrast and polarisator microscopy and H&E histology was performed. The metabolic activity of the hepatocytes was assessed by 3-[4,5-dimethylthiazol-zyl]-2,5-diphenyl tetrazolium bromide (MTT) assay.

Results: $4.4\pm1.2x10^8$ hepatocytes with a viability of 87.5±4.3% were isolated. Only under flow conditions SphA of viable hepatocytes of 50 to 200 μm in diameter were formed. The optimum cell seeding concentration was $20x10^6$ cells per ml with a speed of 52 ml/min yielding the highest ratio of SphA per polymer volume and the largest average diameter of the SphA. The different seeding concentrations had different optimal flow speed settings. Only the hepatocytes within the SphAs showed quick MTT metabolic activity, whereas single hepatocytes showed delayed metabolic activity.

Conclusions: Under flow conditions hepatocytes on a biodegradable PLLA polymer form SphA with a liver like morphology and excellent metabolic activity. These spheroids of hepatocytes may prove useful as a functional unit for tissue engineering of an in vivo liver substitute.

P 3

THE EFFECT OF LIVER BLOOD FLOW AND FUNCTION ON HEPATIC INDOCYANINE GREEN CLEARANCE IN CIRRHOSIS MEASURED DIRECTLY IN A CIRRHOTIC ANIMAL MODEL

Jiao L.R.*, El-Desoky A.A., Seifalian A.M., Habib N.*, Davidson B.R.
University Department of Surgery and Liver Transplant Unit, Royal Free Hospital School of Medicine and *Liver Surgery Section, The Hammersmith Hospital, Imperial College School of Medicine London U.K.

Aims: Direct measurement of hepatic ICG uptake and clearance by near infrared spectroscopy (NIRS) and its correlation with liveer blood flow and function.
Material and Method: Two groups of New Zealand white rabbits (m=12, control and cirrhotic) undeerwent laparotomy for liver exposure. Cirrhosis was induced by feeding animals with a high cholesterol (2%) diet for a duration of 16 weeks. Hepatic blood flow and microcirculation were measured. Hepatic ICG concentration was measured directly with NIRS in these animals. From the ICG concentration-time curve, hepatic ICG uptake ((L)m and excretion rates (B) were calculated by a non-linear least square curve fitting method.
Results: There was a significant reduction in ICG uptake rate (L) (0.30±0.13 vs. 2.04±0.42, p=0.0001) and ICG excretion rate (B) (0.007±0.009 vs. 0.227±0.096, p=0.002 in cirrhotic animals when compared with the normal controls. A significant positive correlation was demonstrated between hepatic ICG rate of uptake (L) and, hepatic blood flow and demonstrated between hepatic ICG rate of uptake (L), and, hepatic blood flow and microcirulation (r=0.81, P=0.002, r=0.92, P<0.0001 respectively). The hepatic ICG excretion rate (B) was significantly associated with the impaired liver function including bilirubin (r=-0.86, p=0.0004), AST (r=-0.81, p=0.001) and LDH (r=-0.83, p=0.0008).
Conclusion: The direct measurement of ICG uptake by NIRS reflects liver blood flow and perfusion in cirrhosis and its excretion correlates with parenchymal dysfunction. This technique has the potential for monitoring organ function during liver surgery or transplantation.

KARGER
Fax +41 61 306 12 34
E-Mail karger@karger.ch
www.karger.com

P 4

A LARGE CIRRHOTIC ANIMAL MODEL

Jiao, L.R.[1], Havlik E.[1], Seifalian A.M.[2], Li Y.[1], Davidson BR[2], Habib N.[1]

[1]Liver Surgery Section, Imperial Collegr School of Medicine, Hammersmith Hospital and [2]Hepatic Haemodynamic Laboratory, University Department of Surgery, Royal Free Hospital and School of Medicine, London, United Kingdom,

Aims: To succesfully establish an experimental model of cirrhosis in a large animal model.

Methods: Large white pigs underwent laparotomy and exposure of the liver: group 1 (n=6) were normal controls, group 2 (m=6) cirrhotic. Cirrhosis was established by ligation of common bile dict. Liver function was assessed with biochemistry liver function test once weekly following ligation of common bile duct. At 4th week, animals underwent second laparotomy for measurement of hepatic haemodynamics and blood gases. Total hepatic blood flow (THBF) was measured by a Transonic Medical Flowmeter system, hepatic gluconeogenesis, alkalisation and indocyanine green clearance (ICG) were also examined in normal and cirrhotic animals.

Results: Following ligation of common bile duct, Cirrhosis characterized by a significant increase in portal pressure (14±3 bd 8±2 mmHg, $p=0.002$, mean ± sd vs controls,) increased total hepatic blod flow (37±10 vs 25±4 ml/min/kg, $p=0.01$) and raised portal vascular resistance ($p=0.03$) was established. There was a grossly abnormal liver function test, a reduced intrahepatic glucogenesis and intrahepatic and systemic metabolic acidosis. Hepatic ICG clearance was also decreased in cirrhotic animals. Histological examination revealed features of portal bridging and regeneration of cirrhotic nodules in ligated animals.

Conclusion: Cirrhosis can be established in porcine model with ligation of common bile duct.

P 5

QUANTITATIVE DETECTION OF HEPATIC TISSUE HYPOXIA WITH NEAR INFRARED SPECTROSCOPY

Seifalian AM, El-Desoky A, Cope M, Delpy DT*, Davidson BR.*
University Department of Surgery and Liver Transplant Unit, Royal Free and University College Medical School, The Royal Free Hospital, London and *Department of Medical Physics and Bioengineering, UCL, London, UK.

Aim: Liver hypoxia occurs during liver surgery and transplantation. The aim of work was to quantify the changes in hepatic tissue oxygenation in hypoxia using Near Infrared Spectroscopy (NIRS).

Methods: Large Landrace pigs (n= 6) underwent laparotomy and liver exposure. NIRS probes were placed on the liver surface to record continuously changes in hepatic tissue oxyhaemoglobin (HbO_2), deoxyhaemoglobin (Hb) and the reduction oxidation (redox) state of cytochrome oxidase (Cyt Ox). Reduction of hepatic tissue oxygenation was achieved by reduction of inspired oxygen (FiO_2). Hepatic venous blood PO_2 measured by direct puncture of the left hepatic vein through the interlobar space between the left central lobe and the left lateral lobe. PO_2 was measured with a blood gas analyser.

Results: With stepwise reduction of FiO_2 a significant reduction of hepatic venous PO_2 from 37 to 4 mmHg. There was significant correlation between hepatic venous PO_2 measured by blood gas analyser and hepatic HbO_2 and Cyt Ox measured by NIRS
($r=-0.936$ & $r=-0.821$ respectively, $p< 0.0001$).

Conclusions: Hepatic tissue hypoxia measured by NIRS correlate well with hepatic venous PO_2 in graded hypoxia. We conclude that, NIRS could be used as a non-invasive method for monitoring hepatic tissue oxygenation.

P 6

SOLUBLE TUMOR NECROSIS FACTOR α – RECEPTOR II (sTNFα–RII) AND ACUTE PHASE PLASMA PROTEINS HAVE SIMILAR KINETICS DURING THE EXPERIMENTAL LIVER REGENERATION IN RATS

Fülöp AK, Pócsik Éva*, Karabélyos Cs, Kiss Á, Dobozy O, Falus A
Department of Genetics, Cell and Immunobiology; Semmelweis University and *National Institute of Haematology and Immunology, Budapest, Hungary

Aims: In the induction of hepatocyte proliferation during liver regeneration — at least partly — the same growth factors (cytokines: eg. IL-6, TNF-α) play crucial role as they do in the control of acute phase plasma protein (APP) gene expression. To induce and stop the hepatocyte proliferation, to avoid the excess cell growth a very fine balance of cytokines is required. In the balancing the cytokine levels the soluble cytokines receptors may take part. These soluble cytokine receptors may act as cytokine antagonists and agonists, depending on the way of action. We hypothesize that the soluble cytokine receptors play role in the cytokine control of liver regeneration. First we intended to carachterize the hepatic acute phase response (APR) during liver regeneration by the investigation of Type I (fibrinogen, α_2-macroglobulin), Type II (haptoglobin) APPs and soluble TNFα-receptors.
Methods: The liver regeneration was induced by partial hepatectomy (HPX) in laboratory rats. The levels of APPs and sTNFα-receptor I and II were measured by ELISA from blood serum/plasma and the transcription induction of APPs was revealed by Northern hybridization at different intervals after HPX.
Results: Type II APPs have similar plasma kinetics after HPX, while type I haptoglobin has a later and higher elevation in blood plasma and liver. Data of sTNFα-RII serum levels and Northern blots of APP mRNAs are also presented.
Conclusions: The regenerating liver produces APR, as the elevation of APP concentrations shows. The positive acute phase plasma proteins as the direct and indirect inhibitors of inflammation may reduce the unwanted consequences the surgical hepatectomy and liver transplantation. The folds of induction, measured from liver were smaller than detected in plasma/serum suggesting a quick secretion of produced APPs. Intrestingly the blood accumulation of haptoglobin was very late comparing with the Type II APPs. The kinetics of sTNFα-RII (p75) closely resembled to that of Type II APPs, suggesting that the same induction factors may contribute in the control of both.

P 7

Angiogenesis in hepatocarcinoma on cirrhosis evaluated by CD 34 immunohistochemistry

*L. Lupo, *G. Marzullo, *A. Gentile, G. Martines, L. Caputi, F. Aquilino, *L. Pollice, V. Memeo* - Chirurgia Gen. e Trapianto di fegato,*Anatomia Patologica, Università di Bari, Italy

Background: Angiogenesis (AG) is essential for cancer growth and has been reported as a prognostic factor in breast and colon cancer.

Aims: To evaluate the extent of AG, its correlation with cancer features and its prognostic value in patients with hepatocellular carcinoma (HCC) and cirrhosis.

Patients & Methods: AG was semi-quantitatively assessed in 35 patients (age: 63y, 32-78) with HCC (O: 6 cm, 2-10) and cirrhosis (Child A 27, B 8), subjected to liver resection, by CD 34 immunohistochemistry on paraffin embedded tissue. During follow up (median: 30 months, 6-48) 19 patients had recurrence and 13 died. Statistics: median, life-tables, c^2, log-rank test.

Results: CD 34 was variably expressed in HCC in all and in the surrounding liver in 24/35 patients. No correlation was found between CD 34 staining and cancer size and grade, presence of capsula and infiltration. Better 3-year survival was found in patients with higher CD 34 level (75 vs 35%, $p<0.05$), and earlier recurrences occurred in patients espressing CD 34 in the liver: 10/14 <12 mths vs 0/5 >12 mths, $p< 0.01$.

Conclusions: The presence of AG varied in HCC and cirrhotic liver tissue. No correlations were found between CD 34 and cancer characteristics and liver disease . Survival was correlated to CD34 level in cancer, and recurrence to CD 34 expressed in the surrounding liver.

P 8

HEPATECTOMY AND COLONIC MUCOSA:AN EXPERIMENTAL STUDY

Çoker A, Aydýn C, Atilla K, Çoker I, Huseyinov A, Özer E, Karademir S, Astarcýoðlu H, Astarcýoðlu I.
Dokuz Eylül, SSK and Ege University Hospitals, Izmir, TURKEY

It is very well known that the long term preoperative fasting for major surgery effects colonic mucosal barrier. In order to prevent mucosal damage it is essential to maintain colonocyte feeding. On the other hand, eicasonoids are the most important indicators of cell viability. Leucocyte originated Leukotriene B4 (LTB4) has a critical role in cell damage in case of inflammation. This study has been designed to assess LTB4 affects on colonic mucosa and a possible role in cell damage. Twenty seven Swiss Albino rats weighing between 110 and 230 gr have been used. Group 1 and Group 2 consist of 6 and 7 rats respectively and fasted 24 hours before surgery. Group 3 and 4, both include 7 rats, received regular diet and high caloric enteral feeding during preoperative period. Rats in Group 2 and 4 had undergone hepatic resection in size of 20% of the whole liver. Colonic mucosal biopsies and colonic mucosal perfusates are taken in all groups. LTB4 levels are measured in both samples by spesific RIA methods. Mean PNL counts are also detected in colonic biopsy specimens. Results are summarized as follows:

	Mucosa LTB4	Perfusate LTB4	Leucocyte
Grup 1	25.50	49.50	66.95
Grup 2	23.14	63.43	75.00
Grup 3	118.28	159.57	40.77
Grup 4	311.14	187.28	41.51

Tisuue levels: pg/mg tissue,
perfusate levels: pg/ml

All values in Group 1 and Group 2 are statistically different from those in Group 3 and 4. We concluded that preoperative fasting and hepatectomy stimulates inflammatory cascade in colonic mucosa. Cessation of enteral feeding caused to increase in leucocyte counts but decrease in LTB4 levels.

P 9

EXPRESSION OF THE E-CADHERIN-CATENIN CELL ADHESION COMPLEX IN HEPATOCELLULAR CARCINOMA

Syrigos K.N.[1], Karayiannakis A.J.[2], Tsioulos D.[1], Papanikolaou Sp.[2], Simatos G.[2], Papanikolaou D.[2], Riza F.[2], Karatzas G.[3]
[1]Third Department of Medicine, University of Athens, Medical School, Athens, Greece
[2]First Department of Surgery, First IKA Hospital, Athens, Greece
[3]Second Propaedeutic Department of Surgery, University of Athens, Athens, Greece

Aims: To evaluate the expression patterns and cellular localization of E-cadherin, α-, β- and γ-catenin in hepatocellular carcinoma.

Methods: The expression of E-cadherin, α-, β- and γ-catenin was investigated immunohistochemically, using the avidin-biotin immunoperoxidase technique, in 55 hepatocellular tumours and in 10 normal liver tissue samples which were used as controls.

Results: All normal liver tissue samples demonstrated membranous localization of all four molecules. On the contrary most of the tumour samples 49/55 (89%) demonstrated abnormal expression (cytoplasmic, heterogeneous or complete loss) of at least one component of the E-cadherin-catenin complex. The most commonly aberration observed was the abnormal expression of β-catenin (43/55, 78%), with 27 of tumours showing nuclear β-catenin localization.

Conclusions: Our findings suggest a regulatory function for β-catenin within the E-cadherin-catenin complex and imply a possible link between signal transduction and intercellular adhesion.

P 10

PROTECTIVE EFFECT OF EXOGENOUS COENZYME Q IN RAT LIVER EXPOSED TO ISCHEMIA-REPERFUSION

B. Nardo, F. Catena, P. Turi, G. Cavallari, M.L. Genova, E. Bonacorsi*, M. D'Aurelio*, G. Formiggini*, M. Merlo Pich*, G. Lenaz*, A. Principe, A. Mazziotti, A. Cavallari*
Clinica Chirurgica II, Dip. Biochimica*, Univ.of Bologna, Bologna ITALY

Aims: The protective antioxidant effect of CoQ_{10} was studied in a rat hepatic ischemia and reperfusion model. In rat the major quinone is CoQ_9 so CoQ_{10} represents a kind of labelling allowing to distinguish endogenous from exogenous CoQ. **Methods**: The rats were divided in group 1 (G1), i.p. injected with CoQ_{10} 1 mg /100g body weight daily and group 2 (G2) treated with the vehicle for 14 days. Thereafter hepatic left and median lobe were occluded for 90 min and reperfused for 30 min (I-R): the remaining tissue utilized as control (C) was removed together with the I-R lobes at the end of the reperfusion; blood was also collected. Antioxidant levels were determined by reverse phase HPLC. Lipid peroxidation was evaluated by determining TBARS; succinate oxidase (S-O) activity was also assayed. **Results**: Our data (expressed in pmol/mg protein) showed that the major CoQ homolog was CoQ_9 both in reduced form (G1: 96± 23 C; 80± 22 I-R; G2: 101± 44 C; 73± 39 I-R) and oxidized form (G1: 158± 54 C; 158± 9 I-R; G2: 240± 78 C; not assayed I-R). The levels of CoQ_9 were lower in I-R lobes than in C lobes in both groups. In G2 the exogenous quinone was incorporated in the liver and became largely reduced in both the I-R and C lobes, so that the total reduced quinone levels were higher in the I-R lobes of G2 than in C lobes of the G2 animals (244 *vs* 110 pmol/mg protein). The ratio CoQ*red*/(total CoQ *ox+red*) was increased in G1 (0.59 C; 0.41 I-R) in comparison with G2 (0.28 C; not assayed I-R). Administered CoQ_{10} doubled the total CoQ content in the C lobes; ischemia and reperfusion in G1 caused 1/3 decrease in the total quinone level. The ratio CoQ_9 red/ CoQ_9 ox was slightly higher in G1 indicating that CoQ_{10} could exert a sparing action. In plasma an high level of reduced CoQ_{10} was find in G1 *vs* G2 (8253±7529 *vs* 0 pmol/ml) while was only in oxidized form in both groups. Low basal levels of lipid peroxidation were found both in C and I-R lobes (min: 149±99; max 376±360 pmol/mg protein). TBARS levels increased after 24h; after 48h were lower in G1 than in G2. The S-O activity was significantly lower in I-R lobes of G2 indicating a mithochondrial damage which was overcome by CoQ_{10} administration. **Conclusions**: Exogenous CoQ_{10} administration under strong oxidative stress conditions induces a normalising effect chiefly due to its large reduction in the body.

P 11

ROLE OF NUTRITIONAL STATUS ON MITHOCONDRIAL INJURY IN A RAT MODEL OF FATTY LIVER.

B. Nardo, P. Caraceni, I. Grattagliano^, , F. Catena, P. Turi, G. Cavallari, M. Domenicali*, M. Dall'Agata*, G.L. Vendemiale^, E. Altomare^, M. Bernardi*, A. Principe, A. Mazziotti, A. Cavallari.*
Clinica Chirurgica II, Medic. Interna*, Univ. of Bologna; Medic. Interna^, Univ. of Bari. Bologna ITALY

Aims: Although fatty liver (FL) is considered a mild and reversible condition the recent finding of an high incidence of graft failure when FL are transplanted has renewed the interest on the intracellular disorders causative of or consequent to fatty liver degeneration. An imbalance of oxidants/antioxidants has been found to occur in several models of FL. The nutritional status greatly modulates the tolerance to oxidative injury in normal livers (NL), but very little is known in the setting of FL. Thus, this study aimed to compare the oxidative stress occurring in mithocondria from fed and fasted rats with FL or NL. **Methods:** FL was induced by feeding male Srague-Dawley rats a choline-deficient diet for 10 days. Histology showed a massive macrovescicolar steatosis without signs of inflammation or fibrosis. The control rats were fed a standard choe diet. Fed and 18h fasted rats with NL or FL were sacrificed to isolate liver mithocondria and to collect serum and liver samples. Mithocondria oxidative injury was assessed by measuring the organelle content of total glutahione (GSH), malondialdehayde 8MDA), protein carbonyl groups (PC), and sulphydryl protein (P-SH). Hepatic injury was assessed by serum ALT and by transmission electron microscopy (TEM). The hepatic ATP was also determined. **Results:** The parameters of oxidative stress were significantly altered ($p<0.05$) in FL compared to NL both in fed and fasted rats. Although fasting enhanced oxidative injury both in FL and NL, the greatest imbalance of oxidants/antioxidants was seen in mithocondria from FL of fasted rats. While no difference was found between the NL rats, serum ALT was higher in fasted than fed FL rats (320±87 vs 93 ±21 U/L; $p<0.01$). TEM showed injury to mithocondria only in fasted FL rats. Finally, the fasting-induced ATP fall was significant only in the FL group (0.93±0.03 vs 0.71±0.05 pmol/mg prot; $p<0.05$). **Conclusions:** These data indicate that: 1) an increased imbalance of oxidants/antioxidants occurs in mithocondria isolated from FL; 2) fasting exacerbates mithocondrial oxidative injury in both NL and FL; and 3) the extent of oxidative stress was greater in mithocondria of fasted rats with FL. The latter finding may contribute to the increased hepatic injury and the ATP decline found in this group.

P 12

Liver regeneration and cancer: what's the role of angiostatin?

Drixler TA[1], Gebbink MF[2], Ritchie ED[1], Aarsman CJ[2], Reyerkerk A[2], Voest EE[2] Borel Rinkes IH
Departments of Surgery[1] and Medical Oncology[2], University Medical Centre, Utrecht, The Netherlands.

Aims: In previous experiments we have confirmed angiostatin (AS) to exert both antiangiogenic and antitumoral effects of in mice. In this study, we examined the effects of angiostatin on *(1) liver regeneration* and *(2) tumor growth* in tumor-bearing mice subjected to 70% partial hepatectomy (PH).
Methods: AS was generated by proteolysis of human plasminogen with pancreatic elastase. Balb/c mice were used (n=3/group). Liver metastases were induced by intrasplenic injection of 10^5 C-26 cells (murine colorectal carcinoma) followed by splenectomy. In the hepatectomized group the left lateral and caudate lobes were removed (about 70%). Tumor growth was evaluated on postoperative days (POD) 7 and 14 by measuring WLW and determination of the tumor/non-tumor ratio on liver slides. Wet liver weight (WLW) and bromodeoxyuridine labeling index (L.I.) were used as parameters for liver regeneration. Mice were treated by continuous (Alzet® pump; sc) administration of AS for up to 14 days to reach a daily dose of 100 mg/kg.
Results: *(1) Effect of angiostatin on liver regeneration.* WLW of control remnant livers increased rapidly after 70% PH and was restored within 7-10 days. L.I. increased from 0.24% (POD_0) to a maximum of 27.3% at POD_2, and decreased thereafter to normalize on POD_7 (0.34%). Mice treated with AS showed a delay in regeneration. L.I. of remnant livers of AS treated mice was still elevated (6.54%) on POD_7, and normal (0.29%) on POD_{14}. In control animals respective WLW values (grams±SD) were 0.43±0.06 (POD_0), 1.2±0.02 (POD_7), and 1.33±0.09 (POD_{14}). In AS-treated animals the WLW were 0.43±0.06 (POD_0), 0.8±0.09 (POD_7), and 1.1±0.13 (POD_{14})($p<0.01$). *(2) Effect of angiostatin on tumor growth in a regenerating liver.* In control mice (tumor-bearing mice followed by 70% PH) WLW increased as a result of tumor growth (grams±SD): POD_0=0.43±0.06; POD_7=4.59±0.49; POD_{14}=5.73±0.74. AS treatment inhibited this phenomenon: POD_0=0.43±0.06; POD_7=2.6±0.16; POD_{14}=3.17±0.44.
Conclusion: In this study, we have demonstrated that angiostatin delays liver regeneration. Furthermore, angiostatin inhibits enhanced tumor growth in regenerating liver. From a clinical point of view these observations suggest that AS might play a role as adjuvant therapy in patients subjected to resection of liver metastases.

P 13

EXPRESSION OF HEAT SHOCK PROTEIN 70 (HSP70) AFTER LASER THERMOTHERAPY OF AN ADENOCARCINOMA TRANSPLANTED INTO RAT LIVER

Tranberg K-G, Ivarsson K, Bruun A, Stenram U
Departments of Surgery, Ophtalmology and Pathology, University of Lund, Sweden

Aim: Heat shock proteins (HSPs) are thought to play a role in the protection of cell structure and to act as chaperones for intracellular transport of peptides. HSP70 is present in tumour cells and may be involved in tumour antigen presentation. It is also involved in thermotolerance and drug resistance. The aim of this study was to find out if interstitial laser thermotherapy (ILT) induces changes of HSP70 in tumour cells.

Method: Experiments were performed in Wistar rats with a dimethyl-hydrazine-induced colonic adenocarcinoma implanted into the left lateral lobe of the liver. 8 days after implantation rats were randomised into three groups: a) ILT at a steady-state temperature of 43°C, 3 mm from the tumour margin, for 30 min, b) sham ILT, and c) no treatment. The thermotherapy system consisted of an Nd:YAG laser and a temperature feedback circuit including an automatic thermometry system and thermistor probes. Rats were sacrificed 5, 10 or 15 h after the end of treatment. HSP70 was determined by an immunohisto-chemical technique.

Results: Following ILT there was an increased expression of HSP70 in the cytoplasm of the tumour cells as compared to tumours undergoing sham ILT or no treatment. The cytoplasmatic concentration of HSP70 was increased already at 5 h after ILT and remained elevated at 10 and 15 h after treatment.

Conclusion: This study showed that ILT induces an early rise of cyto-plasmatic HSP70 in an adenocarcinoma transplanted into rat liver. The possible antigen-presenting role of HSP70 should be explored in further studies.

P 14

PHYSICAL AND PHARMACOLOGICAL INTRAOPERATIVE METHODS FOR THE FINAL HAEMOSTASIS ON THE RAW LIVER SURFACE

Severtsev A., Mironov N., Brekhov E. Ivanova E., Repin I., Merzljakova E., Gaidukova N., Barinov V., Bashilov V., Gribunov Yu., Tupikova E.
MED CENTRE FOR RUSSIAN GOVERNMENT(Moscow, Russia): ① "Volynsky" Hospital; ② Postgraduate & Research Centre (Dept. of Surgery); ③ Central Clinical Hospital

The serious problem of each liver resection is the parenchimatous bleeding and the covering of the raw liver surface at the end of surgery. There are many intraoperative methods for these purposes. All of them could be divided in to chemical (pharmaceutical) and physical methods. From January 1994 till December 1998 we studied the combination of the best and most effective method for the solution of this problem of liver surgery. 142 patients have been treated surgically for this period. During the surgery the haemostasis (intensity; volume, square, stability, time for achievement, additional efforts, subjective impression, postop complications, etc.) was calculated for physical methods (spray-coagulation, CO2-laser, Nd: YAG-laser, argon beam coagulator, plasma flows, US- coagulator) and chemical- pharmaceutical products (collagen fleece, avitene, Surgicel, fibrin glue, gelatin, fibrin glue with collagen fleece) and combinations of these two main methods. Because of uncomparisonable results 56 patients were rejected from the study (final number: 86). All calculated parameters were scored, and the final result was calculated for each method separately and for some combinations too.
Results: In the group of physical methods the best single method was the use of plasma flows. Unfortunately this method had some limits and comments. In the group of chemical methods the maximal scores had fibrin glue and fibrin glue with collagen fleece. The best combination was the double combination: argon beam coagulator (1) and manufactured fibrin glue with collagen fleece (2), but the same score was for triple combination: plasma flows (1) with clear fibrin glue (2) and added in some place collagen fleece (3). Conclusion: The use of five main components of physical and pharmaceutical methods (argon beam coagulator, plasma flows, collagen fleece, fibrin glue, fbrin glue with collagen fleece) could give the best finish of liver resection.

P 15

EXPRESSION OF METALLOTHIONEIN IN THE LIVER AFTER 70% PARTIAL HEPATECTOMY IN RATS.

Theocharis SE, Skaltsas S, Spiliopoulou C, Margeli AP, Koutselinis A.
Department of Forensic Medicine and Toxicology, University of Athens, Medical School, Athens, Greece.

Aims: Metallothioneins (MTs), a set of ubiquitous low molecular weight proteins, are mainly implicated in metal ion detoxification. In the present study, we investigated the expression of hepatic MT during hepatocyte regeneration induced after 70% partial hepatectomy (PH) in rats.
Methods: Male Wistar rats (180-220 g) were subjected to 70% PH and sacrificed at 0, 4, 8, 12, 16, 20, 24, 28, 36, 48, 60 and 72 h after PH. The rate of tritiated thymidine incorporation into hepatic DNA, the enzymatic activity of thymidine kinase in liver tissue and the assessment of mitotic index in hepatocytes, were used as indices of regeneration. Serum and liver tissue Zinc (Zn) levels were also measured by Atomic Absorption Spectro-photometry. MT expression in the liver tissue was detected immunohistochemically.
Results: Tritiated thymidine incorporation into hepatic DNA, hepatic thymidine kinase activity and mitotic index exhibited marked oscillations after 70% PH appearing peaks at 24 and 28 h post-hepatectomy. MT expression became prominent as early as 12 h after PH in the nuclei of hepatocytes. At the time intervals of 20-28 h post-hepatectomy, intense cytoplasmic and nuclear MT expression was noted in all hepatocytes. Liver MT expression was positively correlated to liver tissue Zn content, while negatively to serum Zn levels.
Conclusions: Induction of MT expression was observed in rat liver after 70% PH. The intense expression of MT coincides to the time of maximum hepatocellular proliferation. Our findings also suggest that MT expression correlated with liver tissue Zn content, participating in the accumulation of this metal, involved to DNA replication in the liver.

P 16

THE USAGE OF CRIOPRESERVED BIOLOGICAL MEDICINES IN TBE TREATMENT OF OBTURATION JAUNDICE.

V.I.Mamchich, N.P.Subbota, A.B.Kebkalo, V.I.Palamarchuck. Kiev, Kharkov; Ukraine.

Although there is some progress in modern hepatology there is still an increasing tendency for liver related ailments. The goal of this investigation is to study the efficacy of the use of hemoperfusion through cryopreserved xeuohepatocytes (CX) and fragment samples of the spleen (FS) of patients suffering from mechanical jaundice, the usage of these biological medicines in experimentation as a prevention of the development of acute liver insufficiency in the post operation period.

Three hundred and fifly male white rats, of Wistar breed were used as the objects of investigation during the experimental portion of the project.For the study of the influence of detoxication and the biostimulation e~ect the medicines used in these experiments in the case of experimental mechanical jaundice the laboratory samples, the rats were divided into three groups:
I.Control group rats with mechanical jaundice without treatment. POSter 2.Control group rats with mechanical jaundice was treated surgically. 3.Samples which were operated upon and then injected with CX. 4.Samples which were operated upon and then injected with CX and FS.
Patients with mechanical jaundice were divided into the following groups: I.Patients which were prepared by standard presurgical preparations and then were operated on (control group).2.Patients who were given hemoperfusion through CX in the post operationperiod 3.Patients who were given hemoperfusion through CX and FS in the post operation period.Each group contained 12 to 21 patients.For judging the dynamic progress of biochemical indices (after 24 hours, 72 hours, 5 and 7 days) in the experimental mechanical jaundice, the following parameters were examined in blood samples: bilirubin, alanineaminotransferase, aspartateaminotransferase, cholesterol, malondialdehyde, dien-conjugates, catalaza, quantity of protein and fats; in the liver: malondialdehyde, glutation, superoxidedismutase; in bile: bile acids, cholesterol; morphological changes in the liver as well as parameters of immunity: quantity of phagocytosis, compliment, circulating immune complex. In clinical conditions, judging the efficacy of methods used were done lry clinical biochemical and immunological results.In analysis of the materials presented we draw the following conclusion: 1.Cryopreserved xenohepatocytes and their combination with spleen fragments have expressed anticytolytical, antioxidant and membrane stabilizing effects. 2.Usage of these medicines does not have damaging effects on organs and body systems.3.By the majority of the parameters, usage of cryopreserved xenohepatocytes and spleen fragments is more effective therapeutically than xenohepaticiti alone. 4.Inereased positive resulis of surgeries when preventative acute livernsufficiency in the post operation period have been done by inereasing the detoxicarion function of the liver.

P 17

RISK FACTORS OF VARICEAL BLEEDING IN PATIENTS WITH ADVANCED LIVER CIRRHOSIS

Boulanov K.I.
Department of Liver Surgery & Portal Hypertension
Institute of Clinical & Experimental Surgery, Kiev, Ukraine

Aims: to identify significant prognostic factors for variceal bleeding in patients with advanced liver cirrhosis and to determine an index of risk for first bleeding episode.
Methods: 136 cirrhotic patients (57 women and 79 men, aged 15-67) with histologically proven diagnosis and complications of portal hypertension were studied. According to Child-Pugh criteria, 100 patients were class B and 36 - class C. Twenty-four variables, and among them, general, clinical, haemodynamic and biochemical data, were selected at the entry. The identification of risk factors of variceal bleeding was performed by means of multivariate analysis. Intervariables associations were estimated by multicollinear criteria. Variables showing a significant association with variceal bleeding were analysed further with regression model. To identify groups of high and low risk prognostic coefficients (PC) were calculated using consequent heterogeneous procedure. Three risk groups were classified within PC values interval from -120 to 70: low (-120 to -60), medium (-59,9 to 0) and high (0,1 to 70). Cumulative scoring above 0 indicates the patient who would eventually bleed from varices.
Results: all studied variables taken together determinate hazard of variceal bleeding in 61,2% of cases (R=0,78). Regression model was adequate with the probability >95%. Association with variceal bleeding showed 7 independent variables. Most significant PC values were the following: oesophageal varices ?5 mm in diameter (49,74), prothrombine index <60% (42,42), serum albumin level <30g/l (29,87), clinical signs of encephalopathy (11,07), severe secondary hypersplenism (6,95), refractory ascites (6,90), portal perfusion grade IV (5,29).
Conclusions: presence of large varices along with deterioration in liver function indicates increasing risk of variceal bleeding in patients with advanced liver cirrhosis and make prophylactic treatment reasonable.

P 18

PERCUTANEOUS SCLEROTHERAPY (PS) OF SIMPLE LIVER CYSTS (SLC)

V.N.Polysalov, D.A.Granov, K.V.Prozorovskij, N.V.Oleshchuk
St.Petersburg Research Institute of Roentgenology, Russia

Purpose. Optimization of treatment modalities for SLC.
Materials and methods. Between 1988 and 1998, 49 patients (9 men and 40 women aged 20-72 years) with SLC were treated at our institution. Of them, 23 patients with asymptomatic cysts with the diameter < 4 cm received only clinical and US observation without any active treatment. The remaining 26 patients had symptomatic diseases. Solitary SCL was in 11 and multiple in 15 patients including two with polycystosis. The size of SCL was 4-5 cm in 16 patients, 5-10 cm in 9 patients. The remaining patient had SLC of 13 cm diameter.
In cyst of <5 cm diameter, single session of PS was used. In multiple SLC, successive PS of the largest cysts was performed. In SLC of >5 cm diameter, PS with following drainage of the cyst during 5-20 days was utilized. The one patient with polycystic liver disease occupying more that 80% of the liver and chronic hepatic failure underwent liver transplantation.
Results. In cyst of <5 cm diameter, single session of PS was enough in 13 of 16 patients, the three other patients were treated by repeated PS in 2-3 mo interval. In multiple SLC, good symptomatic effect with was noted in all patients and was followed by obliteration of the treated cysts. In SLC of >5 cm diameter, complete obliteration of the cystic cavity was achieved in 6 and significant decrease with small asymptomatic cavity in 3, the remaining patient was successfully treated with repeated PS. The patient underwent liver transplantation is well in 6 mo.
Conclusion. Patients with asymptomatic SLC of <4 cm diameter need no active treatment. Symptomatic SLC of <5 cm diameter should be treated by single PS, while in SLC of >5 cm diameter, combination of PS and drainage is effective. PS in polycystic liver disease dives a good symptomatic improvement. When the disease is advanced and complicated by liver insufficiency, the possibility of liver transplantation should be considered.

P 19

NEUROENDOCRINE TUMORS METASTATIC TO THE LIVER (NTML): ROLE OF TRANSCATHETER TREATMENT.

A.A.Polykarpov, P.G.Tarazov, D.A.Granov, A.A.Zeadeh
Research Institute of Roentgenology & Radiation Therapy, St.Petersburg, Russia

Aim: To evaluate effectiveness of transcathter arterial chemoembolization (TACE) in the treatment of pts with NTML.

Methods: Between 1987 and 1998, 16 pts with NTLM received TACE (12 pts with carcinoid liver metastases, 3 – metastases of suprarenal tumors and 1 – malignant insulinoma). All pts underwent occlusion of the hepatic artery using 30-80 mg Doxorubicin + 10 ml Lipiodol + Gelfoam and/or Ivalon. 40 embolization was perfomed 1 to 3 times yearly (mean – 2.5 TACE in each pts).

Results: Regression of the neuroendocrine symptoms were seen on 13/16 pts (81%) andlasted for during 6–60(mean 11) mo after the first embolization. At present, 5 pts are alive during 6-127 (mean 66.4±45.6) mo without neuroendocrine symptoms. Mean survival calculated for pts who died was 23.2 ± 14.8 mo.

Conclusion: TACE is effective transcatheter palliation for symptomatic NTLM.

P 20

"Ukrain" in Treatment of the Fatty Liver in Chronic Active Alcoholic Patients.

Zemskova M.V.(1), Zemskov S.V.(2)

1) Kiev Research Center Hepatopancreatobiliary Surgery,
2) Bogomolets National Medical University, Kiev, Ukraine.

Aims: The aim was to study the efficacy of "Ukrain" in treatment of the fatty liver in chronic active alcoholic patients. Compound"Ukrain" is a semisynthetic derivative of thiophosphoric acid and alkaloids isolated from Chelidonium majus L. Its immunomodulating and antiblastic properties are widely described in literature of recent 5 years.
Methods: A double-blind randomized multicenter trial involving 50 chronic active alcoholic patients diagnosed with fatty liver by clinical, biochemical and ultrasonographic criteria was performed. For 1 month 25 patients were treated intrsavenously with 10 mg of "Ukrain" per day and 25 patients obtained placebo. Patients were clinically and biochemically examined every weak. Ultrasonography was performed before and after treatment.
Results: At the end of the study the positive changes were observed in patients treated with "Ukrain", in whom significant changes in serum levels of bilirubin, aminotransferases were already observed after 3 weeks of treatment, and normalization of these parameters was observed at the end. After treatment the percentage of patients with ultrasonographic signs of steatosis was significantly lower in the "Ukrain" group (20%) then in the placebo (80%).
Conclusion: In patients with alcoholic fatty liver "Ukrain" normalized liver function tests and improves ultrasonographic picture. "Ukrain" could be useful of the early stage of alcoholic liver disease.

P 21

Abnormalities of carbohydrate metabolism and immune parameters in patients with hepatitis C and alcohol -related chronic liver disease

M.Pusztay[1], E.Nemesánszky[1], A.Csepregi[1], M.Horányi[2]
[1]Departm. of Gastroenterology and Medicine, Natl.Inst.Rheumatology.
[2]Natl.Inst.Haematology and Immunology, Budapest, Hungary

Background: Hepatitis C virus (HCV) is known to induce a wide variety of extrahepatic syndromes believed to be immune-mediated. Accumulating data support the assumption that diabetes mellitus is one of the extrahepatic manifestations of autoimmun features of virus-induced liver diseases.
Patients and methods: The prevalence of abnormalities of CH metabolism of 94 patients with chronic HCV-induced liver disease (77 CAH, 17 cirrhosis) as well as 100 patients with alcohol-related chronic liver damage (42 steato-hepatitis, 58 cirrhosis) was evaluated.
Thirty two cases from the HCV-CAH group were given interferon-alpha (Intron A or Roferon A in a dose of 3-6 MU TIW) for 12 months.
Of the 32 patients 3 were diabetic (NIDDM) and one had impaired glucose tolerance (IGT) before the interferon treatment. Normal CH metabolism was found in 28 patients.
Immune parameters were detected in 28 patients from the interferon group before and after the treatment. In 17 cases were measured positiv immune parameters (gamma latex, ANF, anti-microsomal antibody, anti- thyreoglobulin antibody) and 6 patients were cryoglobulin positiv before the interferon therapy.
Results: Disorders of CH metabolism was found in 42% of HCV-induced CAH and cirrhosis, whereas only in 25% of alcohol-related chronic liver disease. ($p<0.01$). IGT was proved in 28% of HCV-CAH and cirrhosis, but only 9% in alcohol-related chronic liver diseases ($p<0.01$) Manifested DM was seen in 20% of patients in the first group and 16% of individuals in the second group.
After the end of 12 months interferon therapy one diabetic patient's CH metabolism did not change. Deterioration of CH metabolism was observed in 2 diabetic patients. One patient's IGT turned to a manifested diabetes mellitus. Out of the 28 patients with normal CH metabolism 9 developed IGT.
Cryoglobulin could not be detected after the interferon treatment, and only in 8 cases were found positiv immune parameters. Improvement of immune parameters were independent of virus response.
Conclusions: Presented data suggest that disorders of CH metabolism are more frequent among individuals suffering from HCV-induced chronic liver diseases than in patients with alcohol-related ones. Interferon therapy occasionally has deterious effect on the CH metabolism, but it seems to be reversible impact. Immune parameters and cryoglobulinaemia can improve due to interferon treatment even though the virus could not be eliminated.

P 22

ETIOLOGICAL FACTORS AND TREATMENT OF HEPATIC ABSCESS

Yettimis E, Kalokerinos E, Barsamidakis N, Kourcounakis N, Karagiannis A, Polyzoes C, Dahambre S, Melayes Z, Polymeropoulos Th
1st Surgical Dep., Athen's General Hospital " G Gennimatas"
Athen's, GREECE

The diagnose of hepatic abscess is relative easy but the identification of the underlying cause may in many cases be obscure. The treatment also of these is directed not only to simple drainage of the abscess but to treat the underlying disease. In this work we present our experience of the past 10 years in the treatment of this surgical disease. We had the chance to treat 37 patients (male:58,5% and Female:43,2%) with a mean age of about 60 years. The abscess was single in most cases (right lobe :32, left lobe:3 and multiple :2). The patients had diabetes mellitus in 43,2% of the cases and also hypertension and cardiac disease (19%), pulmonary disease (13,5) and renal insufficiency :1pt. The bile ducts had the major underlying disease : choledochoduodenostomy (11pts), Cholopeptic fistula (7pts), Choledocholithiasis (6pts), Previous CBD operation (5 pts). In one pt there was a Klatskin tumor and in other 3 pts the etiology was obscure ('cryptogenic"). The most common stain from the abscess was E. Coli which was found in 43% cases. The percutaneous drainage failed to treat 3 from the 5 that underwent this procedure and were subsequently treated with laparotomy. Laparotomy was also performed in other 32 pts . the drainage of the abscess was completed with CBD drainage in 31 cases, simple cholecystectomy in 3 pts and cholecystectomy + CBD drainage in a patient. Morbidity was 16% and mortality 0%. Conclusions: (a)The main etiological factors for hepatic abscesses are CBD stone and incomplete bile drainage due to previous CBD operation or cholepeptic fistula . (b) Diabetes mellitus is a common systematic disease that is complicated be biliary sepsis and hepatic abscess formation. (c) The abscess drainage needs further surgical treatment of the coexisting disease to allow free flow of bile to duodenum either by a T-tube or a large choledochopeptic anastomosis

P 23

CHOLECYSTO-JEJUNOSTOMY AS A SUBSTITUTE FOR CHOLECYSTECTOMY IN PORTAL VENOUS THROMBOSIS

PENTEADO S, MACHADO MCC, JUKEMURA J, CUNHA JEM , MONTAGNINI AL.
Hospital das Clínicas . Universidade de S.Paulo . Brazil.

Mortality rates related to cholecystectomy are very low nowadays. Postoperative deaths of elective procedure are related to patients with portal hypertension, mainly in those with portal venous thrombosis . In these , bleeding from dissected is difficult to control and contributes to aggravating coagulation disorders , surgical infection and other post-operative complications. In order to avoid dissection a different surgical strategy can be the removal of the stones and construction of a cholecystojejunostomy.
AIM To study the safety and effectiveness of cholecystojejunostomy in the treatment of symptomatic gallbladder stones in patients with portal hypertension .
METHOD : Three patients complaining of biliary colic with associated portal hypertension due to portal thrombosis and preserved liver function were submitted to open surgery . Stones were removed by opening a 2 cm incision in gallbladder fundus , this opening was anastomosed to proximal jejunum , in an omega loop (Braun fashion) . All the sutures were made by hand with absorbable material . Bleeding was monitored by hematocrit determination.
RESULTS: Surgical procedure was uneventful , none patient required blood transfusion.
Biliary leak was not observed . Pre and post operative hematocrit deteminations showed no difference. Patients were discharged from day 5 to 7. They are being followed up for 6 mo to 1 year, without biliary related problems.
CONCLUSION : Cholecystojejunostomy is a safe procedure and can be used as an effective procedure for the treatment of symptomatic gallbadder stones in patients with associated portal thrombosis.

P 24

ENDOSCOPIC LIGATION OF ESOPHAGEAL BLEEDING VARICES PREVIOUSLY TREATED BY ENDOSCOPIC SCLEROTERAPY.

Caputi Iambrenghi O., Pannarale O., Scardigno A., Simone M., Verzillo F., Memeo V..
3rd Division of General Surgery - University of Bari - ITALY

Background and aims
Endoscopic variceal ligation (EVL) is widely used to treat esophageal varices (EV), and has been adopted in recent years to substitute for endoscopic injection sclerotherapy (EIS) in managing bleeding esophageal varices.
Most controlled studies, comparing EVL with EIS, favoured EVL in terms of sessions required to achieve variceal obliteration, rebleeding rate and complication rate.
In this study the results of EVL in patients with recurrent bleeding varices, previously treated with EIS, are reported.

Patients and methods
Twenty-one consecutive pts, previously treated by EIS for variceal bleeding who experienced recurrent haemorrage from F3 EV , were enrolled for the study from January 1997 to July 1998. EVL has been carried out with a multiple ligating device (*Saeed Six-Shooter, Wilson-Cook*). All pts were treated within 24 hrs from the bleeding episode and 7 (33%) of them in emergency.

Results
Primary success rate (bleeding stopped for 72 hours) was 100% and all patients received further treatment (median 3: range 2-5) at intervals ranging from 10 days to 8 weeks, with the long-term goal of variceal eradication or a marked reduction of bleeding risk signs.
There were no major acute complications; only one patient experienced a minor bleeding recurrence one week after the first session.
Median follow-up was 6 months (3-10). In all pts a marked reduction of variceal size was achieved (18 pts F1 and 3 pts F2) and no patient rebled during the follow-up period.

Conclusions
It's concluded from this non-randomized experience that EVL allows an adequate lenght of bleeding free interval and therefore should be the choice-treatment in those patients with enlarged varices, in whom EIS failed. Further studies with longer period of follow-up are required.

P 25

HEPATIC VENO-OCCLUSIVE DISEASE CAUSED BY ORAL CONTRACEPTIVES

Borka K., Illyés G., Fischer M.*
2nd Department of Pathology, 1st Department of Medicine*, Semmelweis University of Medicine, Budapest, Hungary

Aims: Veno-occlusive disease (VOD) is characterized by fibrous occlusion of small hepatic veins with secondary hepatic congestion. Human toxicity is mainly due to ingestion of pyrrolizidine alkaloids of herbal teas or occurs in epidemics caused by contaminated grain. VOD is also reported as a common complication of hepatic radiation and intensive chemotherapy preceding bone marrow transplantation. Budd-Chiari syndrome is a well known complication of oral contraceptives, but simultaneous or isolated small hepatic vein occlusion are rare findings.
Methods: A review of autopsy records of 2nd Department of Pathology revealed two cases of VOD secondary to oral contraceptive intake. The clinical findings and histopathology correlations were analyzed in those cases.
Results: Oral contraceptive Marvelon was used for more than 5 years in both cases. One patient died in stroke caused by arterial thrombosis. She developed hepatomegaly and laboratory sings of slight liver function alterations shortly before death. The other patient, after having had an uncomplicated pregnancy, continued to take the contraceptive pills, and developed a Budd-Chiari syndrome, but hepatic vein thrombosis was not identified. She died in hepatic failure 6 month later. On histology hepatic vein fibrotic occlusions starting from the central veins were the main alterations in both cases. Secondary centrolobular congestion and necrosis, subacute atrophy and nodular regeneration were also found.
Conclusions: Oral contraceptives may cause progressive hepatic veno-occlusive disease, which could be fatal, or is associated to other concurrent vascular complications.

P 26

PATHOLOGY OF LIVER INVOLVEMENT IN NON-HODGKIN'S LYMPHOMAS

Markovic M., Basic H., Nikolic D.,Lazarevic V.
Clinic of oncology, Nis, Yugoslavia

Aims: We investigated liver tissue from cases Non-Hodgkin's Lymphomas (NHL) with aim of determining incidence and pattern of liver involvement in malignant lymphomas.

Methods: The seven autopsy cases of NHL were investigated. The liver tissue was fixed in formalin, embedded in paraffin and stained with hematoxylin and eosin. Sections were also immunostained by APAAP method with following antibodies: L26 (CD 20), 4KB5 (CD 45 RA), UCHLA (CD 45 RO), OPD4 (CD 45 RO). The topographic distribution of the infiltration was classified according to whether it involved the portal triads, sinusoids or formed tumour nodules.

Results: The neoplastic infiltration of liver was conformed in five cases, the portal triads were predominantly involved. Greater degrees of infiltration were associated with hepatomegaly. Nodular infiltration was presents in two cases of high-grade NHL. Subtyping into B cell and T cell lymphomas was possible in all cases.

Conclusions: In our investigation of autopsy cases, neoplastic infiltration's of portal triads were presents predominantly, nodular destructive infiltration also was presents. Immunohistochemical investigations are necessary to determinate whether the infiltrates of liver are reactive or neoplastic.

P 27

THE SURGICAL TREATMENT OF THE HEPATIC HYDATID CYST IN SURGICAL CLINIC No. III. TG.-MURES

Bara T., Bancu S., Esianu M., Zamfir D., Butilca F., Marian D., Borz C., Jimboreanu O., Butiurca A., Danieal Frandes
Surgical Clinic No. III., TG.-Mures, Romania

Aims: We discuss 23 hepatic hidatid cysts (HHC) treated in our clinic between 1 Oct. 1996 (when the clinic was founded) and 31 Dec. 1998. The surgical treatment of HHC is difficult to codify but there are some rules to follow: 1. isolation of the peritoneal cavity to prevent innoculation when the cysts are fertile. 2. parasitic inactivation. 3. cystotomy with extraction of proliger membrane and daughter vesicle. 4. treatment of the residual cavity. 5. the management of the biliary complications.

Methods: The distribution of cysts of our 23 cases was: 14 in the right lobe, 7 in the left lobe and 2 in both lobes, the cysts were superficial in 16 cases and profound in 7 cases. The surgical treatment was: partial pericystectomy with flatten-12 cases, partial pericystectomy with closure (3 cases), closure with drainage (3 cases) and omental-patch (1 cases), 'ideal' cystectomy (in fact atipical liver resection-4 cases, associated simple cholecystectomy-5 cases, cholecystectomy with the drainage of the common bile duct-7 cases.

Results: In 16 superficial cysts we perform 'ideal' cystectomy or partial pericystectomy with flatten and the medium hospitalization time was 7 days. In profound cysts the management of residual cavity is more difficult to treat: we perform suture of the biliary leaks with and closure the cavity (3 cases), omental patch (1 cases) or closure with drainage of the cavity (3 cases) and the medium hospitalisation time was 16 days. We associate simple cholecystectomy for tactical reason or in case of gllstone. In other cases along with cholecystectomy we perform drainage of common bile duct.

Conclusions: 1. The hidatid cyst is parasitose with a main localisation on the liver. 2. The surgical treatment depend on the biliary three involvement and how deep is located the cyst. The medium hospitalisation time was 9,7 days without major complications and/or mortality we haven't mortality or major complications.

P 28

WAS IT A SIMPLE CYST OR A LETHAL LESION? AN UNUSUAL PRESENTATION OF PELIOSIS HEPATIS.

Karademir S, Astarcıoğlu H, Sağol H, Ak D, Çoker A, Astarcıoğlu İ.
Dokuz Eylül University Hospital,Izmir, TURKEY

Peliosis hepatis is a rare and highly lethal liver lesion in which numerous blood-filled cavities or cystic spaces are dispersed throughout the hepatic parenchyma. The cause is unknown, although the condition is associated with several disease states and medications. Here, we report an unusual case of fatal peliosis of the liver in a 43-year-old man who had been previously operated (6 mon.ago) with the clinical diagnosis of hydatid cyst of the liver. However, the lesion (16x14cm) was found to be a septated cyst filled with clear fluid. The cyst was unroofed and biopsy from the cyst was pathologically interpreted as a simple cyst. Five months later, the patient was readmitted with a big cystic lesion almost occupying the whole right liver lobe (23x18x13cm). His physical examination was significant for shortness of breath and right pleural effusion and huge palpable mass on right upper abdomen. Right hepatectomy was planned. In surgery, mobilization of the right liver lobe was so difficult due to dense adhesions. During dissection blood filled cysts were ruptured. Without any control on suprahepatic IVC, Pringle manœuvre alone could not prevent massive blood loss and subsequent transfusions. Following a stormy postoperative course, the patient died 3 days after operation with multiorgan failure. On pathologic examination, multicystic blood filled lesion measuring 18x15x10 cm with cysts ranging between 0.5 and 4 cms. On microscopic examination, the hepatic parenchyma was replaced with multiple cystic cavities filled with erythrocytes and lined by flattened endothelium like cells in some areas. The lesion was diagnosed as peliosis hepatis. Here, we aimed to present an unusual manifestation of lethal peliosis hepatis.

P 29

SUCCESSFUL REVASCULARIZATION OF THE LATE HEPATIC ARTERIAL THROMBOSIS BY INTERPOSITIONAL SAPHENOUS VEIN GRAFT IN LIVING RELATED LIVER TRANSPLANTATION.

Astarcıoğlu H, Karademir S, Koçdor MA, Akgür F, Olguner M, Çoker A Astarcıoğlu İ
Dokuz Eylül University Hospital, İzmir, TURKEY

A 23-month-old girl underwent living related liver transplantation (LRLT) with left lateral segments from her mother. She has had Kasai's operation for biliary atresia at her 4 months of age. End-to-end arterial anastomosis was performed under microscope with 9/0 Prolene® between the left hepatic artery of the donor and the right hepatic artery of the recipient, which were both 3-mm in diameter. Despite postoperative adequate anticoagulation, she developed hepatic artery thrombosis (HAT) 19 days after LRLT, which presented with peak enzyme levels. Attempted urokinase therapy did not reinstitute the arterial flow. Mild improvements in her clinical and biochemical progress made us think about possible existence of collateral arterial neo-vascularization to the graft. However, her clinical course necessitated arterial revascularization which was done a week after HAT. After resection the segment of thrombosed vessel including the primary anastomotic site retrograde bleeding was obtained and rearterialization of the graft was established with saphenous vein interpositional graft. Her postoperative course was uneventful and she was discharged 2 weeks after her secondary operation. At 24 months follow-up, her hepatic artery was patent and her growth as between normal ranges. As a result, late arterial thrombosis (about 3 weeks postoperatively) can be treated with interpositional grafts (even after 7 days of thrombosis). As the collateral neovascular arterial circulation after HAT is never sufficient to vascularize the biliary tree; the risk of late graft lost due to biliary complications will be high. Therefore, it is reasonable to revascularize these liver grafts with preferably arterial or venous interpositonal grafts.

P 30

THE KIDNEYS AND ALCOHOL - WHAT IS THE RELATIONSHIP IN LIVER CIRRHOSIS ?

Apetrecheoaie C. , Diculescu M., Pitigoi D., Tudor C, Jinga M., Oproiu A
Fundeni National Gastroenterology Center, Fundeni Hospital, Bucharest, ROMANIA

Aims : Hepatorenal syndrome represents one of the most severe complications of liver cirrhosis. It represents functional kidney insufficiency in the absence of morphological changes to the kidney. The aims of our study were to assess weather there are relationships between alcohol and kidney involvment in the cirrhotic patients.
Methods : We made two cohorts of patients with liver cirrhosis admitted in Fundeni Gastroenterology Center in one year (1.01.1997 - 1.01.1998) the first with alcoholic liver cirrhosis (ALC) of 185 patients, the other with viral liver cirrhosis (VLC) of 185 patients ; the two cohorts were matched by sex , and age, in a longitudinal study.
Results : Hepatorenal syndrome was present in 13 % of the patients with ALC and in 11,2 % of patients with VLC. All patients had ascites at presentation; 42 % of the patients with ALC had ascitis refractory to diurrhetics, 38 % of those with VLC hat refractory ascitis.. All patients had also other signs of portal hypertension. Porto-systemic encephalopathy was present in 75 % of patients with ALC and at 67.5 % of the patients with VLC. For the ALC patients the median of serum sodium concentration was of 139 mEq / l, lower then the rest of the group (142 mEq / l. The difference had statistical significance (p = 0.004) . the synthesis function of hepatocytes was significantly lower at the patient with hepatorenal syndrome. The median value of Prothrombine activity was of 51 % , versus the other patients with a median value of 67 %. Icteric syndrome was much more important at patients with hepatorenal syndrome (with a median value of total bilirubin of 4.5 mg / dl versus the other patients who had a median value of 2.3 mg / dl. The Child - Pugh score was C for 87.5 % of the patients in the ALC group. For 75 % of the patients it was found a consumption of diurrhetics prior to installation of hepatorenal syndrome. Of the ALC group 37.5 % of the patients had deceased while admitted in the hospital.
Conclusions : 1. Hepatorenal syndrome is one of the most severe complications of alcoholic liver cirrhosis with portal hypertension and ascitis 2. Hyponatremia is an important risk factors for hepatorenal syndrome in patients with alcoholic liver cirrhosis 3.The use of diurrhetics may be another risk factor for the hepatorenal syndrome in patients with alcoholic liver cirrhosis

P 31

DIAGNOSIS OF PORTAL HYPERTENSION-ENDOSCOPY OR ULTRASOUND? WHAT IS THE BEST?

Diculescu M., Apetrechioaie C, Tudor C., Pitigoi D., Oproiu A.
Fundeni National Gastroenterology Center, Fundeni Hospital, Bucharest, ROMANIA

Aims: assessing the value of the two non-invasive methods in evaluation of the portal hypertension.
Methods: We accomplished a retrospective case-control study, including 180 patients admitted in Fundeni National Gastroenterology Center during 1997 with hepatic cirrhosis. All these subjects performed during their clinical surveillance an abdominal sonographic evaluation (including duplex Doppler) and endoscopy. There were 2 groups of patients: group A (117 subjects) with alcoholic cirhosis and group B (153 subjects) with nonalcoholic cirhosis. The statistical study was realized with the aid of Epi Info 6.04 programs.
Results: Both groups did not differ statistically regarding the endoscopic or ultrasonographic signs of portal hypertension, except for portosystemic encephalopathy, whose prevalence was more than twice higher among patients included in group A (33.3%) comparing with M group (13.3%). We found a high incidence of normal spleen diameter, similar for both groups: 36,7%. Presence of splenomegaly (longitudinal diameter of spleen >12 cm) was the sole ecographic parameter wich correlated well with the advanced grading of endoscopic signs of portal hypertension for all patients ($p=0.03$) and especially for group M ($p=0.02$). Only for group M the degree of dilation of portal vein correlated well with the advanced signs of portal hypertension ($p=0.05$). The severity of endoscopic signs (increased size of varices, presence of "red wale markings", severe portal gastropathy) correlated well with the presence of bleeding at the admission or in the past ($p=0.04$), but the correlation wasn't available for the following ultrasonographic signs: splenomegaly ($p=0.5$) and the degree of dilation of portal vein ($p=0.2$). The presence of ascites and portosystemic encephalopathy doesn't correlate with the severity of portal hypertension evaluated endoscopically.
Conclusions: 1.Endoscopy is the cornerstone for the evaluation of portal hypertension, not only diagnostic, but also therapeutic. 2. The severity of endoscopic signs of portal hypertension correlates well with splenomegaly, especially for nonalcoholic cirrhosis. 3. The presence of ascites and portosystemic encephalopathy doesn't correlate well with the grading of endoscopic signs of portal hypertension.

P 32

THE MANAGEMENT OF INTRABILIARY RUPTURED HYDATID DISEASE OF LIVER

Koksal N, Muftuoglu T, Uzun M.A, Gunerhan Y, Kurt R.
Haydarpasa Numune Hospital, Istanbul, Turkey

Aim : To evaluate outcomes of patients with intrabiliary ruptured disease of liver.

Patients and methods: Two hundred and eleven patients were operated between 1990 and 1998. Twenty four patients were reviewed retrospectively for intrabiliary ruptured hydatid diseaese of the liver. We performed partial cystectomy + omentoplasty + transduodenal sphincteroplasty for 18 patients (75%), partial cystectomy + omentoplasty +choledochoduodenostomy for 2 patients (8%) and partial cystectomy + omentoplasty + T-tube drainage for 4 patients (17%). The commmon bile duct was explored in all patients. Daughter cysts, hydatid debris were found in 8 patients (33%). Cholecystectomy was done for all patients underwent choledochododenostomy and transduodenal sphincteroplasty.

Results : Morbidity rate was 12 per cent. Wound infections developed in two patients, one intraabdominal collection was seen and recovered uneventfully. One patient died of unrelated causes. Average hospitalization period was 6.7 days.

Conclusion:
Transduodenal sphincteroplasty can be preferred in the management of intrabiliary ruptured hydatid disease because of shorter hospitalization period, lower morbidity and to decompress intrabiliary pressure.

P 33

EVALUATION OF ULTRASOUND GUIDED ASPIRATION BIOPSY OF FOCAL LIVER LESIONS

Tarján Z, Winternitz T*, Járay B**, Haj H, Forgács B,Tóth G, Galgóczy H,
Dept. of Radiology, *1st Dept of Surgery and **2nd Dept. of Pathology, Semmelweis Univ. Budapest, Hungary

Aims: To evaluate the diagnostic value of Ultrasound Guided Percutaneous Fine Needle Biopsy (US-FNAB) in diagnosing focal liver lesions.
Methods: During the last 6 years 552 US-FNABs were performed in patients with suspected neoplastic involvement of the liver with 22-gauge Chiba needles. In 223 cases the results were compared with final diagnosis based on postoperative histology (54), operation detecting primary tumour according to the metastasis (97), autopsy (22) or clinical and radiological follow up methods (for benign lesions, 60).
Results: Sufficient material for cytological analysis was obtained in 93% of the cases. The biopsies confirmed malignancy in 39.3%, 9% were suspected of malignancy and in 29.7% benign lesions were diagnosed. Considering suspicion of malignancy as a diagnosis of malignancy, FNAB diagnosis had 95.8% sensitivity, 97% specificity and 96.1% overall accuracy. In characterising malignant lesions FNAB was found to be 98.4% accurate for metastases, and 96.4% accurate for HCCs. There were no false positive cases with undoubtful malignancy FNAB diagnosis. No noteworthy complications were observed.
Conclusions: US-FNAB is a highly reliable, safe, inexpensive diagnostic procedure. Based on our experiences we advise US-FNAB as a routine, first level tool for the diagnosis of focal liver diseases.

P 34

Factors associated with hepatic cirrhosis development in chronic hepatitis C

A Constantino MD, F Ramalho MD, F Serejo MD, N Fatela MD, H Glória MD, J Lopes MD, R Marinho MD, M Raimundo MD, J Velosa MD, MC Moura MD. Liver Unit - Santa Maria Hospital, Lisbon, Portugal

Background: The HCV infection, once established, persists in the vast majority (>80%) of patients. The progression of disease is largely silent. Available prospective studies indicate that at least 20-30 years of infection are required to develop clinically significant disease. **Aim**: To evaluate the factors that may be associated with progression to cirrhosis in chronic HCV infection. **Material**: We studied 117 patients (87males/30 females), and each one was assessed to risk factors for hepatitis C infection. **Results**: The mean age at entry was 35,6 years (16-70) years. Sporadic form was the predominant risk for HCV infection (n=53), whereas 41 were drug-addicts and 24 had received blood transfusions. The mean duration of HVC infection was 6,3 years (1-19 years). Of 52 patients with no reliable data regarding the time of infection, 78,9% were alcoholic. Forty-two patients (36%) have been infected at 40 years of age or older. No patients was HBsAg+, whereas 26 (50%) were HBcAb+, and 38,4% had alcohol abuse. HVC genotypes determined in the first 90 consecutive patients, showed genotype 1 the most prevalent (n=63; 1b=57), followed by genotype 2c (n=20) and 3a (n=7). The histopathological examination revealed the majority of patients had either mild (n=13), moderate (n=29) or severe (n=35) chronic hepatitis, and cirrhosis in 40. **Conclusion**: In multivariate logistic regression analysis, duration of infection (HR-0,864; 0,959-98% CI, p=0,006) and age of entry in the study (HR-1,049; 1,074-95% CI, p<0,0005), were independent determinants of progression to cirrhosis in patients with HCV chronic infection.

P 35

LITTLE-INVASIVE SURGERY IN THE TREATMENT OF ECHINOCOCCOSIS OF LIVER AND LUNGS.

M.Aliev, M.D.,Ph.D., M.Seysembaev,M.D.,Ph.D., C.Adylkhanov,M.D., B.Narzhanov,M.D, A.Kenzhebaev,M.D.
Scientific Center of Surgery, Almaty, Kazakstan.

Aims: Since 1993 we developed the method of endosurgical intervention for hydatid cysts of the liver and in 1996 the one for the hydatid cysts of lungs. We have an experience of 27 laparoscopic and 14 thoracoscopic echinococcectomies in patients with echinococcosis aged between 3 and 57 years.

Methods: Solitair cysts 3,5-8 cm. in diameter located in approachable segments. Diagnosis was made using ultrasonic and CT-investigation. Cyst area was surrounded by gauses soaked in formaldehid solution or sterile glycerin. After aspiration of the content of the cyst the cavity was processed by "running steam". Steam exposure time was 3-5 min. After fibrous capsule was opened the elements of the cyst were put in a polyethylene container and removed, then the fibrous capsule was maximally excised. By echinococcosis of the liver remained cavity was liquidated using peritonisation or abdominisation, by echinococcosis of lungs it was done by clipping.

Results: After echinococcectomy from the liver patients were followed for 5 years and for 2 years after echinococcectomy from lungs. There were no cases of recurrence of the disease.

Conclusions: On the base of obtained clinical experience we suppose that endovideosurgical echinococcectomy is an effective method of the treatment of echinococcosis of liver and lungs. This method can be successfully applied in patients with small cysts located in approachable for this manipulation segments.

P 36

SURGERY OF PORTAL HYPERTENSION.

N.Arynov M.D., Ph.D., B.Shirtaev M.D, Dh.Nashanov M.D.
Scientific Center of Surgery, Almaty, Kazakstan.

Aims: The aim of the research was to study the results of surgical correction of portal blood flow block since it is an actual and discussed problem of hepatology.

Methods: In the clinic 45 patients with the syndrome of portal hypertension were operated on. Among them there were 32 boys and 13 girls aged between 1,5 and 15 years. In 21 patients extrahepatic form of portal hypertension (in 5 of them segmental form) in 20 patients intrahepatic form, and in 4 cases miscellaneous form was revealed. In 5 patients with segmental form splenectomy was performed. In the rest of patients with extrahepatic form variants of elective portocaval shunts (splenorenal "side-to-side","H-type", "end-to-side", mesocaval) combined with denervation of the common hepatic artery were done. In 13 patients with intrahepatic and miscellaneous form liver tunnelisation along with gastrorenopexy in 2 cases, common hepatic artery denervation in 10 cases, and pericholedocheal denervation in 2 cases was done.
In 14 patients with III degree esophageal varices the variants of elective portocaval shunts were performed.

Results: The efficacy of surgical treatment was evaluated by changes of morphology, intra- and extrahepatic hemodinamics. Satisfactory results were obtained in 93,3% of cases, and non-satisfactory results were obtained in 6,7% of cases.

Conclusions: Surgical treatment must be aimed on decrease of portal pressure by elective portocaval shunting and improvement of hepatic regeneration.

P 37

ANEMIA IN CIRHOTIC PATIENTS

Ditoiu AV*, Motoi O*, Stoica V**
*Fundeni Hospital, Medical Clinic ; ** Cantacuzino Hospital, Medical Clinic, Bucharest, Romania.
Aim : evaluation of red cells alterations and their relationship with the evolution of liver cirrhosis (LC)
Methods : the study was made on 332 patients with LC successively admitted in clinic. All patients were investigated to establish the diagnosis of LC, of digestive tract hemorrhages (UDE, rectoscopy, occult faecal blood test), peripheral blood smear, reticulocytes, medular bone exam. In this group we individualized 4 subgroups: A = hepatoma on LC, B = hepatorenal syndrome; C = hepatic encephalopathy; D = LC with anemia.
Results : anemia was found in 25.30% patients; mean value of hemoglobin = 10.68 g/dl $\pm$2 g/dl; average MEV = 108.27 $\pm$ 10.68μ^3 in lot D macrocytosis was noted in 58.33% cases , microcytosis in 16.66%. In LC without anemia MEV was 98.6 $\pm$ 8,8 μ^3, and macrocytosis was found in only 21.42% patients. Hypersplenism (anemia $\pm$ trombocitopenia $\pm$ leucopenia without any loss of blood) was noted in 48.8% patients in lot D, vs. 15.66 % in whole group of patients. As etiology of anemia we found hemorrhagia in 31.09 % cases (22.61% digestive hemorrhagia); anemia was normoregenerative in 71.42% patients, hyporegenerative in 19.04% cases and hyperregenerative in 9.52% patients. Anemia was found in 55.80% cases in lot C, 62.06% in lot B, 76.4% in lot A.
Conclusions: anemia is noted in 25.35% patients with LC, loss of blood is found to be responsible in 25.30% cases, and hypersplenism in 48.8% patients. Anemia is usually macrocytic and normoregenerative, much more frequent in LC with hepatorenal syndrome, hepatoma with LC or hepatic encephalopathy.

P 38

PALIATIVE TRANSCATHETER HEMOEMBOLIZATION IN TREATMENT OF HEPATIC CARCINOMA

D. Ma{ulovic, M. Mili}evic, @. Markovic, Dj. [aranovic, Lj.Borota, Z.Bo`ovic, P.Anojcic

Clinical center of Serbia,
Dept. of Interv. Radiology, Policlinics
Ul. Dimitrija Tucovi}a 162/3
11000 Belgrade, Serbia

The authors report their experience with chemoemboliyation (CE) as a form of palliation in the manayenant of unresectable hepatocellular carcinoma (HCC).
In the procedure was applied in 19 patients. Thirteen patients received more than one chemoembolic therapy. 38 treatments were perfomed ina all. The stages were defined according to Occuda's method. Most of the tumors (14) were classified as stage I. Liver cirrhosis was present in 17 patients, and abnormal levels of alpha fetoproteins were found in 68% of cases. The initial diagnosis was established by echotomography and laboratory studies, while Doppler sonography, CT and angiography were used for staging.
The catheter was placed transfemorally to apply a mixture of lipiodol and chemoiotherapeutic agents into the a. hepatica propria and its branches. CT scan a neoplasm necrosis in 90%, while alpha lipoprotein values were reduced in all.
All patients survived three and six months, and 68% survived a year. Not a singl case of fatal outcome occurred during the procedure, and the overall morbidity rate was 19%.
The effects of the relatively safe procedure probobly improved both survival and the quality of life, particularly if proper patient sel ection was done.

P 39

UNUSUAL CASE OF BUDD-CHIARI SYNDROME (A CASE REPORT)

Szántová, M., Kupčová, V., Rajková , M., Kolníková , M., Janík, P., Belan, V., Turecký, L . 3rd Depart. of Medicine, Pathol. Depart., Medical faculty of Comenius University, Bratislava, Slovakia.

A 34-year-old woman was addmitted to hospital for gradually developed ascites, weakness, jaundice, nausea, vomitus, anorexia and fever in the last 2 months following on the episode of diarrhea. Laboratory parameters showed leukemoid reaction with leukocytosis , high thrombocytemia , hypocoagulative state (severe hypoprothrombinemia and slight hypofibrinogenemia) with high hyperbilirubinemia. There was 100-times elevation of transaminases with 10-times elevation of cholestatic enzymes at admission with gradually decrease to 10-times of normal value of enzymes with rapid increase of hyperbilirubinemia to 660 umol/l within last week . Severe hypoproteinemia and hyperamonia were found . Virologic examination was negative. Salmonelosis and urinary infection were found . Hepatomegaly and ascites with slow portal vein flow, splenomegaly and cholelitiasis were found on ultrasonography . CT found hepatosplenomegaly with massive infiltrate inflammatory or neoplastic process, ascites, fluidothorax, retroperitoneal and intraperitoneal lymphadenopathy and suspicion on ovarian tumor . Nonvisualisation of hepatic veins and narrowing of vein cava found on US and CT could not exclude Budd-Chiari syndrome. Cavography could not be done for the severe hypocoagulative state. Esophageal varices P. II. were found with following hematemesis . Cultivation of ascites showed presence of Acinetobacter, cytologic examinations were repeatedly negative. Because of suspicion on gynecologic or urologic malignancy (under CT, US , positive CA 125, CA 19-9, B2M, NSE), clinical and laboratory picture there was non considered liver transplantation as a treatment procedure. Recurrent torpid hematemesis ocurred and the patient died. Post mortem microsopic examination showed acute flebithis of hepatic veins with Budd-Chiari syndrome. Cholestatic syndrome was caused by stenosing of bile ducts by chronic fibrosing pancreatitis. In the literature described inflammation-induced cholestasis participated in our case, too . Disseminated hemorrhage from the whole gastrointestinal tract, lung, heart and urinary bladder was present despite slight anticoagulative and substitution treatment .
Nonvisualisation of hepatic veins is often present in liver cirrhosis. Inflammation of hepatic veins and disseminated intravascular coagulation caused their thrombosis in our patient . The cause cf infammation could be salmonelosis with the following bacterial peritonitis . Liver transplantation could be the only therapeutic option .

P 40

LIVER HEMANGIOMAS : IMPORTANCE OF DYNAMIC CONTRAST-ENHANCED MR IMAGING

Benkő K., Tóth J., Péter M.

Univ. Med. School of Debrecen, Department of Radiology, Hungary

Aim: Our objective was to study whether conventional spin-echo sequences could define alone the diagnosis of liver hemangiomas.

Materials and methods: 325 patients (104 male/221 female, age 8-93 years, mean age 47,8 years) with focal liver lesions were examined at 1.0 Tesla using conventional SE sequences (T1, T2-weighted) in axial, sometimes coronal and sagittal planes. In 97/325 cases dynamic MR imaging was performed by breath-hold gradient-echo fast low angle shot (FLASH) technique following intravenous gadolinium-DTPA (0,1-0,2 ml per kilogram body weight).

Results: In 104 of 325 cases (32 %) common hemangiomas with „light bulb sign" (calculated T2 value above 100 msec) were found by conventional SE sequences. 48 patients of 104 were examined by dynamic MR paralelly. Hemangiomas shown „iris phenomenon" could determinated using dynamic MR imaging even in further 16 patients.

Conclusion: If the appereance of the hepatic lesion detected by conventional SE sequentes is not characteristic for hemangioma (calculated T2 value below 100 msec) dynamic MR have to be done. Thus the noncommon hemangiomas also could be evaluated.

P 41

ROLE OF VIRAL AND HOST FACTORS IN THE PATHOGENESIS OF HEPATITIS C VIRUS (HCV) INFECTION AND IN THE RESPONSE TO INTERFERON TREATMENT.

A. Pár, M. Paál, M. Horányi, G. Pár, B. Gasztonyi, J.Szekeres-Bartho, Gy.Mózsik.
University Medical School, Pécs, National Institute of Hematology and Immunology, Budapest, Hungary

Aims: To asses the role of viral and host factors in the pathogenesis of HCV infection, virological and immunological studies have been performed.

Patients and methods: 48 patients (pts) with chronic hepatitis C and 36 symptomfree, HCV-positive blood donors were investigated. Serum HCV-RNA bDNA , anti-HCV, HBsAg, anti-HBc, lymphocyte subset, lymphoproliferative response, natural killer cell activity and HLA determinations were done.

Results: serum HCV-RNA levels were significantly lower in symptomfree HCV-positive individuals, than in HCV pts. (1.886 ± 2.881 vs 4.620 ± 5.000 MEQ/ml $p < 0.05$). Similarly, responders to IFN showed lower HCV-RNA load than non-responders (1.433 ± 2.581 vs 6.610±3.400 MEQ/ml, $p < 0.05$). Previous HBV infection occurred only in chronic hepatitis pts. IFN non-responders had more frequent HBV+HCV coinfection than responders (18% vs 82%, $p < 0.05$). NK cell activity decreased in HCV pts. (3.44 ±1.10 vs 122.0± 52.0 %, $p < 0.05$).HLA DR3 was found with higher frequency in HCV pts compared with normal control (56.0% vs 20.7%). Non-responders to IFN showed higher HLA DR3 occurrence than responders (89% vs 44%, $p<0.05$). Prevalence of HLA DR5 was lower in chronic HCV infection as compared with healthy controls (16% vs 39%, $p <0.05$).

Conclusion: serum HCV-RNA as viral factor and HLA as host factor may determine the the course of HCV infection and the response to antiviral treatment. HLA DR3 is a marker of susceptibility and negative predictor of therapeutic response, while HLA DR5 may play a protective role in HCV infection.

(Supported by grants from ETT 031/96 and OTKA T 023476).

P 42

AN ORIGINAL PORTO-SISTEMIC SHUNT USING ADRENAL VEIN.

Jovine E, Masetti M, Cescon M, Ercolani G, Pierangeli F, Grazi GL, Mazziotti A, Cavallari A. Second Department of Surgery. University of Bologna (Italy)

AIMS: Management of gastrointestinal hemorrhage from rupture of esophageal and gastric varices due to portal hypertension remains a debated question. In patients with sclerotherapy-resistant esofago-gastric varices, and preserved hepatic function, a surgical shunt is considered the treatment of choice. The distal spleno-renal shunt (warren procedure) seems to offer the best results The authors present the first case in the english literature of successful spleno-adrenal shunt, utilizing a left adrenal vein of unespected, considerable diameter after having planned a Warren procedure.
METHODS: a 63 year old caucasian male was admitted in our Department, with a diagnosis of idiopatic hepatic fibrosis, portal hypertension, esophageal and gastric varices and previous history of variceal bleeding. Esophageal varices with high risk of bleeding and gastric varices were detected at EGDS; An hepatic angiography showed patency of splenic, mesenteric and portal veins with intrahepatic barrage,due to cirrhosis. A distal spleno-renal shunt was planned. During the isolation the left renal vein, a large diameter (8 mm) left adrenal vein was identified. The splenic vein was isolated up to the confluence with the superior mesenteric vein and divided as in Warren procedure. The adrenal vein was clamped and interrupted at one centimeter far from the the renal vein. An end-to-end anastomosis with distal splenic and proximal adrenal stump was performed, using a 5/0 polipropilene running suture. After revascularization, the anastomosis appeared patent and tension-free. Finally, the left gastric and gastroepiploic veins were ligated as in the Warren original technique. RESULTS The procedure was technically uneventful and didn't required any blood transfusion. An ultra sound color Doppler on the 3rd p.o. day, showed normal intrasplenic resistence index (R.I.= O.59), demonstrating the efficacy of the shunt. A splenic angiography carried out on the 8th p.o. day showed the complete patency of the spleno-adrenal shunt, with exclusive caval flow during the venous phase.
DISCUSSION Sclerosis of the esofago-gastric varices in patients with portal hypertension is the treatment of choice. Patients with sclerotherapy-resistant esofago-gastric varices, and preserved hepatic function, a surgical shunt is considered the treatment of choice. Spleno-adrenal shunt, utilizing a left adrenal vein represent an excellent option .
The adrenal vein has the advantage of an autogenous conduit, which is the best solution according to the principles of vascular surgery.

P 43

Experiences with surgical therapy of hepatic echinococcosis

Bakula B, Rašić Ž, Zoričić I, Košuta D, Anić T.
University Department of Surgery, "Sveti Duh" General Hospital
Zagreb, Croatia

Human echinococcus is still endemic in some areas of the world, including Mediterranean countries, like Croatia. Because there is no effective medical therapy, surgery remains the principal mode of treatment. Between January 1990 and December 1998 145 patients 68 male (46,8%) and 77 female (53,2%), aged 16 to 75 years (mean 46) with hydatid liver disease were treated surgical at our Department. Diagnosis was made using clinical criteria, serology and imaging techniques liver ultrasound and CT. The right lobe of the liver was affected in 106 (76%), the left lobe in 29 (20%) and both lobes in10 (4%). Patients with hydatic cysts in ader sites than liver were excluded from the study.
Our surgical procedure were:

PARTIAL RESECTION		87	(60,00%)
PARTIAL RESECTION WITH "T"–TUBE INSERTION		13	(8,96%)
LIVER RESECTION	ATIPICAL	24	(16,56%)
	RIGHT HEPATECTOMY	13	(8,97%)
	LEFT HEPATECTOMY	7	(4,83%)
EXTERNAL DRAINAGE		1	(0,68%)
TOTAL		145	(100,00%)

Fatal complication did not occur. Two patients developed hepatic abscess, three wound infection and one massive bleeding after hepatic resection.

P 44

Contemporary principles of conservative treatment of esophagi–gastric hemorrhages in patients with portal hypertension.

Ashrafov A.A., Mamedli Z.Z.

Azerbaijcan Medical University
Department of Surgery, Baku.

This work is a report of result of Conservative treatment of esophagi hemorrhages in 100 patients with portal hypertment aged between 17 and 79 years old. There were 68 male and 32 female patients, Conservative measures included endoscopic electrocoagulation and sleazing of varies in esophagus and cardiac part of stomach. We used trombovarum, 66% solution of glucose, 70° ethanol for endoseopic selesoring of esophageal varicose.
In course of medical treatment in 49 patients homeostasis was obtained in 30 cases. In 23 patients medical treatment was coupled by balloon tamponade with a senstaken-blakemore tube for esophageal varicose blooding. The blooding was managed in 18 patients. In 10 patients medical treatment was associated with endoscopic sleazing of esophageal varicose. In 6 cases thrombosis was induced. In. course of endoseopic selerosinf of esophageal varicose if the blooding was continuing we modified this procedure. When the endoscopic and electrocoagulation failed. We changed it with inserting of polyethl tube having pnuimoballoon. Greeting a pressure of 100-150 cm air we pulled the balloon, managed to tamponade cardiac varicose, and get thrombosis. Then we again placed endoscope, aspirated blood from esophagus and injected sclazosing medicines Endo- and paravasally.
This method helped to manage in 17 cases with in 18 patients. This in 100 patients with continuing blooding we had a success by holding conservative measure in 71 cases, but in 6 cases the blooding relapsed. Conservative medical therapy did not undue reliable homeostasis in 35 patients 22 of them Died because of recurrent blooding against a hepatic failure background, the severity of which was a contraindication for emergency surgical procedures. 13 patient underwent surgery at the top-level of bulging.
In conclusion we think that conservative treatment of patients with esophageal, gastric varicose should be complex, and associate endoscopic selerosing of blooding vans with their balloon tamponade what increases the effectiveness of homeostasis.

P 45

TREATMENT OF HEPATO-CELLULAR CARCINOMA: RESULTS ON 12 SURGICALYY RESECTED CASES

Techniques of hepatic surgery quickly improved in the last two decades. Is now possible to perform safe minimal resections of hepatic tissue in patients affected by Hepato Cellular Carcinoma (HCC) even in presence of coexisting hepatic cirrhosis. In presence of higher perioperative risk, alternative therapies have been recently validated. At our Institution in 1995 a multimodal protocol was established. It included surgical (excision or transplant) and non surgical (alchool injection or, more recently, thermoablation) therapies. Surgical excision was attempted only in presence of certain malignant (αFP> 200 and/or positive biopsy) monolateral lesions in Child-Pugh A patients. From November 1995 through December 1998 we observed 22 patients with HCC. Performance status was evaluated in all patients using ASA classification. In presence of cirrhosis (20 patients, 90.9%) hepatic function was evaluated by the use of Child-Pugh classification. In 54.5% of the cases (n° 12 patients, M: 10 F: 2, mean age: 60.9 years) surgical treatment was indicated. Cirrhosis was present in 10 patients (83.3%). Lesions were multiple in 4 cases (33.3%) and single in 8 cases (66.7%). Mean size of the lesions was 3.1 cm (1-8 cm); they were located in the right and left lobe in 10 cases (83.3%) and 2 cases (16.7%). All but one patients belonged to the class A of Child-Pugh classification. All patients underwent laparotomy; In one patient an under-staged 18 cm lesion was not removed for the presence of hypotrophy of the contro-lateral lobe. All remaining patients were radically resected. One patient underwent surgery twice (first and second (after 17 months) wedge resections of a 3.3 and 1 cm right lobe lesions). Two right- and 1 left-side hepatectomies, 3 segmentectomies and 6 wedge resections were performed. Partial inflow occlusion was performed in 4 cases (36.4%). Mean blood loss consisted of 400 ml (200-2000 ml). A 10 mm margin from the tumour was always preserved. Intra operative mortality was absent. Perioperative mortality was present in a 78 years old patient (8.3%) for the postoperative occurrence of an acute necrotic-haemorrhagic pancreatitis. Major post-operative morbidity was present in 3 patients (30%). We encountered two cases of transient hepatic failure and one case of cerebral hemorrhage. Minor morbidity rate was observed in 2 patients (20%) Patients were discharged after a mean time of 13.9 (8-50) days. According to a prospective strategy nor neo-adjuvant or adjuvant treatments were performed. After a mean follow-up of 10.5 (1-27) months 1 patient died for hepatic failure and 1 died for a pulmonary primitive tumor; in one patient multiple malignant hepatic lesions were present at MRI after 4 months by surgical excision. This patient is now waiting to be treated by thermoablation therapy. Six patients (66.7%) are alive and free of disease. The experience in hepatic surgery of HCC at our Institution is still limited. Nevertheless it can be confirmed that the use of minimal resections in Child-Pugh A patients affected by single or monolateral tumours, is a safe, effective and potentially radical treatment with accettable mortality rate. In our experience a careful assessment of perioperative risk and a correct perioperative management, significantly reduce the risk of hepatic failure. Our experience finally seems to confirm that alternative therapies can be conveniently considered in case of multicentric Child-Pugh B-C patients or in presence of tumour recurrence after surgery.

P 46

BENIGN HEPATIC TUMORS. ANALYSIS OF 19 CASES.

*L. Vlad, *S. Duca, **M. Grigorescu, ***S. Cotul
*Clinic of Surgery No. 3, **Clinic of Internal Medicine No. 3, ***Department of Nuclear Medicine, University of Medicine Cluj, Romania

Among 93 patients operated in the period 01.01.1992-30.11.1997 for primary liver tumors, we found 19 benign hepatic tumors (20,4): 15 hemangiomas, 1 adenoma, 2 hamartoma, and 1 focal nodular hyperplasia. Hepatic hemangioma was the most frequent 978% of benign tumors), in 4 cases being located to one segment, in 5 cases extended to 3 segments, 1 case to right lobe and in 5 cases to the left lobe. The preoperative diagnosis was based on the hyperechoic pattern at the Ultrasonography and the intense peripheral enhancement after the administration of contrast agent bolus, as well on HPI (hepatic perfusion index) by means of hepatic scintigraphy. The clinical examination found a palpable hepatic mass only in 5 cases - giant hemangioma occurred in 1 case (in this case the surgical exploration demonstrated the definitive diagnosis). The laparotomy was done in all cases: in 10 cases we performed only the exploration and biopsy, in 3 cases left lobectomy, in 1 case left hepatectomy and in 1 case the resection of the quadrant lobe. All patients with hemangioma had a good postoperative outcome, without complications.
One patient presented hepatic adenoma. In this case because the intratumoral bleeding, the preoperative diagnosis suggested cavernous hemangioma. The operation consisted in segmentectomy of the segment IV, the final diagnosis has been demonstrated by the histologic examination of the resected parenchyma.
The hepatic hamartoma was found in two cases, both being operated (hepatic excision - 1 case and left lobectomy - 1 case) and the diagnosis was made after the histologic examination of the resected specimen. One patient with focal nodular hyperplasia was cured by segmentectomy (segment VI) and the postoperative histologic examination pointed the type of the tumor.
In conclusion the heterogeneous appearance of these tumors require surgical exploration and biopsy to avoid the confusion with various malignant hepatic lesions. Finally we discuss the various imaging patterns of the benign hepatic tumors.

P 47

INTRAOPERATIVE ULTRASONOGRAPHY OF LIVER ECHINOCOCCOSIS.

S.A.Dadvani, A.N.Lotov, G.H.Musaev, O.S.Schkrob, Y.V.Kulezneva, V.N.Avakian,

Moscow Medical Academy, Surgical clinic № 1, Moscow, Russia

Aims: improvement of diagnostics and results of surgical treatment in patients by a liver echinococcosis.
Materials and methods: In Surgical clinic N 1 Moscow medical Academy between 1986 and 1999 102 patients were examined by means intraoperative ultrasound during operative treatment of the liver echinococcosis cysts. In 78 supervision the echinococcosis cysts were solitary, in 24 - multiple. The sizes of cysts have made from 56 up to 220 mm, age of patients from 13 to 58 years.
The intraoperative ultrasound enabled to estimate extent of a defeat, anatomo-topographical ratio of a cyst's brood capsule and liver's vessels and bile ducts, to reveal not diagnosed fine cysts in 7 supervision with the subsequent choice of optimal operative volume. 13 patients with high risk of radical operation and multiple cysts in liver parenchyma underwent the intraoperative punction of the deeply located liver cysts under the US-control during operation with lavage of a cavity 20 % NaCl (9 patients) or 86 % by a glycerin (4 patients).
Results of research: the intraoperative ultrasound has allowed in 7 supervision to reveal the fine echinococcosis cysts, not diagnosed up to operation, in thicker of a liver parenchyma. At supervision from 6 months to 13 years recidivation of disease (including with an intraoperative punction and antiparasitic lavage of echinococcosis cysts) are marked in 6 (5,8%) supervision.
Conclusions: the intraoperative ultrasound allows to increase efficacy of operation, reduces risk of occurrence postoperative bile- and hemorrage in residual cavities, to reveal not diagnosed echinococcosis liver cysts and if necessary to execute of intraoperative minimally invasive intervention.

P 48

THE RIGHT HEPATIC LOBE FOR LIVING RELATED GRAFTING: BENEFITS AND PROBLEMS

S.Gautier, O.Tsiroulnikova, A.Filin, A.Semenkov, J.Kamalov
National Research Centre of Surgery, Moscow, Russia.

The traditional use of left lateral segment (II and III C.Couinaud segments) of living donor doesn't fit the requirements of recipients with body weight more than 20 kg. In such cases the hole left lobe for living related grafting is still problematic and depends on survival of the IV segment. So, the right hepatic lobe in spite of being a half of the organ is very attractive from the point of view of living related liver transplantation (LRLT) perhaps in elder children. Benefits of the right lobe in comparison with the left lobe are being presented by more permanent anatomy and more convenient configuration and immobility in orthotopic position. Besides this our anatomical research in 170 cadavers revealed right hepatic artery to be thicker than the left in 86% of cases even being transected distally from the IV segment's arterial branch if any. The right hepatectomy in donor saves the median hepatic vein with no problem for graft while the left lobe replacement dictates the removal of median vein with the graft. So, the right hepatectomy appears to be less harmful for donor if to perform it precisely. The mismatch of vertical and sagital sizes of donor's and recipient's right fossa hepatica as well as big accessory hepatic veins from the right lobe must be predicted before surgery.

Among 5 LRLT for the period from March 1997 to November 1998 performed in children with 12 – 25 kg. body weight we used right lobes in 2 recipients of 20 and 25 kg. body weight. The indications were cryptogenic cirrhosis and Byler's disease. In both cases the graft volume ratio of donor's left lateral segment was less than 0.3 and arterial blood supply of the IV segment from the right hepatic artery ruined the possibility to use the left lobe. In the same time the graft volume ratio of the right lobe was near 1.0 (0.93 and 1.02, respectively). Donors' blood loss during right hepatectomy was no more than 500.0 ml and returned by cell-saver. No allohaemotransfusion was used. Both mothers were discharged after 10 days with no complications. The grafts' conservation was performed with HTK-solution (CUSTODIOL®, Dr.Franz Kohler Chemie GmbH). The recipients' postoperative course was uneventful. The use of living donor's right hepatic lobe can provide new good facilities for liver replacement in elder children and small sized adults in the cadaver organs shortage or absence.

P 49

HEMODYNAMIC STABILITY AND ADECUATED OUTFLOW IN LIVER TRANSPLANTATION WITH PIGGYBACK TECHNIQUE AND END-TO-SIDE CAVO-CAVA ANASTOMOSIS

Moneva ME, Muñoz L, Arranz J, Barrera M, Varona A, Soriano A.
"N<u>tra</u> S<u>ra</u> de Candelaria" Hospital. Santa Cruz de Tenerife. Spain

Aims: The piggyback technique with preservation of the caval flow provides hemodynamic stability during the anhepatic phase and avoids venous bypass. Nevertheless, in 9% of cases, the common cuff of the left and middle hepatic veins seems to be too small and with inadequate outflow. We adopted the end-to-side caval reconstruction as routine procedure and we have studied our results.

Methods: 30 Liver Transplantations in 28 patients were performed consecutively with preservation of the inferior vena Cava (IVC), longitudinal partial clamping of the native vena Cava, and end-to-side caval reconstruction.

Results: In all cases, the recipient's IVC was only partially clamped and the caval flow was preserved. Patients remained hemodynamic stable, with preserved diuresis at all stages of the procedure (table). Venous bypass was avoided in all cases. Warm isquemia time and transfusion requirements were 75 ± 10 min and 9,8 ± 4,3 U of packed RBC, respectively. There were no specific complications or death due to the technique. No cases of graft congestion were observed neither postoperative acute renal failure.

	Pre-IVC clamping	Post-IVC clamping	P
MAP (mmHg)	82.5 ± 2.6	86.4 ± 2.5	NS
IVC pressure (mmHg)	9.7 ± 1.1	8.7 ± 1.1	NS
Cardiac index (l/min/m^2)	5.6 ± 0.5	4.9 ± 0.3	NS
SVRI (dyn·s·cm^{-5}/m^2)	1228 ± 89	1353 ± 98	NS

MAP mean arterial pressure, *IVC* inferior vena cava,
SVRI systemic vascular resistance index, *NS* not significant

Conclusions: End-to-side caval reconstruction, with a wide caval anastomosis ensures adequate venous drainage of the graft avoiding the development of postoperative ascitis and Budd-Chiari acute. Longitudinal partial clamping of the native vena Cava provides hemodynamic stability throughout the procedure, obviating the need for venous bypass.

P 50

THE REGENERATIVE ACTIVITY IN LIVER REMNANT AND GRAFT

O.Tsiroulnikova, J.Kamalov, A.Filin, G.Sheremet'eva, M.Morozova, D.Semenov and S.Gautier
National Research Centre of Surgery, Moscow, Russia.

The success of trisegmentectomy and more advanced major hepatic resections as well as segmental liver transplantation in cases of "small for size" grafts is based on famous ability of liver parenchyma to restore the necessary volume. The aim of research was to estimate the intensity of regenerative process depending on liver remnant or graft mass compared to ideal liver mass for patient. Postoperative course was studied after 70 major liver resections (LR) in 67 patients of 1 – 62 years old (mean age 34,9±2,3 years) with remnant volume ratio (VR) 0.2 – 0.5; 21 cadaver orthotopic liver transplantations (OLT) in 20 adults (mean age 24,3±3,2 years) with graft VR 0.8 – 1.1, and 9 living related liver transplantations (LRLT) in children (mean age 6,3±1,2 years) with graft VR 0.5 – 1.0. To estimate the liver function and regeneration the laboratory tests, sonography, axial computed tomography and morphological investigations with electronic microscopy were used. The most active regeneration was found during the first 3 months after operation in spite of the kind of procedure. In this period hyperplastic process was being provided by hepatocyte hypertrophy with nuclear enlargement and doubling correlated with rising of protein synthetic activity in hepatocytes. Karyometry revealed different degree of nuclear enlargement. In all cases of OLT and in 2 cases of right lobe LRLT in children with body weight 20 and 25 kg (VR 1.0 and 0.93, respectively) the mean nuclear volume in the end of the first week was 266.1±21.8 μm^3 that meant 50% more than just after surgery. The mean hepatocyte nuclear volume after resection was 311.6±16.5 μm^3 (80%). The most dramatic hypertrophy of hepatocyte nuclei with mean volume 495.6 ± 82.7 μm^3 that was 2.8 times more than initial size was found in 7 cases of LRLT of the left lateral segment. These changes were followed by the growth of hepatic blood vessels' pool mainly by portal and hepatic veins widening. So, the regenerative processes were expressed in living related grafts most of all while regenerative activity was minimal in unresected cadaver grafts and living related right lobes. The regenerative mechanisms of transplanted and/or resected liver are quite similar and depend on liver graft or remnant VR.

P 51

ORTHOTOPIC LIVER TRANSPLANTATION: IMPACT OF IMPROVEMENT IN SURGICAL TECHNIQUE ON ARTERIAL AND BILIARY ANASTOMOTIC FAILURE RATES

BJ Ammori, R Prasad, JPA Lodge, SG Pollard
Departments of Hepatobiliary Surgery and Anaesthesia[1], St. James's University Hospital, Beckett Street, Leeds LS9 7TF, UK

AIMS: To describe the operative techniques and results of hepatic artery and biliary anastomoses in patients undergoing orthotopic liver transplantation.

METHODS: Our experience with 400 consecutive orthotopic liver transplants was reviewed. The operative technique involved shortening of the hepatic artery as much as possible to avoid subsequent vascular kinks, with sacrifice of the classically advised aortic or splenic patch. A fine (6-0 to 8-0) prolene or Gore-Tex suture was utilised to effect the vascular anastomosis. Low-dose heparin was routinely introduced as soon as the coagulation has returned to normal. The donor bile duct was shortened as much as possible to reduce ischaemia to its distal end and risk of anastomotic failure. The biliary anastomosis was fashioned with a direct duct-to-duct anastomosis (94%) or a Roux-en-Y hepaticojejunostomy (6%). It was constructed using interrupted 5-0 PDS with all knots placed outside.

RESULTS: Arterial thrombosis and biliary complications occurred in 1.9% and 5.5% of cases. Bile leaks complicated 0.7% of transplant procedures, and were effectively managed by endoscopic stenting. Biliary strictures presented 'early' after transplantation in 2.9% of cases and 'late' in 1.8% of transplants. No biliary complications developed in the hepaticojejunostomy group.

CONCLUSIONS: Improvements in surgical techniques for the construction of the arterial and biliary anastomosis in patients undergoing orthotopic liver transplantation can lead to low anastomotic failure rates.

P 52

MONITORING INTRAMUCOSAL PH DURING LIVER TRANSPLANTATION

T. Mándli, T. Gondos
Semmelweis Medical University Transplantation and Surgical Department, Budapest, Hungary

Aims: Application of a sensitive examination method to establish the early graft function among patients underwent liver transplantation.

Patients and methods: The Hungarian liver transplantation program was started in 1995 at Semmelweis Medical University, Transplantation and Surgical Department. Early and quick establishing of the graft function is important of deciding the retransplantation indication. Such way can be the continuous measurement of intramucosal pH with air-tonometer (Tonocap TC-200, Datex). This method has been practised at transplantation of 25 patients since 1996. The hemodynamic, oxygenation and liver function parameters of the recipients and the intramucosal pH (pHi) and the pressure of regional mucosal CO2 (PrCO2) were monitorised in the perioperative period. Patients have been classified into two groups according to the early graft function. Good function were in 18 patients (Group 1) and deterioration of graft function had been noticed in 7 patients in the perioperative period (Group 2).

Results: Group 1: pHi value was mainly above 7.3 in the perioperative phase. The worst pHi value was 7.0 and PrCO2 70 mmHg. All patients survived the early postoperative phase.
Group 2: The measured pHi values were permanently below 7.1 in the perioperative period. The worst pHi value was 6.6 and PrCO2 97 mmHg. One patient died on the 2nd postoperative day due to primary non-function graft, another died on the 1st postoperative day due to primary poor graft function. One patient died on the 1st day because of insufficiency of circulation.
There is a significant difference in the pHi and PrCO2 values between two groups from the phase of hepatectomy until the postoperative 24th hours.

Conclusion: Regarding to our experiences the application of intramucosal pH measurement in the perioperative period can be a good indicator of the early graft dysfunction, and may help to decide the adequate diagnostic and therapeutic steps.

P 53

ARE REDUCED SERUM LIPIDS IN POSTALCOHOLIC CIRRHOSIS A HIGHER RISK OF NEUROLOGIC EVENTS AFTER LIVER TRANSPLANTATION?

Talaulicar R., Lorf Th., Hanack U., Binder L[1]., Canelo R., Ringe B.
Klinik für Transplantationschirurgie und Klinische Chemie[1] der Georg-August-Universität Göttingen, Germany

Aims: Reduced serum lipids in liver graft recipients may be associated with higher risk for neurologic complications in the postoperative course. Aim of our study was to evaluate the impact of the kind of cirrhosis on serum lipids and the frequency of postoperative neurologic complications.
Methods: 13/83 patients underwent liver transplantation because of postalcoholic cirrhosis, 70/83 because of other diagnoses (posthepatitis B=6, posthepatitis C=21, others=43). Initial immunosuppression consists of cyclosporine A, ATG or BT 563, or tacrolimus and prednisolone. Liver function, cholesterol, triglycerides and neurologic events (pareses, seizures, prolongated respiration therapy, guillain-barré-like syndrom) were monitored before and up to 6 months postoperative.
Results: In the postalcoholic-cirrhosis-group significant reduced serum lipids with 155+/-38,6 (median+/- SD) mg/dl cholesterol vs 243+/- 25,4 mg/dl in the non-postalcoholic-cirrhosis patients, and 95+/-58 vs 189+/-47 mg/dl triglycerides were observed at the time of transplantation. These differences were detected during 3 month. In this period we had to treat severe neurologic complications in 3/13 (23,1 %) postalcoholic-cirrhotic patients vs 3/70 (4,3%) non-postalcoholic-cirrhotic patients.
Conclusions: Liver graft recipients with postalcoholic cirrhosis have significant reduced triglycerides and cholesterol serum levels at time of operation.These patients seems to have a higher risk of neurologic events. Further investigations are necessary to improve the lipid deterioation and to analyse the impact of immunosuppressive regimen on neurologic events.

P 54

SELECTIVE BOWEL DECONTAMINATION VERSUS FIBRE CONTAINING ENTERAL NUTRITION PLUS LACTOBACILLUS OR PLACEBO TO PREVENT BACTERIAL INFECTIONS AFTER LIVER TRANSPLANTATION

N Rayes, S Hansen, AR Müller, G Staffa, WO Bechstein, P Neuhaus
Department of Surgery, Charité, Campus Virchow, Berlin, Germany

Aims: During the last years we used SBD (selective bowel decontamination)to decrease bacterial translocation but it has some disad-vantages like high costs, elimination of the protective gut flora and minor effectiveness for grampositive bacilli. A new concept tries to prevent translocation by feeding enterocytes with fibre and adding lactobacilli. We present preliminary results of a randomised prospective trial comparing the rate of bacterial infections using SBD and a conventional enteral diet with a fibre containing enteral solution plus lactobacillus plantarum or placebo after liver transplantation.
Patients and Methods: Up to now, 45 liver transplant recipients have been enrolled in the study. All patients received enteral nutrition via feeding tube from POD 1 to POD 11 additionally to their normal diet. Urine and stool samples, swabs from the T-drainage, abdominal catheters and wounds were sent regularly to our microbiology institute. Immunosuppression consisted of cyclosporine A and prednisolone (n=27), 24 together with an IL2-receptor antibody (SDZ), 3 with mycophenolate mofetil, or of tacrolimus and prednisolone (n=18). SBD contained tobramycine, amphotericin B and colistin.
Results: *Group 1* (n=15): Pts received SBD from POD 0 to POD 28 and 2 liters of a fibre free enteral diet. In this group 6/15 pts (40 %) had the following infections: cholangitis (n=3), urinary tract infection (n=3), pneumonia (n=1) and wound infection (n=1), Serratia marcescens, enterococci, pseudomonas and staphylococci were isolated from the specimen. The mean hospital stay was 37 days.
Group 2 (n=15): The enteral diet (2 liters per day) contained 1,5g fibre/100 ml. Twice a day lactobacillus plantarum 299 was added through the feeding tube. In one patient each, cholangitis with isolation of E. coli and urinary tract infection with enterococci and pseudomonas was noted (13 %). The mean hospital stay was 31 days.
Group 3 (n=15): The same enteral solution was given as in group 2 but placebo (inactivated lactobacilli) was added. The infection rate was 4/15 (27 %): cholangitis (n=2) and urinary tract infection (n=2). E. coli, streptococci and pseudomonas were isolated. The mean hospital stay was 36 days.
Conclusion: Although the study is still ongoing and numbers are very small, the concept of restoring the normal gut flora instead of eliminating potentially pathogenic bacilli does not increase the rate of bacterial infections after liver transplantation.

P 55

SEVERE PORTAL HYPERTENSION IN LIVER TRANSPLANT CANDIDATES.

Grazi GL, Mazziotti A, Ercolani G, Pierangeli F, Ravaioli M, Quintini C, Cavallari A
Dept of Surgery and Transplantation, Sant'Orsola Hospital, University of Bologna, Bologna, Italy

Severe portal hypertension (SPH), as defined as large oesophageal varices and/or intractable ascites, is a major clinical problem in patients under evaluation for orthotopic liver transplantation (OLT).

Methods: A retrospective study was performed with 202 pt. carrying clinical problems related to SPH out of 546 (38.8%) evaluated for OLT since 1990. There were 143 (70.8%) man and 59 (29.2%) female. Mean age was 48.8 ± 8.9 years (range 20 - 67). Postnecrotic cirrhosis was the leading indication for surgery (131 pt., 64.9%). 129 (63.9%) pt. had large oesophageal varices, 51 (25.2%) massive ascites and 22 (10.9%) both. Forty-two (20.8%) pt. received different treatments: sclerotherapy 24 (11.8%), TIPSS 8 (3.9%), varices binding 5 (2.4%) and surgical shunt 5 (2.4%).

Results: At the time of the study, there were 27 (13.4%) pt. still on evaluation, 120 (59.4%) received OLT while the remaining 55 (27.2%) deceased. Of these latter, 7 (12.7%) died due to uncontrollable bleeding from ruptured oesophageal varices. Among pt. with varices or ascites 28.7% died before OLT, while this figure increased to 52.6% in the group of pt. with both symptoms ($p < 0.05$). After 2 years from the original evaluation, 119 pt. (58.9%) received OLT, 44 died (21.7%) and 23 (11.3%) were still alive. There was an higher rate of deaths among those pt. which did not receive any pre-OLT treatment (33.3% vs. 10.7%, $p < 0.05$). Consequently, a significantly higher rate of OLT was recorded among treated pt. (89.3% vs. 66.7%). Only in 2 cases preoperative therapy gives raise to technical difficulties during OLT: in these pt. TIPSS was displaced in the main trunk of the portal vein and in the inferior vena cava respectively.

Conclusions: SPH still represents a major clinical problem for pt. evaluated for OLT: it enforces the establishment of a very strict clinical and endoscopic follow-up. The presence of both large varices and massive ascites represents a significant risk factor for death during the period before OLT. During the first 2 years after evaluation, pt. that for any reasons received treatment for SPH have greater chance to undergo OLT. Treatment should be considered for the high risk group of pt. with both ascites and varices.

P 56

IMPORTANCE OF RADIOLOGICAL AND SURGICAL TREATMENT OF RUPTURED PSEUDOANEURYSM FOLLOWING NECROTISING PANCREATITIS. (CASE REPORT)

A. Paszt, Gy. Farkas, E. Nagy

Albert Szent-Györgyi Med. Univ., Szeged, Hungary

Aims: The pesudoaneurysm of different abdominal arterys is rare complication of necrotising pancreatitis or pseudocyst. The clinical symptoms, US and CT scan can suggest this serious complication.

Methods: We can report a 44 years old male patient, who had ruptured pseudoaneurysm of mesenteric artery following necrotising pancreatitis. The diagnosis was confirmed by US, contrast enhanced CT scan and select angiography. The first intervention was the special non-operativ radiological procedures (occlusion of pseudoaneurysm). Six weeks later surgical procedure was performed: cysto-Wirsungo-jejunostomy.

Results: The postoperative course was uneventful, no rebleeding was noticed.

Conclusions: CT scan and select angiography is mandatory to achive correct preoperative diagnosis. Nowdays the presence of a pseudoaneurysm is not itself an indication for surgical treatment. Treatment should be special non-operarative radiological intervention and occasionly if it necessary in the second step surgical therapy is advisable.

P 57

PERCUTANEOUS ETHANOL INJECTION THERAPY (PEIT) OF LIVER MALIGNANCIES

***P.G.Tarazov**, V.N.Polysalov, N.V.Oleshchuk*
Sr.Petersburg Research Institute of Roentgenology, St.Petersburg, Russia

Purpose. To evaluate results of PEIT in primary and metastatic liver cancer.
Materials and Methods. Between 1992 and 1997, PEIT was performed in 20 patients aged 32-80 years. Of them, 4 had hepatocellular carcinoma (HCC) and 16 liver metastases from colorectal cancer (9), carcinoid tumor and gastric carcinoma (2 each), tumor of the breast, oral cavity, and corpus uteri (1 each). All patients had 3 to 6 tumor nodules of 1 to 6 cm diameter in both lobes of the liver. We performed PEIT sessions one or two times a week using 96% ethanol and US guidance. The treatment was repeated when tumor recurrence was detected and was stopped when recurrent tumor was inaccessible for image-guided punction. Prior to PEIT, all patients except two received transcatheter hepatic artery chemoembolization (TACE) with 30-80 mg doxorubicin-in-Lipiodol and gelatin sponge.
Results. The following CT and US showed an excellent local effect of PEIT in 18 of 20 patients. No recurrence of tumors underwent PEIT was detected. However, recurrence of the tumor in other liver segments or other organs developed in 5 to 12 mo after the treatment. Of 4 patients with HCC, one is alive for 14 mo, and three died in 24, 30, and 42 mo after the beginning of treatment. The patient with carcinoid liver metastases is alive for 10 years. Of the remaining 15 patients with liver metastases, 4 are alive in 10 to 14 mo, and 11 died from tumor progression in 5-23 (mean 10 ± 5) mo. These results were very close to that after TACE.
Conclusion. In our group, PEIT was effective in unresectable HCC < 5 cm diameter. In liver metastasis, unlike complete tumor necrosis, PEIT did not prevent following tumor progression in the liver or other organs and is why does not improve the survival of patients.

P 58

METASTASES IN A LIVER AND PREVENTION OF COLOSTOMA

Sulyma Volodymyr, Ukraine

Aims: The requirements to increase of quality life after treatment in modern medicine have also relation to the patient by Rectum Cancer, with which the formation of permanent colostoma is planned in connection with non-operattive of a tumour or presence metastatic of the centers in a liver. The prevention of formation of a various kind of permanent colostoma at the patients with metastases in a liver with Rectum Cancer was studied in this work.
Methods: Carried out by us of the ANTICOLOSTOMA® *International Medical Programme* includes various aspects of interaction of the surgeons-proctologists, gastroenterologists, oncologists by development of techniques of the prevention of formation permanent of colostoma, including at the patients with a Rectum Cancer with inoperable of metastases in a liver. The technique, offered us, consists of local introduction in a layer at a tumour of the photo-sensibilizer haemoporphirin of a line with the subsequent influence He-Ne low level laser radiation on the tumour and realization of operation of „stool drain" of a tumour by an elektroknife. In postopration a period the realization y-beam and chemical therapy in possible.
Results: Performance of the offered technique of treatment of the patients with a Rectum Cancer, at which available of metastases in a liver do not allow to carry out radical surgical intervention, will warm formation of palliative of the permanent colostoma, will restore progress stool by a natural way, and also will allow to lower of intocsication influence of the left tumour or its parts - will be a long of the life a patients..
Conclusions: The anticolostoma® *International Medical Programme* part, submitted by us, which allows to warn formation of the permanent of colostoma at patients with a Rectum Cancer, with which inoperable of metastases in a liver interferes with peerformance of radical operation, shows, that co-operation of the doctors of different specialities and development of new techniques of treatment, promote not only prolongation of life the patient oncological of a structure, and keep or even raise, in some cases, quality of life of such patients after treatment. Is considered, the ANTICOLOSTOMA®*Inteernational Medical Programme* and, its component, technique of treatment of the patients with of metastases in a liver for the prevention of formation of the permanent colostoma should actively be used by the doctors at the patients of the given category.

P 59

TREATMENT OF THE SINHRONOUS HEPATIC COLO-RECTAL METASTASIS

Milosevic Z., Milosevic K., Cvijanovic R., Zoricic D.

Clinical Center Novi Sad, Institute for Surgery, Clinic for Abdominal and Endocrine Surgery, Novi Sad, Yugoslavia

Aims: Purpose was to establish algorithms of the synchronous colorectal hepatic metastases treatment.
Methods: From 1990-1998 at our Clinic there was 28 patients operated on from colo-rectal carcinoma who had hepatic metastases simultaneously. Treatment of hepatic metastases depended on intraoperative surgical judgment. Postoperative findings compared with preoperative findings of the US and CT showed lack of the latter – in sense of presence, localization, or number of metastases.
Results: Number of the revealed metastases at operated patients were 1-6, while in 4 patients there was diffuse involvement of the right (3), or left (1) hepatic lobe. Two patients had peritoneal carcinosis. Treatment depended on few factors: 1. Local status of the primary colorectal carcinoma; 2. Presence of the extrahepatic spreading of the carcinoma; 3. Number, size and localization of the hepatic metastases; 4. Experience of the surgeon in hepatic surgery. If intraoperative surgical estimation was that there is condition for metastasis elimination during primary operation (1-2 metastases, locally surgical curable colorectal tumor, absence of the extrahepatic spreading) resection methods was done: wedge resection, segmentectomy, bisegmentectomy. If metastasis elimination demanded larger procedure (lobectomy, hepatectomy) operation effected one month after primary operation. If simultaneous operation was impossible because of the size and localization of the metastases, patients was treated by chemotherapy protocol and after that if there is reduction of the metastasis and there is no evidence of the extrahepatic spreading, patient was consider for operation.
Conclusions: Final decision on manner and extension of the synchronous hepatic metastasis of colo-rectal carcinoma lies on surgeon who depends on intraoperative findings and overall situation.

P 60

RESULTS OF RADICAL OPERATIONS IN PATIENTS WITH LIVER METASTASES

V. Vishnevski , A. Chzhao , R. Ikramov, N.Nazarenko

Institute of surgery , Moscow , Russia .

Aims: Analyzing long term results after operations for liver metastases (MTS)
Methods: 100 (M= 50, F=50) pts were operated for liver metastases (37 major and 63 minor resections) In 2 pts right hepatectomy was performed in one month after portal embolization
Results: Postoperative mortality was 8%. The 1-,3- and 5 yr. actuarial survival was 79.5%, 53.0%, and 41.7% respectively. Factors significantly favoured survival included : male sex, < 3 MTS lesions, high level of differenciation of the primary . Pts. age, time of diagnosis of MTS, size of MTS lesions, location of MTS (in right or left lobe) and extent of liver resection did not significantly affect pt. survival. The best results were observed in pts with carcinoid (3) and colorectal metastatic tumors (94).
Conclusion : Liver resection approves in cases of colorectal and carcinoid metastatic tumors.

P 61

COMBINED RADIOLOGICAL TRETMENT OF INOPERABLE RECTAL TUMORS AND THEIR LIVER METASTASES

Z. Vigváry, Zs. Tarján, E. Makó, H Galgóczy, Dept. of Radiology Semmelweis Univ. Budapest, Hungary

Aims: To asses the alternative interventional treatment results for rectal tumours and liver metastases.

Methods: sixty-one patients with inoperable lumen restricting rectal tumours, were treated with the combination of selective (ADM and/or MMC + Gelaspon) chemoembolisation, intraluminal cryotherapy and LDR Cs-137 irradiation. The catheter was placed into the superior rectal artery or into the hypogastric arteries. In 29 pts having liver metastases additional selective hepatic artery chemoembolisation was performed in altogether 55 cycles. For response assessment rectal and abdominal US and CT examinations were carried out. Survival times and quality of life were assessed.

Results:

I. Rectal tumours: acute bleedings were stopped and tumour volume was reduced in all cases. CR: 0, PR: 36, MR : 23, P: 2.

II. Multiple liver metastases (n=29): CR: 0. PR, 13, MR: 12. P: 4.

Conclusions: Combined chemoembolisation, intraluminal cryotherapy and LDR Cs-137 after-loading interventional radiological treatment proved to be efficient as palliative treatment in inoperable rectall tumours and their hepatic metastases.

P 62

CLINICAL OUTCOME OF LOCAL LIPIODOL CHEMO-EMBOLISATION IN LIVER MALIGNANCIES

András Cs., Csiki Z., Szűcs Zs., Takács I. and Péter M.
3rd. Department of Internal Medicine, Department of Radiology, 2nd Department of Surgery, Debrecen Medical University, Hungary

Aims: Regional intrahepatic chemoembolisation therapy may be beneficial for selected subgroup of patients with liver metastasis and primary liver tumor. Our therapeutic goal was the improvement of the overal patient survival, of the life quality and if possible the achievment of operability.
Methods: 20 patients treated between 1996 and 1998 using local lipiodol chemoembolisation were evaluated. After the selective catheterisation of the hepatic artery 1000 mg 5-FU, 20-50 mg Doxorubicine, 8 mg Mitomycin-C suspended in 4-10 ml Lipiodol Ultrafluid was injected. The treatments were repeated after every 4-6 weeks. The biological parameters (liver function, blood count, serum bilirubine, tumor markers - CA 19-9, CEA, AFP) and patient subjective status were continuously monitorized.
Results: 10 patients had primary liver carcinoma, in 10 patients the primary tumor was: 1 stomach, 2 rectum, 4 colon, 1 lung, 1 pancreas, 1 gallbladder. 18 patients were staged Child class A, 2 patients Child class B. Partial tumor response was seen 4 patients (20%), stabil disease was achieved in 10 patients (50%), progression in 6 patients (30%). Side effects observed: 1 transient cholangio-hepatitis, 1 gastritis, 34 occasions of abdominal dyscomfort, hematemesis, vomiting grade I-II.
Conclusions: in well selected cases of primary and secondary liver cancers the lipiodol chemoembolisation is a well tolerated, low side effect intervention which leads to mild improvement in the patient's life quality and offers temporary disease control.

P 63

METASTATIC LEIOMYOSARCOMA IN LIVER CASE REEPORT AND LITERATURE REVIEW

Crema,E; Lupinacci, R.A.; Farah,F.; Meneses, A .C.O.; Marçal, M.V.L..; Junqueira.,V.C.N. Department of Digestive Surgery of Federal School of Medicine of Triângulo Mineiro, Uberaba – MG, Brazil.

Malign tumors of small bowel are rare constituting about 3% of all malign neoplasms in the digestive tract, and less frequently involving the ileum. Among them the most common are the gastrointestinal stroma tumors (leiomyosarcomas), however no ganglion or hepatic metastases have been found.
We report a case of leiomyosarcoma with metastasis to liver and mesoileum ganglia ten years following ileum resection. The patient was a 24-years-old female with past history of mild abdominal pain, in the right hypochondrium. She had undergone enterectomy due to "benign tumor of the small bowel. During clinical assessment it was found a non-painful palpable mass in the liver right lobe. US and CT showed a great solid cystic tumor in the liver right lobe. The patient underwent laparotomy through right subcostal incision aiming hepatectomy, and 3 ganglion masses were found, the largest being 7.0 x 5.0 x 2.5cm, in the mesoileum. Deep-frozen anatomopathologic study of the masses showed metastatic adenocarcinoma and that of the hepatic lesion depicted hepatic cyst.
Because of these results, hepatectomy was not performed. Nevertheless after staining and special techniques it was proved that the ganglion masses and the solid cystic lesion wall were gastrointestinal stroma tumors (leiomyosarcoma). Then the patient underwent right lobe hepatectomy through bi-subcostal incision and widened by a right thoraco-freno-laparotomy.
Outcome was uneventful, the patient being discharged 9 days after the surgery. Clinical assessment, US, CT and laboratory exams have been normal for 23 months. Although CT findings of tumoral mass with extensive necrosis or cystic changes are non-specific, the surgeon should consider diagnosis of leiomyosarcoma.
Primary tumors of gastrointestinal stroma are uncommon and its metastatic spreading to liver and ganglion have not been reported in the literature to our knowledge. Surgical resection of these lesions extends the patient survival.

P 64

A NEW CONCEPT REGARDING IMPLICATIONS OF CARBONIC ANHYDRASE II AND IV IN THE MECHANISM OF ACTION OF INTERFERON α-2b, USED AS THERAPY IN THE PROLIFERATIVE PROCESSES.

I.Matyas, Nicolita Mayas, Carmen Puscas*, I.Herea*, M.Mihăescu** The County Hospital Simleu Silvaniei, *Center for Research & Medical Assistance, Simleu Silvaniei, **The County Hospital Zalau,Romania.

Interferons are glycoproteins that have a variety of biological actions; they are potent cytokines that posses complex antiviral, immuno-modulating and antiproliferative effects. Endogenous production and release of interferon occur in response to viruses, especially and other inducers, including bacterial exotoxins, polyanions, certain low-molecular-weight compounds and microorganisms capable of intracellular growth. Our research have proved that anticarcinogenic substances increase carbonic anhydrase (CA) II activity (*D.D.W., San Francisco, 1996, A579)*, while those cancerigenic ones decrease it (*D.D.W., San Diego, A912, 1995*). **AIM:** Having known the antiproliferative properties of interferon (INF) α-2b we followed-up its effect on CA II and CA IV, *in vitro* and *in vivo*, in animals and in humans. **MATERIAL AND METHOD:** *In vitro*, we followed INF α-2b effect on purified CA I, II and IV, between 10^{-9}-10^{-6} M, according to dose-response relationship. *In vivo*, we performed an acut experiment on two groups: Gr.1(N=27) - chronic hepatitis B volunteers, who received 3 million I.U. INF α-2b; Gr.2(N=29) - rabbits, which received 600.000 I.U. INF α-2b. Erythrocyte CA II was assessed before and 2 hours after a single i.v. dose of INF α-2b perfusion. CA activity was determined by stopped-flow method (*Khalifah, 1971*) using a rapid kinetic apparatus HI-TECH (England). Rabbit hepatic cells CA IV was isolated by Maren technique (1993). **RESULTS:**

In vitro	10^{-8} M	10^{-6} M	*In vivo*: Human	Rabbits
CA II	94%	182%	174%	191%
CA IV	89%	168%	-	184%

DISCUSSION AND CONCLUSIONS: INF α-2b activates cytosol CA II and membrane CA IV while it seems to not modify significantly CA I activity. The results suggest that pH changes produced by membrane CA IV activation would contribute to INF α-2b binding to its specific membrane receptor, followed by information transmission within the cell. Cytosol CA II activation might be needed for information transmitting to effector. Intracellular pH changes induced by the very strong CA II activation could be involved in the INF α-2b immuno-modulating effect in chronic hepatitis and in its antiproliferative effects.

P 65

ERCP FINDINGS IN PATIENTS WITH CHRONIC ALCHOCOLIC PANCREATITIS

Nagorni A, Mitrovic D, Jeremic M, Pejcic V, Petrovic-Nagorni S, Benedeto-Stojanov D, Popovic N, Radovanovic B, Stojanovic M, Raicevic-Sibinovic S
Clinic for gastroenterology and hepatology and Clinic for surgery Clinical Centre Nis, Clinic for digestive disease Clinical Centre Serbia, Belgrade

Aims: The aim of our study was to evaluate findings of endoscopic retrograde cholangio-pancreatography (ERCP) in patients with chronic alchocol consumption.

Methods: After laboratory and ultrasound examinations of patients with chronic alchocol abuse, duodenoscopy with side view endoscope and canulation of papilla of Vateri with contrast injection was done in all patients. Findings of pancreatic ducts morphology were classified according to Cambridge classification.

Results: There were 56 patients (40 males and 16 females, aged 25-67 years, mean age 47,8 years). In 20 (35,7%) patients Wirsung duct was unchanged with changes in less than a three side branches (equivocal changes). Mild ductular changes, three or more side branches are altered, the main duct is normal, were found in in 18 (32,2%) patients. Moderate ductular changes (three or more side branches are alterated with irregularities of the main duct) were obtained in 10 (17,8%) patients, but severe ductular changes were diagnosed in 8 (14,3%) patients (in addition to moderate ductular chaneges, one or more of the following findings: large cavities, obstruction, intraductular filling defect, mild dilatation, or irregularity of the main pancreatic duct).

Conclusions: In patients with chronic alchocol abuse ERCP visuelize pancreatic ductal system with changes in the main pancreatic duct and side branches. More than 60% patiens had at least changes in more than a three side branches with or without changes in the main pancreatic duct. ERCP is important diagnostic method in evaluation of patients with chronic alchocol consumption.

P 66

FREE RADICAL STATE AND TUMOUR MARKERS: COMPARISON EXAMINATIONS IN GASTROINTESTINAL TUMOURS

Szilvás,Á.., Székely, Gy., Blázovics, A[*]
1 st Dept. of Internal Medicine and Gastroenterology, St. János Hospital, 2 nd Dept. of Medicine, Semmelweis University Medical School[*], Budapest, (Hungary)

Aims: The change of free radical state is well known in tumorous processes. The authors examine the radical state and the tumour markers in gastrointestinal malignancies. They try to find which parameters indicate the tumour stage well.

Methods: The authors examined the liver, gallbladder and pancreatic tumorous patients in different stages. The free radical state is characterised by detection of plasma and sera Relative Light Unit (RLU%), and SH levels. For the detection they applied Berthold Lumat's equipment and chemiluminescent method. The results are compared with the tumour parameters (CEA, CA 19-9, AFP, TPA, CA72-4).

Results: The RLU plasma changes from 1,19-47,92 the RLU sera from 11,69-35,38, the SH plasma 0,22-0,33, and the SH sera 0,21-0,35 RLU%. The results were compared to healthy control patients and the data marked the difference between the two groups.

Conclusions: The data show, that the detection of free radical state is a useful parameter for the definition of gastrointestinal tumour-stages. In some cases they indicate the progression of malignant diseases better and earlier than the tumour markers. Sometimes specific markers are not useful in the progressive stage.

P 67

CARCINOID TUMOUR SPREADING: A FOLLOW UP

Szilvás, Á.., Székely, Gy., Sági, S[*]*, Rajnai, V.*[*]*, Szilvási, I.*[**]*., Jakab, F.*[***]
1 st Dept. of Internal Medicine and Gastroenterology, Dept. of Radiology[*] St. János Hospital, Dept. of Radiology, Imre Haynal University of Health Sciences[**], Dept. of Surgery, Uzsoki Municipal Hospital[***], Budapest, (Hungary)

Aims: The authors introduce the possibilities of examinations in a case of carcinoid tumour. From 1990. they followed up the patient, and in different stages used laboratory, ultrasound, angiographic, scintigraphic and three-dimensional ultrasound methods for the diagnosis. The optimal treatment depends on the follow-up strategies.

Methods: The 64 years old man underwent chemoembolisation and partial hepatic resection because of a metastatised carcinoid tumour in 1990. For 6 years he had no symptoms to report. The tumour marker and ultrasound examinations proved the metastatised tumour in 1996. The octreoscan scintigraphy showed a large number of octreotide-receptors in the liver. The authors treated it with a combination of octreotid and interferon.

Results: During the three years period the authors detected the decreased of 5-HIAA level in urine, and the patient'symptoms receded. In the last year beside slight complaints they found sludge in the gallbladder and showed a well circumscribed lesion in the abdomen by ultrasound detection. CT and selective enterography proved the diagnosis of new metastasis surrounded by bowels. Surgical treatment beside the pharmacological therapy dissolved the complaints.

Conclusions: The authors showed by a case demonstration the importance of the follow up strategy. Right examination methods can help choose the therapy in the metastatised cases too.

P 68

THE INFLUENCE OF HEPATOPANCREATOBILIARY PATHOLOGY ON THE TOLERANCE OF ANTIHELICOBACTERIAL THERAPY

Vyortkin A.L., Bezborodniy S.D., Masharova A.A., Barmina A.A.
Moscow Medical Institute, Moscow, Russia

15 patients with ulcer associated with Helicobacter pylor (H.p.) and the concomitant pathology of hepatopancreatobiliary system were under examination. 10 cases were diagnosed as cholelithiasis and chronic cholecystitis, 3 cases as chronic pancreatitis with the alcohol history and 2 cases as chronic hepatitis in the phase of remission. The control group was comprised of 15 patients without any concomitant pathology. The Helicobacter pylor diagnostics was carried out on the basis of 13C urea breath tests and histological tests. All the patients were administered a triple therapy with ranitidin (150 mg twice in 24 hours), metronidazol (250 mg four times in 24 hours) and cyproflocsacyn (20 mg once in 24 hours). The maximum concentration of ranitidin and cyproflocsacyn in the blood was evaluated during the first 4 days of treatment, the evaluation was done on the automatic analyser of drugs concentrations - REMEDi HS Drug Profiling System (Bio-Rad, USA).

The concentration of ranitidin and cyproflocsacyn in cases of the concomitant pathology manifested the significant increase from the first test to the fourth one and came to 0,129+/-0,4 - 0,865+/- 0,8 accordingly for ranitidin, and 2,4+/-0,05 - 10,2+/-0,3 mkg/ml for cyproflocsacyn ($p<0,1$). On the 5th-7th day of treatment the side effects like dyspepsia, anorexia, diarrhea developed in 6 cases and in 4 cases antibiotics treatment had to be given up. At the same time, the concentration of ranitidin and cyproflocsacyn in cases without any concomitant pathology did not significantly change in the process of treatment and came to 0,140+/- 0,6 - 0,328+/- mkg/ml for ranitidin and 1,9+/-0,07 - 3,4+/-0,04 mkg/ml for cyproflocsacyn ($p>0,1$). All the patients from the control group tolerated the treatment well and no side effects were registered in these cases.

Thus, the concomitant pathology of the hepatopancreatobiliary system aggravates the tolerance of antihelicobacterial therapy due to the disturbance of hepatic metabolism of anti-ulcer drugs which leads to the increase of their concentration in the blood and the development of side effects.

P 69

DISPOSITION OF THE TIP OF THE HEPATIC ARTERY CANULE INTO THE LUMEN OF THE DUODENUM

Lukovich P.[1], Kupcsulik P.[1], Papp A.[1], Kiss K.[2], Sipos B[3]

[1]1st Dept. of Surgery, [2]Dept. of Radiology, [3]Dept. of Pathology Semmelweis Medical University of Medicine, Budapest, Hungary

58 years old male was admitted in our department 4 months after resection of the VI. segment of the liver and an implantation of the hepatic artery canule into the superior pancreatico-duodenal artery because of primary hepatocellular carcinoma. Endoscopic examination of the upper GI tract , which was made owing to abdominal discomfort appearing after the 2nd postoperative chemotherapy, have found the tip of the hepatic artery canule into the lumen of the duodenum. Stomach contrast X-ray showed a 3x3 cm diameter additional filling at the head of the pancreas. Bacause of the patient's poor general condition we only remove the canule from a small incision of the skin without exploration of the abdominal cavity. But on the 7th day massive gastrointestinal bleeding started, therefore we reoperated the patients. We have found extensive necrosis at the head of the pancreas, with particularly necrotized wall of the portal vein at the bottom of the cavity. There were no any possibility for any reconstruction, we could only close the surrounding tissue over the cavity with gasto-jejunostomy after closing the antrum of the stomach. The postoperative period except of 3 days of transient and idiopathic confusing of the consciusness of the patient was uneventful. The patient 2 months after the last operation is without any complains and sign of the bleeding of the GI tract.

P 70

ENKEPHALINERGIC MODIFICATION PHENOMENON OF MACROMOLECULAR STRUCTURE FOR PANCREACYTES SECRETORY PROTEINS.

G.M.Mogilnaya, A.N.Kurzanov
Republic Centre of Functional Surgical Gastroenterology, Krasnodar,Russia

The mechanisms of previously founded effect of inhibition for pancreatic exosecretion under leu-enkephalin influence have been studied in dogs. All experiments were carried out in conformity with "Guiding Principles in the Care and Use of Animals" of American Physiology Society.
Leu-enkephalin was intramuscularly injected in dose 50 mkg/kg body weight three times a day during 7 days. The pieces of pancreatic tissue were fixed in Hamperl solution , embedded in paraffine wax and then examined. The control samples were taken from intact animals and prepared in the same fashion.
Cytochemical study for determination of total protein in sections stained according to Danielli, cationic protein (stained with bromphenol blue at pH 8,2), bisulphide groups of cysteine, amino acid residues of lysine,arginine,histidine was performed.
Histochemical investigation of distributive character of protein-containing biopolymers in exosecretory pancreatic cells after leu-enkephalin injection revealed that distribution of total protein in experimental conditions hadn't any differences from control group. However, these cells had another level of cationic protein content. There was cationic protein accumulation in apical portion of pancreacytes. It can be the feature of synthesis increasing or mucus extrusion decreasing. However, the evaluation of nature of cationic proteins produced by pancreacytes allowed to establish high content of amino acid residues of histidine and poor content of amino acid residues of lysine in these proteins. There were also amino acid residues of arginine in cationic protein. It is interesting to note that the level of cationic protein content was changed when peptide was injected, but not at protein's with high histidine content expense. It is likely that the character of protein's cationic charge changed first when enkephalin was injected.
The data obtained witnessed that leu-enkephalin injection affected not at synthesis and extrusion rate of secretory pancreacytes product but at its macromolecular structure. It leads to release of marked quantities of cationic groups with high screening properties: The character of bisulphide cysteine groups distribution confirmed the phenomenon of modification for zimogenic granules macromolecules. Arising of bisulphide groups quantities pointed to zimogen macromolecules stabilization that can lead to reducing of their fermentative activity.

P 71

HUMAN PANCREATIC LEIOMYOSARCOMA (PZX-7) GROWING AS A SERIALLY TRANSPLANTABLE XENOGRAFT IN IMMUNOSUPPRESSED MICE

Zalatnai, A., Bocsi, J., Csákány, T., Fekete, T., Lásztity, J.
First Institute of Pathology & Experimental Cancer Research, Semmelweis University of Medicine, Budapest, HUNGARY

Aims: Several human leiomyosarcoma xenografts are available in the literature but pancreatic smooth muscle sarcomas have never been serially transplanted and investigated. We have established a morphologically and biologically stable leiomyosarcoma line derived from a primary pancreatic tumor.
Methods: Immunosuppression on CBA/CA mice was achieved by thymectomy, whole-body irradiation and bone marrow reconstruction. Tumor fragments were subcutaneously implanted from a Grade III pancreatic leiomyosarcoma and serially passaged for more than 24 months. The xenografted tumors were characterized by morphological, morphometrical, biochemical and flow cytometric methods.
Results: The tumor has retained its original characteristic morphology and no further differentiation occurred. The mitotic counts, the amount of the connective tissue all remained constant. The calculated volume doubling time was 11.3 days. The DNA index and the proliferation indexes did not change significantly with the time (mean D.I.: 1.65, range: 1.561 - 1.70; mean P.I.: 17.9 %, range: 15.3 - 20.7 %). LDH-isoenzyme electrophoresis evidenced a retained human pattern of the tumor even after 2 years of transplantations.
Conclusions: The first human pancreatic leiomyosarcoma xenograft (PZX-7) growing in immunosuppressed mice is described and characterized.

P 72

FLOW CYTOMETRIC EVIDENCE OF APOPTOSIS IN PANCREATIC CARCINOMA XENOGRAFTS BY OCTREOTIDE (SANDOSTATIN)

Bocsi J., Zalatnai, A.,
First Institute of Pathology and Experimental Cancer Research, Semmelweis University of Medicine, Budapest Hungary,

Aims: Sandostatin (a synthetic analog of somatostatin) is an approved hormone for treatment of gastro-entero-pancreatic neuroendocrine tumors, however, pancreatic adenocarcinomas have rarely been treated with this drug. Earlier studies indicated a moderate beneficial effect (alone or in combination with tamoxifen) in these patients, however, the exact mode of action is not known. Our aim was to evaluate the apoptosis-inducing effect of Sandostatin in a human pancreatic carcinoma xenograft (PZX-5) by means of flow cytometry.
Methods: Experiments were performed on a newly established, well--characterized PZX-5 human pancreatic carcinoma growing in immunosuppressed mice (Int J Pancreatol., 23, 51, 1998.). Animals were treated by 500 μg/kg b.w. Sandostatin i.p. twice a day. After four weeks they were sacrificed and tumours were processed for histologic and flow cytometric studies. Morphologically, the histologic signs of regression and the mitotic count were evaluated, and the apoptosis was assessed by flow cytometric DNA content measurements on cell nuclei suspension (Becton Dickinson - FACStar). The rationale of this method is that the apoptotic cells display a so called sub G_1 population on DNA histogram.
Results: Nine controls and eighteen Sandostatin treated PZX-5 xenografts were studied. In the treatment group regressive histological signs were seen in 10 of 18 tumors (56 %). The mitotic counts (number of mitotic figures per square mm) proved to be unchanged in these animals (18.8 ± 4.4 vs. 16.1 ± 6.3), however, the apoptotic ratio measured by flow cytometry has doubled (3.6 ± 1.3 % vs. 7.2 ± 2.2 %, $p < 0{,}001$).
Conclusions: These data reinforce the earlier observations that Sandostatin may induce a tumor-inhibiting action on ductal pancreatic adenocarcinoma and its effect is mediated by accelerating the process of apoptotic cell loss.

P 73

ISOLATION OF ISLERS OF LANGERHANS BY DIGESTION OF PANCREATIC TISSUE WITH COLLAGENASE TYPE V. EXPERIMENTAL STUDY IN DOGS

Waisberg, J., Bromberg, S.H., Concalves, J.E., Zanotto, A., Speranzini, M.B.
Faculdade de Medicina do ABC - Santo André

Aims: The autotransplantation of Langerhans is a methode used in the prevention, correction or diminuition of pancreatic diabetes. One of the critical points for the success of this event is the separation's method and the enrichmen of the pancreatic islets tissue.

Methods: In order to research the action of collagenase 23 dog's pancreas were obtained by total pancreatectomy.After properly prepared, they were incubated with collagenase type V, at the dosage of 600 units/gram of pancreatic tissue. It was also gathered a control group of 15 dogs on which we used the same methodology, but we didn't use the enzyme.

Results: The results disclosed that the insulin content of pancreatic tissue was bigger and the amtlase content of pancreatic tissue was smaller on the pancreatic tissues treated with collagenase. The counting of histological items showed that the pancreatic tissue treated with collagenase had a smaller content of collagenous tissue (p 0,0001) and greater content of endocrine tissue (p 0,0001).

Conclusions: We concluded that the preparstion of pancreatic tissue with collagenase increases the endocrine tissue concentration, causing the islets to keep more isolated from the remaining pancreatic parenchyma. Moreover the diminuition of the amylase content of pancreatic tissue as well as of the other pancreatic exocrine ferments, by analogy, would reduce the effective action of the pancreatic exocrine secretion upon the islets. These results recommend an accurate action of collagenase type V in the isolation and concentration of pancreatic islets.

P 74

CARCINOEMBRYONIC ANTIGEN LEVELS IN GALLBLADER BILE OF PATIENT WITH COLORECTAL CANCER: PRELIMINARY RESULTS

Bromberg, S.H., Waisberg, J., Pradal, M.G., Menezes, A.M., Barretto, E. & Godoy
Hospital ab Seervidor Punlico Estadual - Sao Paolo, Brazil

Aims: The autoshave studied the carcinoembryonic antigen (CEA) levels in the gallbladder bile of patients with colorectal adenocarcinoma and other 10 patients with cholelthiasis without acute inflamatory conditions evidence of biliary obstruction.

Methods: The gallbladder bile samples were obtained during operation by gallbladder funds puncture. The CEA levels in serum and in the gallbladder bile were assayed using solid phase, two-side fluoroimmunometric method base on the direct sandwich technique with two monoclonal antibodies.

Results: In 13 cases with no evidence of liver metastases, the mean serum CEA level was 6.08 ng(ml (1.0 to 22.8 ng(ml), the mean CEA level in gallbladder bile reached 101.43 ng/ml (0.2 to 571 ng/ml). In three with liver metastases the mean serum CEA level was 44.6 ng/ml (37.5 a 51.3 ng/ml), the mean CEA level in gallbladder bile reached 13.811 ng/ml (9.230 to 17,520 ng/ml). In patients with cholelithiasis, the mean serum CEA level was 1.94 ng/ml (1.0 to 3.2 ng/ml), the mean CEA level in gallbladder bile was 1.25 ng/ml (0.3 to 2.9 ng/ml).

Conclusions: These findings suggest that patients with clorectaladenocarcinoma, who lack evidence of distant metastases of the time of primary colorectal resection, but who do have increased CEA level in gallbladder bile, should be followed with specific attention for the future appearance of hepatic metastases.

P 75

CARBONIC ANHYDRASE INVOLVEMENT IN THE GLUCAGON AND INSULIN MECHANISM OF ACTION.

Carmen Puscas, I.Herea, Nicolita Mayas*, I.Matyas*, Ioana Mihăescu**
Center for Research & Medical Assistance, Simleu Silvaniei, *The County Hospital Simleu Silvaniei, **The County Hospital Zalau,Romania.

Glucagon (Glucag) is one of the most important hyperglycemia-induce hormone secreted by pancreatic A cells which antagonizes the insulin-induced hypoglicemia effects. The receptors existence for these two hormones was described. The main glucagon mollecular mechanism of action known so far consists in adenilat cyclase activation with consecutive rising of intracellular cAMP levels. **AIM:** We studied the relationship between glucagon and carbonic anhydrase (CA), as well as the insulin effect upon this association. **METHOD:** *In vitro*, we followed-up the effect of glucagon alone and associated to insulin upon purified CA II and on pig pancreatic membrane cell CA IV. Assessments have been performed using the dose-response relationship, at concentrations between 10^{10}-10^{-5} M. In *vivo*, we selected 32 male healthy volunteers, who received a single i.v. dose of 1 mg glucagon. For 2 hours they have been monitorized and to every 10 minutes erythrocyte CA II activity and glycemia values were measured. CA activity was assessed by stopped-flow method (Khalifah,1971), using a HI-TECH apparatus (England). **RESULTS**:

IN VITRO	Glucag 10^{-5} M	Glucag+ Insulin 10^{-5} M	*IN VIVO*	CA II (EU/ml)	Glycemia (mg/dl)
			Before Glucag	1.016±0.2	78 ± 12
CA II	155 %	63 %	After 20 '	2.330±0.3	224 ± 19
CA IV	138 %	54 %	After 120'	1.010±0.1	71 ± 14

DISCUSSION AND CONCLUSIONS: Our in vitro results prove that glucagon powerfully activates CA II and CA IV after dose-response relationship and this activating effect is antagonized by insulin. In vivo, the strong and significant CA II activation glucagon-induced in humans is paralel with glycemia increase, and the return of glycemia to normal values is also paralel with the falling of enzyme activity to initial values. Our findings prove that glucagon activates not only adenilat cyclase but also CA by a direct mechanism of action. These data suggest that glucagon-induced pancreatic membrane CA IV activation produces pH changes that favourize information transmission within the cell. These effects are antagonized by insulin. The same pH changes induced by CA II activation (a cytosol enzyme) may contribute both to hormone signal transduction into the cell, as well as to adenilat cyclase activation, known as a pH-dependent enzyme. Our results also prove that glucagon acts dually, meaning on its specific receptor and also on CA, enzyme functionally coupled to these receptors.

P 76

DECREASE OF ANTIOXIDANT ENZYMES IN ACUTE BILIRUBINEMIA AND UREMIA WITH RATS

TAN A., ÇELİK T., ÇETİNER S., YAKUT M., KAYMAKÇIOĞLU N., TUFAN T.
Gülhane Military Medical Academy, General Surgery
Ankara – TURKEY

Aims: To examine whether acute liver failure, uremia and bilirubinemia influence the status of the oxidant-antioxidants systems.

Methods: We investigated the erythrocyte cooper zinc superoxide dismutase (CuZn SOD) and selenium dependent glutathione peroxidase (Se GSH-Px) activity in the animal model. Sprague–Dawley Rats were divided into four groups, 20 rats in each. Bilirubinemia was performed with common bile duct ligation and resection as Acute Cholestasis (AC) model in group I . Uremia was perormed with ureter ligation and resection as Acute Uremia (AU) model in group II. The model of Acute Liver Failure (ALF) was induced by thioacetamide in group III. In SHAM group, laparotomy was performed without ligation and resection The results were compared with control group.

Results: The erythrocyte Cu, Zn SOD activity was found significantly higher in ALF group than the controls but not in bilirubinemia and uremia groups. In these groups it was found significantly lower than the controls. Plasma and erythrocyte levels of GSH-Px activity was decreased in both bilirubinemia and uremia groups while it was normal in ALFI group.

Conclusions: Acute liver failure enhanced the oxidative stress, whereas uremia and bilirubinemia decreased the erythrocyte cooper zinc superoxide dismutase and selenium dependent glutathione peroxidase activities which are the enzymes of antioxidant systems.

P 77

PRO-METASTATIC EFFECTS OF CHEMOTHERAY AGENTS MODULATED BY ADHESION CHANGES IN MODEL ENDOTHELIAL CELLS

K. Seymour, E. O'Flaherty, B.K. Shenton, R.M. Chamley, J.A. Kirby
Department of Surgical and Reproductive Science, Medical School, University of Newcastle upon Tyne

Framlington Place, United Kingdom

Aims: Recent reports of changes in the expression of adhesion molecules on the endothelial cell undergoing apoptosis prompted us to examine the effects on tumour-endothelial cell adhesion under normal conditions and those that promote apoptosis. Of the various methods available, we chose to utilise agents known to induce apoptosis and used in experimental regional chemotherapy, Mitomycin C (MMC) and tumour necrosis factor-L (TNF-L).

Results: At the doses used MMC and TNF-L lead to increased endothelial cell apoptosis compared to normal EC cultures ($p<0.01$and $p=0.04$ respectively). There is no statistically significant difference in the rates of apoptosis with either agent ($p=0.27$). COLO205 cells show significantly increased adhesion to EC exposed either apoptosis stimulant as compared to control medium HT29 cells show reduced binding to apoptopic endothelium. For TNF-L the binding ratio for COLO205 was 1.5 ($p<0.01$), the binding ratio HT29 was 0.5 ($p<0.001$). For MMC the binding ratio for COLO205 was 1.5 ($p<0.01$), the binding ratio for HT29 was 0.8 ($p=0.068$). Similar results are demonstrated for additional doses of MMC used. EC expression of VCAM-1 is significantly up-regulated in response to both TNF-L ($p<0.01$) and MMC ($p<0.01$). EC expression of ICAM-1 is significantly up-regulated by TNF-L ($p<0.01$) but unchanged by MMC. EC exspression of E-selection is not significantly altered with either agent at 24 hours.

Conclusions: We have shown that both TNF-L and the commonly used chemotherapeutic agent MMC induce endothelial apoptosis, furthermore, it is demonstrated that this treatment has profound modulatory effects on the subsequent adhesion of colorectal cancer cells and adhesion molecule expression. Whether this is a pro- or anti-metastatic effect is determined by the phenotype of the tumour cell.

P 79

METABOLIC DISORDERS IN SYNDROME OF ENDOGENIC INTOXICATION ON SEVERE PANCREATITIS

Chooklin S, Perejaslov A, Detsyk Y.
Medical University, Lviv, Ukraine

Aims: Increase of lipid peroxidation and protein nature toxic substances (middlemolecular olygopeptides) obviously influenced on endotoxicosis development.

Methods: Influence of lipid peroxidation products and middle mass molecules on endogenic intoxication on severe acute pancreatitis was studied.

Results: It was noted, that during intoxication increasing and intensifying the pathological processes' severity (purulent-septic complications' development) the quantities of malonic dialdegid, dienic conjugates and middle molecules were increased in blood, on the background of catalase activity decrease. Accumulation of the intermediate and terminal products of free radical oxidation leads to the lysosomas membrane disintegration, right up to its full rupture, activation of the system of complement, what promotes disseminative intravascular coagulation development. These disorders intensify the tissue hypoxia also (increased lactate and pyruvate concentration).

Conclusions: Thus intensification of lipid peroxidation processes and middle mass molecules plays an important role on endotoxicosis during the severe pancreatitis, what, on the background, of obvious depression mechanisms of antioxidant defense can give the process an unreversible character.

P 80

THE ROLE OF CYTOKINES IN DISORDERS OF CIRCULATION ON ACUTE PANCREATITIS

Perejaslov A, Chooklin S, Detsyk Y.
Medical University, Lviv, Ukraine

Aims: Disorders of circulation both systemic and regional are observed on severe acute pancreatitis. In the own turn the, the disturbances of the microcirculation led to the progressing of the pancreatic necrosis extend. The several factors, such as IL-1, IL-8 and TNF, play an important role in the pathogenesis of these disturbances.
Methods: The levels of the IL-1, IL-8 and TNF were studied in 35 patients with acute pancreatitis of the different degree of severity.
Results: Already, on the first day of the disease onset the level of IL-1 increased, particularly in cases of necrotizing pancreatitis. IL-1 stimulates the synthesis of tissue factors of coagulation, platelet activated factor and inhibitor of plasminogen activation. IL-8 is an important neutrophil-activating cytokine and its level increased during the first days of severe pancreatitis also. IL-8 stimulates the neutrophiles, what leads to the intensifying of its adhesive properties, stimulating arachidonic acid metabolic cascade and synthesis platelet activated factor. The increasing levels of all these mediators were observed in all patients. The serum concentrations of TNF were below the level of detection in 29 of 35 patients on the first day of admission Besides the determination of cytokines, the condition of blood circulation on vessels of pancreatic area was studied. The investigations were performed with the help of pulse color doppler (Acuson XL). The disturbances of circulation of various degrees were observed in all patients. The blood speed was increased to 1-1.5 m/s (N<0.6 m/s) in the system of portal vein, what indicates on the vessels compression. The whirlwind flow in vessels was noted also. The similar picture was noted in v.lienalis and v.mesenterica superior.
Conclusions: Applying of the cytokines-antagonists (IL-1ra, pentoxyphillin), antiinflammatory cytokine IL-10 can decrease the negative influence of cytotoxic cytokines, improves the blood rheologic properties and prevents the microthrombosis formation.

P 81

JEJUNAL FEEDING WITH SOMATOSTATIN FOR PLEURAL AND PERITONEAL EFFUSIONS ASSOCIATED WITH ACUTE PANCREATITIS

J. Hamvas, Á. Pap
Gastroenterologia, MAV Hospital, Budapest, Hungary

It is generally accepted that pancreatitis and/or pseudocysts associated with pleural and/or peritoneal effusion is a serious complication indicating surgical intervention with high mortality rate.
We report on two cases of pleural fluid collection caused by pleuroabdominal pancreatic fistula, and two other cases with pancreatic ascites. In all cases diagnoses was based on biochemical analysis of peritoneal and pleural fluids. Extremely high levels of amylase (12000-43000 U/L) and protein (35-44 g/l) indicated pancreatic origin. Four patient were treated with jejunal feeding combined with somatostatin (Sandostatin, Sandoz 50-100 ug, three times a day or Stilamin, Serono 800 ug/day) for 10-21 days. The pleural and peritoneal fluid diminished in every patients, a consecutive drainage and continuous pleural aspiration was necessary in 1 case. In 1 case remaining pancreatic pseudocyst was decompressed surgically and in 1 case the pseudocyst was drained by endoscopic cystoduodenostomy.
Conclusion: pleural and peritoneal effusion associated with acute pancreatitis is a rare but severe complication. A complex intensive therapy is necessary to achieve regression of this entity. Somatostatin alone or in combination with jejunal feeding might play an important role in the favourable outcome of our cases and it can be proposed for treatment of this severe disease.

P 82

DUODENAL INJURIES

Djordjevic R., Kitanovic A., Zajic S.

Surgical Department Health Center Kruševac

This artical presents our expiriences in surgical treatment of duodenum injuries caused by blunt and penetrating abdominal trauma.

Within the period 1988-1997, 9 patients were surgically treated having abdominal trauma and duodenum injuries. Clinical picture analysis elaborated the mechanisms of injuries, diagnostic procedures, the ways of surgical care as well as postoperative complications. In the same period we had 617 patients with abdominal organs injuries.

In 7 patients the injury was caused by blunt and in 2 patients by penetrating abdominal trauma. In only one patient the injury of duodenum was differentiated and all others were associated by the pancreas, mesocolon transversum, stomach, spleen and liver injuries. Injury diagnostic was established during the operation when bile-stained duodenal contents was found and mobilisation of duodenum by Kocher manuver was effected. In 3 patients duodenal lesions were solved by only suture of perforation. Another 2 duodenal lesions were solved by suture with pyloric exclusion and side to side gastrojejunostomy, and in 4 cases injuries were solved by covering of lesion with Roux-en-Y duodenojejunostomy. After the operations decompression with nasogastric tube was usually continued until bowel function return. Five lesions were localised at the second portion, and 5 of them at the third and fourth duodenum portion.

As for postoperative complications we have had 4 wound infections. Average hospitalization used to be 17 days.

Duodenum injuries are rare, but inspection of the whole duodenum is important during the abdominal exploration. We have had the bes results with Roux-en-Y duodenojejunostomy.

P 83

PANCREATIC INJURY

Djordjevic R., Kitanovic A., Zajic S.

Surgical Department Health Center Kruševac

The aim of the article is to present our experience in surgical treatment of trauma to the pancreas due to blunt ant penetrating injury.

In the period from 1989 to 1998 we treated 630 patientes with abdominal trauma. In 8 patients we found injured pancreas (7 males and 1 female). We observed mechanismus of the injury, diagnostical procedures, surgical tereatment, associated other organs injuries and postoperative complications.

All patients in observed group had a blunt abdominal injury. Pancreas trauma was associated with other abdominal organs injuries in all cases (liver, duodenum, vena cava inferior, transversal colon, lien). All patients peroperatively had an US-abdominal scans. In 5 patients we assesed the diagnosis with percutaneous peritoneal lavage. According to Lucas classification of pancreatic injuries (1977) two patients had gradus I pancreatic injury, four patients gradus II and two patients gradus III. Bouth gradus III injuries were without ductal disruption and in one case associated with duodenal injury. After thorough abdominal exploration (Kocher manuver, exposing bursae omentalis/lesser sac cavity), we performed distal pancreatectomy with splenectomy in two cases and exact hemostasis and abdominal drainage in the rest of the patientes. In all cases pancreatic bed drainage was done. Postoperative serum amilase level was assesed. We had no mortality. Avarrige hospital stay was 15 days, and the mean age of the operated patients was 34 years.

Pancreatic injuries are rare, but exact assesment of the traumatized organ is of the outstanding importance in other to perform a right surgical procedure.

P 84

OMENTHAL BURSOSCOPY IN THE MANAGEMENT OF ACUTE NECROTIZING PANCREATITIS

I. Gagauz, G. Ghidirim, E. Gutsu

State University of Medicine and Pharmacy "N. Testemitanu", Department of Surgery "N. Anestiadi", Chisinau, Republic of Moldova

Methods: Four hundred twenty four patients with the difference forms of acute pancreatitis (AP) have been admitted in the City Emergency Hospital of Chisinau during the period 1996-1998. Treatment was started initially with conservative measures in everybody of them. Routine laporoscopy was performed in 74 patients and in 20 patients of them omenthal bursoscopy (OB) was carried out.

Results: On the basis of our own experience indications for OB were considered as follow:

- Disaccordance of laparoscopical "findings" and clinical manifestations of AP.
- Estimation of spreading of the pancreatic tissue lesion.
- Necessity of necrozectomy and drainage of lesser sac.

Various endoscopic operative procedures were performed: laparoscopical omenthal bursoscopy - in 9 cases and "opened" omenthal bursoscopy – in 11 cases. Conversion to "opened" OB is caused by: severe adherent process in gastrocolicum ligament as well as in the lesser sac, in order to debride devitalized tissues and when a scheduled necrozectomies and repeated lesser sac visualization in postoperative period are evident. During OB infected pancreatic necrosis was established in 12 cases (all of these patients underwent surgery), necrotic non-infected pancreatitis – in 5 cases, severe edema of pancreas – in 2 cases and paraneoplastic pancreatitis – in 1 case. After exudate elimination and necrozectomy, operative procedure was finished with external drainage of lesser sac. If the postoperative repeated visualization of lesser sac and scheduled necrozectomies are necessary – omenthal bursostomy was formed.

Conclusions: OB allows to assess objective a spreading of the destructive process in pancreas, to perform a numerous miniinvasive interventions and to decrease a number of early laparotomies in destructive pancreatitis.

P 85

ECHOGRAPHIC CHANGES OF THE PANCREAS IN PATIENTS WITH CHRONIC LIVER DISEASES

Tîrnăveanu Amelita, Lenghel A, Frăţilă O, Drăgan Graţiela, Ţîrlea Felicia, Frăţilă Simona

4th Medical Clinic, University of Oradea, Romania

Aim: **To evaluate the pancreatic sonographic changes in patients with chronic liver diseases.**

Methods: **Our study included 238 patients with chronic liver diseases (69.4% males and 30.6% females) with alcoholic liver - 74 % and viral liver diseases - 26 %. We evaluated: a) sonographic changes of chronic pancreatitis based on alterations of shape, echostructure, Wirsung duct dilatations > 2 mm and visualisation of ther duct over a distance longer than 20 mm, calcifications, cysts; b) urinary amylase > 64 UW and c) blood glucose level > 110 mg/dl.**

Results: **1) echographic changes of the pancreas were found in 65 % of cases: volume-size alterations – 18 %, shape alterations – 7 %, hyperechogenity – 81%, unhomogeneous pancreas – 26 %, dilated Wirsung duct – 46 %, pancreatic calcifications – 1.2 %; 2) echographic changes were found in 50 % of the patients with alcoholic liver steatosis, in 70 % of the cases with chronic alcoholic hepatitis, in 80 % of those with alcoholic cirrhosis; 3) we evidenced changes in 42 % of the cases with viral chronic hepatitis and in in 63% of the cases with viral cirrhosis; 4) urinary amylasis levels were increased in 61 % of the patients and they were related to the hyperechogenic pancreas (60 %), to the unhomogeneous pancreas (13 %), to the dilated Wirsung duct (10 %), to the pancreatic size (9 %) and shape (5 %) changes; 5) diabetes mellitus was detected in 30 % of the patients with pancreatic echographic alterations, as follow: 50 % with hyperechogenic pancreas, 27 % with dilated Wirsung duct, 14 % with unhomogeneous pancreas, 4 % with shape changes, 3 % with calcifications and 3 % of the patients with pancreatic size changes.**

Conclusion: **1. Pancreatic echographic changes in patients with chronic liver diseases are frequent. 2. The dilatation of the Wirsung duct highly suggests the presence of the chronic pancreatitis in 46 % of the chronic liver diseases. 3. The incidence of the chronic pancreatitis associated to the chronic liver diseases increases with the severity of the latter. 4. The pancreatic echographic changes are related to high urinary amylase levels in 61 % of the cases. 5. Diabetes mellitus was found in 30 % of the cases with echographic pancreatic changes and chronic liver disease.**

P 86

SURGICAL TREATMENT OF INFECTED PANCREATIC NECROSIS

Wajda Z., Gruca Z., Reszetow J., Dobosz M.
II Dept. of General, Gastroenterological, Endocrinological Surgery
Medical University of Gdańsk, Poland

We analysed retrospectively 44 cases of infected pancreatic nectosis (IPN).
All the patients (29 male and 15 female) were treated operatively at the I[nd] Dept. of General, Gastroenterological and Endocrinological Surgery, Medical University in Gdańsk, Poland.
The diagnosis of IPN was establised prior to the surgery by means of contrast enhanced computed tomography and fine needle aspirate of the infected pancreatic and peripancreatic tissue. Microbiological findings of infected tissue showed most common E.coli (22 cases) and Klebsiela pneumoniae (13 cases). Candidiasis was observed in 5 cases.
All the patients were stratified according to APACHE II score (2-21 pts, average 12 pts.) within 24 hours after the admission to the ward. Wide surgical exploration of the omental sac and retroperitoneal space, gentle necrosectomy of necrotic tissue and open packing (laparostomy) according to Bradley's technique was carried out within the period of 4-22 days (mean 10 days) from the onset of the disease. Closure of the abdomen was performed within 14-34 days (mean 23) after the primary laparotomy.
Fifteen patients died (mortality rate 34%) during postoperative period due to multisystemic organ failure accompanying septic shock. The most common postoperatively observed complications were : respiratory insufficiency requiring mechanical ventilation (10 cases) colonic fistula (8 cases) and pancreatic fistula (6 cases). Incisional hernia was noticed in 11 patients leaving the hospital. Hospital stay period of the survivors ranged between 26-52 days (mean 36 days).
IPN is still associated with high mortality and morbidity rate. It is correlated with high APACHE II score estimated during the first 24 hours after the admission. Accurate early diagnosis upon - enhanced CT and bacteriological examination of necrotic aspirate together with proper surgical treatment, including wide repeated debridement and laparostomy, in author's opinion is management of choice, and may improve the results of the treatment.

P 87

Pancreatic pseudocysts : Retrospective evaluation of 32 patients treated by surgical intervention

S. Yüceyar, S. Çarkman, S. Ertürk, D. Yıldırım, Y. Kafadar
Istanbul University, Cerrahpaşa Medical Faculty, Department of Surgery, İstanbul, TURKIYE

In This study, records of 32 patients with pancreatic pseudocyst treated by surgical intrevention in Cerrahpaşa Medical Faculty Department of Surgery between December 1989 - December 1998 were reviewed .

Male/ female ratio was 15/17 and age of the patients ranged from 17 to 74 years . Most patients (11 case) were in fourth decade . Abdominal pain was encountered in 26 patients (% 81) . Nausea-vomiting (% 31) and dyspepsia (% 28) were other frequently seen symptoms . Interestingly, in one case , initial clinical sign was upper gastro-intestinal bleeding from an ulcer located on gastric corpus near the pseudocyst. Biliary and alcoholic pancreatitis were found in 18 (%56) cases. In one (%3) patient, etiology was blunt abdominal trauma . In other 13 (% 41) cases , we were not able to detect any primary etiologic factor causing pancreatitis. The main diagnostic imaging studies were abdominal ultrasonography (US) and computed tomography (CT) . US was used in 10 (% 31) and CT in 6 (% 19) cases . In other 16 (% 50) cases , US and CT were used together . Pancreatic resection was made in 7 (% 22) and cysto-digestive anastomosis in 25 (% 78) patients . Among the latter , 14 were cysto-gastrostomy , 10 were cysto-jejunostomy and 1 was cysto-duodenostomy . One patient was died from generalize peritonitis due to anastomotic leakage.

As a conclusion , in pancreatic pseudocyst which may have complications like infection , rupture , bleeding and intestinal obstruction , if spontaneous resolution do not occur surgical treatment must be considered

P 88

HOW TO GET BETTER RESULT IN THE TREATMENT OF ACUTE NECROTIZING PANCREATITIS

Szentkereszty Zs., Kerekes L., Boland MG., Hallay J., Sápy P.
2nd Department of Surgery, University Medical School of Debrecen, Hungary

Aims: The good effects of new methods in the treatment of acute necrotizing pancreatitis were investigated by authors.
Methods: Authors studied the results of treatment in 25 operated patients with acute necrotizing pancreatitis from 1st. January 1997 to 31st. December 1998. During this period in our practice we routinly used prolonged necrectomy with peripancreatic drainage, nasojejunal tube nutrition, epidural canulation and wide spectrum antibiotic therapy e.g. imipenem.
It was necessary to prolonge the first operation with the use of ultrasound guided percutaneus drainage in two cases.
Results: The mean hospital stay was 52,3 days at this very high risk group. Eleven patients had only one operation, six of them had a second operation and four patients had two reoperations. Two patients had four and the other two had five operations respectively. Bleeding due to necrosis occured four times in three patients. We found perforation of the transverse colon in one case.
The mortality rate was 12 %.
Conclusions: The mortality rate can be decreased by
1. prolongation of the first operation,
2. use of wide spectrum antibiotic therapy
3. early use of nasojejunal or catheter jejunal nutrition.

P 89

OUR EXPERIENCE IN THE TREATMENT OF THE SEVERE ACUTE PANCREATITIS AND IT'S COMPLICATIONS

A.Papakonstantinou ,S.Drakopoulos, P.Alfaras, V.Vougas, A.Poultsidi, F. Hadjidimitriou, I.Terzis, C.Stratopoulos, C.Rammos, E.Hadjiyannakis.
1st Surgical Dept –Transplant Unit, Gen Hospital "Evangelismos of Athens", Greece.

Aim: We present our experience in the treatment of severe acute pancreatitis and it's complications.
Methods : During a period of twelve years (1987-1998), 104 patients with severe acute pancreatitis (0,67% from a total number of 15384 patients) treated in our department.
In 69 cases cholelithiasis coexisted (therefor the pancreatitis was characterized as gallstone – associated).
In 9 cases the pancreatitis was alcoholic, in 6 traumatic and in 20 idiopathic or of other origin.
In all cases the treatment was conservative initially. In 89 cases (85,5%) a surgical intervention was required. Of those 89 patients, 62 underwent cholocystectomy, 14 underwent pancreatic drainage and in the last 13 a thorough debridement and peritoneal lavage was performed.
Results : The postoperatively course of those 89 patients was the following : 60 patients were curent, 14 expired and in 15 patients a pancreatic pseudocyst was formed. From those 15 cases with the pancreatic pseudocyst, 14 had to be reoperated (the cyst was drained to an adjacent hollow organ such as the stomach) while in the last case the cyst was drained under gastroscopy. The results were entively satisfactory.
Conclusion : Severe acute pancreatitis should be conservatively treated initially. Surgical intervention is indicated only in cases where patient's life is threatened or complications have supervened.

P 90

THE EVOLUTION OF ACUTE PANGEATITIS TREATED WHITH SANDOSTATINE

Megalokonomos K., Paizis B., Bliuras N., Theodorakopulu M., Saritzoglou I., Panetsos G., Sikiotis K.
Surgical Department, Hippokration Hospital, Athens, Greece

Aims: The treatment of acute pancreatitis it is mainly conservative and cases who need surgery treatment have been significantly limited last years. The aim of our study was the description of this tension which noticeable increased since somatostatine has been used for the treatment of acute pancreatitis and also we tried to show the direct relation between batter prognosis of acute pancreatitis and somatostatine.
Material-Methods: Between 1988-1997 in our clinic have been treated for acute pancreatitis 199 patients, 92 M and 107 F (M/F 1:1,16) with middle age 61,5 years old, with the youngest one 17 years old and the oldest one 91 years old. Estimation of clinical stage of those patiens has been done by using the criterions of Ranson at the admission of them to the hospital.
We compare period A (1988-1991) in which treatment didn't conclude somatostatine with period B (1992-1998) in which period our clinic used somatostatine for the treatment of acute pancreatitis.
Results: Comparing the period A (1988-1991) in which from 91 patients 16 needed operation at period B (1991-1998) from 108 patients (+18,7% patients) only 5 patients have been operated. Mortality decreased 46,4% at period B compared with period A (Mortality period A: 12,9. Mortality period B: 6,48).Mortality has been improved comparing the middle period of nursing of period A (26,4 days) with middle period of nursing of period B (20,57 days).
Conclusions: Somatostatine decrease mortality and morbidity of acute pancreatitis and also decrease the proportion of those patients who need surgery treatment. Somatostatine as treatment of acute pancreatitis at the admission to the hospital improves and keeps lower the prognostic pointers of Ranson, pointers we use 48 h after the admission for the estimation of clinical stage of acute pancreatitis.
Patients with severe acute pancreatitis the use of somatostatine didn't decrease their morbidity or their mortality.

P 91

PARTICULARITY OF POSTOPERATIVE DEVELOPMEN OF ACUTE PANCREATITIS AT OBESITY PATIENTS

Gh.Contu, I.Mahovici, S.Domente
State University of Medicine and Pfarmacy "N.Testemitanu", Departement of Surgery "N.Anestiadi", Chisinau, Republic of Moldova

In our study we evaluate the association between acute pancreatitis and obesity.

Patients were classified according to the body mass index (BMI) as obese: 22 (32,8%) patients (BMI > 25 kg/m2) and nonobese: 43 (64,2%) cases (BMI < 25 kg/m2). Morbid obesity was observed at 7 (10,4%) patients (BMI > 40 kg/m2), wich have been associated with serious metabolic, cardiovascular and pulmonary co-morbid conditions.

Cardiovascular complications (pancreatic shock, thromboembolism of pulmonary artery), pulmonary complications (acute respiratory failure, pancreatic pleurisy, pulmonary edema, pneumonia) and the incidence of infectious complications was more frequent at obesity patients. Hyperglycemia and ketoacidosis have contributed to the encephalopaty, which occurred in particular at the severe obese category.

Postoperative mortality was 6,6% in nonobese patients and it was highly (13,3%) at patients with BMI>25 and <40 kg/m2. In the same time postoperative mortality was highest (57,14%) in cases of severe obesity.

Conclusion: The risk for acute pancreatitis increased according to the degree of obesity.

P 92

Ethanol Injection Therapy Application in the Complex Treatment of Pancreas Cancer

I.A. Kovalskaya, V.S. Zemskov

Ukrainian National Medical University, Center of Liver and Pancreas Surgery

Aims: Cancer is the most often met pancreas tumour. However, at present the surgical treatment of pancreas cancer is characterized by the low resection ability, acceptable nearest and nonsatisfactory remote results. The main goal of this study was to determine the efficiency of the ethanol injection therapy of nonoperable tumours of pancreas (by analogy with the metastatic foci in the liver).

Materials and methods .We have selected a group of patients (17) with this pathology whom the injection of ethanol into the primary foci in the pancreas was made to simultaneously with alcoholization of metastases in the liver. The volume of the injected ethanol was determined by the formula 3\4 π(r+0.5cm), where r is the focus radius.

Results. The first positive results (improvement of the life quality and its duration) permitted us under nonoperable primary foci and performance of drainaging operations to carry out alcoholization of the primary tumour of pancreas independently of their localization in the pancreas tissue. It was found a decrease of the tumour focus volume by 30-55%, their destruction and aseptic necrosis. Complications were observed in 18.7% of patients which were manifested by the flowing of bile along drainages, moderate hepatic insufficiency in the postsurgical period. There were no deceased. At present the duration of life in this group of patients is on the average 9.2 months.

Conclusions. The results presented allow us to speak about possibility to apply ethanol injection into the primary focus of pancreas cancer in combined treatment in case of nonresection ability of the primary tumour independently of the site of its localization in the pancreas tissue. In this case the application of biliodigestive anastomosis and stabilizing destructive action of ethanol on the tumour make it possible to prepare a patient to the second radical stage of the operation as well as to improve the life quality of patients with this pathology and to prolong their life.The volume of the introduced ethanol is determined by the formula 3\4 π(r+0.5cm), where r is the focus radius.

P 93

PANCREATODUODENECTOMY FOR CANCER : EXPERIENCE WITH ANASTOMOSIS OF THE PANCREATIC DUCT

Yettimis E, Kalokerinos E, Costopanayiotou E, Metrou S, Karayiannis A, Matziaras D, Polymeropoulos Th

1st Surgical Dep.of Athen's General Hospital "G. Gennimatas"
Athen's, GREECE

Pancreotoduodenectomy (PDM) is being performed in a small percentage of suitable patients with pancreatic cancer (15-25%). The operation offers the pts the chance for longer survival but the quality of life is disturbed due to the operation . One of the problems that seem to contribute to this is the way the surgeon repairs the continuity of the Main Pancreatic Duct (MPD) to the gastrointestinal tract. During the last nine years we operated on 52 patients with Pancreatic cancer (P.head:32, P. body and tail:10, Vater papillae:10). The operations we performed were: Pancreatoduodenectomy: 41 pts, Distal Pancreatectomy: 9 pts, local excision of Vater: 1 pt, Total pancreatoduodenectomy: 1 pt. Of the 42 pts that underwent PDM in the 13 (31%) the pylorus was preserved and the 29 pts (69%) had an antrectomy. Ligation of the MPD and the pancreatic remnant was performed in 13 pts (31%) and these had complications in 23% of the cases. Pancreatojejunal was performed in 55% of the cases and was accompanied by complications in 22% of the cases. Pancreatojejunal dunking was performed in 6 pts (14%) with a complication rate of 33%. In all cases of pancreatic anastomosis the MPD was stent with a PVC tube which was brought to the skin through a jejunal loop. The stent was removed about 14 days from the operation. The whole postoperative morbitity was 24% and mortality 3,8% (2pts died). Conclusions: A. Pancreaticojejunal anstomosis is a safe way to offer the patients with PDM the exocrine function of the pancreas improving their quality of life. B. The postoperative morbidity and mortality in PDM is low enough to enable the surgeons to extend the indications for PDM to more patients with pancreatic cancer.

P 94

MR- venoportography in malignant lesions of the liver and pancreas

Tutin L.A.,Chelkoplias E.N., Yakovleva E.K., Stoukov L.A.
Research Institute of Roentgenology and Radiology,
St.Petersburg, RUSSIA

Purpose: to study diagnostic possibilities of the contrast MR-angiography for a visualization of the vein portal in liver and pancreas tumor.

Materials and methods: Total number of the observed patients was 26. The study has been performed with Magneton "Vision" MR-tomograph of Siemens make with a voltage of magnetic field of 1,5 T and with the use of the built-in Body coil.

Magnevist Shering has been used as a contrast. All the patients have undergone a conventional X-ray abdomen angiography. Total amount of the contrast was 15 ml (3 ml for a bollus test and 11 - 12 ml in order to contrast the area in question. . T2 Haste, T2 Firm and MRA 3D bh timescout sequences for a bollus test have been used.

Results: Thrombosis of the main trunk of the vein portal has been revealed in 4 patients with a primary liver tumor (stage 3-4), thrombosis of the branches of the vein portal has been observed in 12 cases with a multiple metastatic liver lesion and in 8 cases with a primary liver tumor.

Conclusion: A comparative analysis of the diagnostic efficiency of MR- venoportography and of conventional X-ray angiography has shown similar diagnostic possibilities. Thus, out of 10 cases of the tumoral lesion in 7 cases a complete coincidence has been seen; in 1 case MRA turned out to be more effective; in 1 case more out of 2 the lesion, previously observed by a conventional X-ray angiography, was not proved by the MR-angiograms.

P 95

PARTIAL PANCREATICODUODENECTOMY (WHIPPLE PROCEDURE) FOR PANCREATIC MALIGNANCY: OCCLUSION OF A NON-ANASTOMOSED PANCREATIC STUMP WITH FIBRIN SEALANT

A.P.MARCZELL, Hanusch Medical Center, Department of Surgery, Heinrich Collin-Str. 30, A-1140 Vienna, Austria

Following partial pancreaticoduodenectomy for periampu lary and pancreatic cancer, the complication and mortality rates are particullarly high. Various approaches have aimed at improving the postoperative result, with less than complete success. The discouraging results of others, and our own dissatisfaction, led us to evaluate an atraumatic, sutureless method for management of the residual gland.

Following head resection, the remaining pancreas is occluded with a fibrin sealant (Tisseel, Immuno AG, Vienna) via injection into the pancreatic duct - which is then ligated and left free in the peritoneal cavity.

Among 104 patients treated with this method, there were no perioperative deaths. 7 patients developed local complications (6 fistulae, 1 pancreatitis) due to technical errors that presumably resulted in incomplete occlusion. Evaluation of patients after 3 to 4 years indicates that the endocrine function of the pancreas has been largely conserved despite ductal occlusion.

In the 104 patients in whom we have used this occlusion method, we were able to reduce significantly the perioperative mortality as well as the postoperative complication rate. We continue to see satisfactory long term results due to less interstitial reaction and fibrosis with this physiologic substance which doesn't induce a foreign body reaction.

P 96

MORPHOLOGICAL AND IMMUNOHISTOCHEMICAL EXAMINATIONS OF PREBLASTOMATIC LESIONS OF THE PANCREAS

Györffy H., Járay B., Harsányi L.
2nd Dept. of Pathology, 1st Dept. of Surgery
Semmelweis University of Medicine, Budapest, Hungary

Background: Due to technical difficulties in reaching pancreas for clinical and pathological work-up we have limited informations about its preblastomatic lesions.

Materials and methods: Randomly selected 10 cases of chronic pancreatitis and 6 pancreatic adenocarcinomas were examined for cellular and structural characteristics. Chronic pancreatitis and „normal" tissue adjacent the tumour revealed preblastomatic lesions (eg. ducectasia, ductal proliferation, papillary intraductal epithelial proliferation, mucinous and epithelial metaplasia, dysplasia). In addition to conventional staining PAS reaction and immunohistochemical reactions (chromogranin, carcinoembryonic antigen, smooth muscle actin, p53, Ki67, c-erB2, bcl2) were performed on each specimen. The findings were compared in cases of chronic pancreatitis and those of the tissues surrounding the invasive tumours.

Results: Preneoplastic lesions, found in chronic pancreatitis, have given the same immunohistochemical reactions as invasiv tumours although with less frequency and lower intensity.

P 97

PAPILLARY AND SOLID EPITHELIAL NEOPLASM OF THE PANCREAS (PSEN) - A STUDY OF 6 CASES

L. Madaras, J. Kulka, G. Mózes, Z. Király *

2nd Department of Pathology and *1st Department of Surgery, Semmelweis University of Medicine, Budapest, Hungary

Aims: Papillary and Solid Epithelial Neoplasm (PSEN) is a relatively rare tumour of the pancreas with a good prognosis and controversial pathogenesis occurring almost exclusively in adolescent girls and young women. Because of its gross and histologic features PSEN is also known as papillary cystic tumour or solid and cystic tumour or papillary epithelial neoplasm. In the 2nd Department of Pathology of the Semmelweis University of Medicine we have seen 6 cases between 1996 and 1998. We have examined them to compare their clinical, histological and immunhistochemical features.
Methods: Clinical study was performed, macroscopic descriptions and photos of the tumours and routine HE sections were examined. We have made immunhistochemical reactions for vimentin, alpha-1-antitrypsin, NSE, synaptophysin, chromogranin, cytokeratin and progesterone receptor.
Results: All the 6 were female patients ranging in age from 14 years to 44 years. They presented with abdominal pain, or the tumour was found on routine ultrasound examination and in one case a huge retroperitoneal mass was revealed during gynaecological surgery. The tumour was localised in different parts of the pancreas. The diameter of the tumour varied between 2 and 21 cm, it had a fibrous capsule in every case, solid and cystic areas were seen in every tumour. On microscopic examination the relatively uniform tumour cells were arranged in several layers around a fibrovascular core, forming solid areas.Degenerative changes were observed. Invasion of the capsule, vascular or local invasion, metastases were not found. Immunhistochemistry revealed positivity for vimentin, NSE, synaptophysin, chromogranin, alpha-1-antitrypsin.
Conclusions: Like in other studies, our cases also revealed a good prognosis, the patients are well after 10-26 months, no recidive tumour or metastases were found.

P 98

THE USE OF MUFF-LIKE PANCREATOJEJUNAL ANASTOMOSIS IN PANCREATODUODENAL RESECTION

V.V.Ershov, M.V.Kukosh, A.D.Rybinsky
Nizhegorodsky State Medical Academy, Nizhni Novgorod, Russia

Aim. To improve the reliability of pancreatojejunal anastomosis.

Methods. There were operated 18 patients(age ranging from 41 to 72 years) for cancer of pancreatic head (12) and gasric cancer with involvement of pancreatic head(6). Pancreatogastroduodenal resection was done in 13 patients and pancreatoduodenal resection with gastectomy - in 5 patients. Pancreatojejunal anastomosis was performed in accordance with the methods developed by the authors.

Results. One patiens died of acute cardio-vascular insufficiency.No adverse effects of pancreatojejunal anastomosis were noted.

Conclusion. The developed methods of muff-like pancreatojejunal anastomosis makes it possible to improve the results in the surgical treatment of the pancreas

P 99

NON-FUNCTIONING NEUROENDOCRINE PANCREATIC CANCER =96 THREE CASES.

J. Kostro, M.I. Pirski, Z. Cledzinski.
I Department of Surgery Medical University of Gdansk, Poland

Aim: Neuroendocrine cancer is a rarely reported neoplasm of the pancreas. The aim of this study is to present three cases of them. Methods: Three cases presented were diagnosed for pancreatic cancer. Gastrointestinal disturbance and abdominal pain were the most frequent presented symptoms. Diagnostic procedures were carried out according to adequate protocole, which comprised of the following: standard and endocavital USG, ERCP, CT, Doppler Ultrasound. In all patients examination confirmed existing tumor of the pancreas. None of them presented positive examination for functioning islet cell tumor. Resective procedures were done in all cases. Postoperative, all tumors proved histologically to be neuroendocrine in origin. Immunohistochemical staining showed positive reactivity for neuron-specific enolase (NSE), chromogramin (CgA) and synaptophysin. As an adjuvant chemotherapy we administrated 5-Fluorouracil by intravenous bolus injection at an injection dose of 500 mg/m2/day for 5 days each month, for 6 months.
Results: The follow-up period was 5-12 months. Control USG and CT revealed normal structure of pancreatic stump. All patients are alive and do not have any symptoms nor progress.
Conclusions: Although this group of patients is small we conclude that:
1. Non-functioning neuroendocrine tumors of the pancreas have similar symptoms to adenocarcinoma which makes them difficult to differentiate.
2. In our material neuroendocrine cancer of the pancreas seems to have better prognosis then adenocarcinoma.

P 100

ASSOCIATION BETWEEN SERUM LEVELS OF TUMOUR NECROSIS FACTOR AND CACHEXIA IN PANCREATIC CANCER PATIENTS

Karayiannakis A.J.[1], *Syrigos K.N.*[2], *Simatos G.*[1], *Papanikolaou Sp.*[1], *Papanikolaou D.*[1], *Bogris S.*[1], *Karatzas G.*[3]
[1]First Department of Surgery, First IKA Hospital, Athens, Greece
[2]Third Department of Medicine, University of Athens, Medical School, Athens, Greece
[3]Second Propaedeutic Department of Surgery, University of Athens, Athens, Greece

Aims: To evaluate serum levels of tumour necrosis factor-α (TNF-α) in patients with pancreatic cancer and to investigate the relationship between TNF-α levels and cachexia in these patients.
Methods: Serum levels of TNF-α were determined with an enzyme immunoassay specific for human TNF-α in 43 patients with pancreatic cancer and were correlated to body weight, body mass index, total protein, albumin, hematocrit and hemoglobin.
Results: Twenty four (56%) of the patients had detectable serum levels of TNF-α. Patients with elevated TNF-α levels had significantly lower body weight, body mass index, total protein, albumin, hematocrit and hemoglobin compared to patients with undetectable serum TNF-α levels. There was also a significant inverse correlation between TNF-α levels and body weight, body mass index, total protein, albumin, hematocrit and hemoglobin, respectively.
Conclusions: These findings suggest that TNF-α is possibly involved in the development of cachexia in patients with pancreatic cancer.

P 101

The effect of prophylactic somatostatin or octreotide in patients undergoing pancreatic surgery

Milonaki D., Katsaragakis S., Gomatos I.P., Treptov M., Manouras A., Apostolidis N., Konstadoulakis M.M., Androulakis G.,

1st Departement of Propaedeutic Surgery, Hippocration Hospital, Athens Medical School

Aims: Increased mortality (10%) and complication rates (35%) follow pancreatic tumor resections. Among the most common complications are pancreatic fistulas and abscesses which are closely related to the exocrine pancreatic function. The aim of this study was to investigate the effect of prophylactic somatostatin or octreotide in patients undergoing pancreatic surgery.

Methods: We have studied 57 patients who were submitted to pancreaticoduodenectomy, distal pancreatectomy, pancreatic biopsies and by-pass procedures. Twenty-one patients received somatostatin (somastin) from the day of surgery until the fifth postoperative day. Another 19 patients received octreotide (sandostatin) and 17 patients were the control group.

Results: The hospital stay for the three groups has been 21 days (somastin) vs 17 days (sandostatin) vs 28 days (controls). We have also studied the incidence of pancreatic fistulas, abscesses and leakages, as well as other complications in each group of patients.

Conclusions: The perioperative administration of somatostatin or its analogue can significantly reduce the incidence of postoperative complications in patients submitted to pancreatic surgery. Additionally, patients who receive this pharmaceutical regimen have a shorter hospital stay.

P 102

IDIOPATHIC MASSIVE ASCITES FOLLOWING WHIPPLE PROCEDURE

Papastratis G. M.D. , Zografos G. M.D. , Koliopanos A. M.D. , Korkolis D. M.D. , Nikolakopoulou Z. M.D. , Orfanos A. M.D.

Third Department of Surgery , General Hospital of Athens , Greece .

We present a rare case of prolonged massive ascites following Whipple procedure in a 65 – year – old man , suffering from a large pancreatic head adenocarcinoma . The procedure lasted 6 hours . Gastrointestinal continuity was established with end – to – end pancreatojejunostomy , end – to – side choledochojejunostomy and side – to – side gastrojejunostomy , with the same jejunal loop . He had uneventful recovery in the wards , but 12 hours following the procedure , large amount of clear yellowish fluid appeared in the drained bags . The amount of this ascitic fluid was 5 – 7 liters per day , necessitating large volume of fresh frozen plasma , human albumin and crystalloids , to maintain haemodynamic stability . Repeated biochemical studies of the fluid showed :
Amylase : 17 – 22 I.U. / lt , LDH : 73 I.U. / lt , Albumin:13 – 26 mg/dl , Glucose : 209 mg / dl . Lipids were not found and cytology was negative for malignant cells . The fluid was found sterile and total cell concentration was 140 / ml with 90 % lymphocytes . Elevated levels of alkaline phosphatase and γ - GT were noticed , whereas the virology profile for hepatitis was negative . Abdominal CT scan showed liver enlargement . Visceral and MRI angiography demonstrated patency of the splenic , portal and hepatic veins .
The duration of this massive ascitic fluid production was 3 weeks . The patient was also treated with protein – rich diet , furosemide and spironolactone . He was discharged on the 25th postoperative day , with a small amount of remnant ascitic fluid , in a perfectly well physical condition .
To the best of our knowledge , this case is the first ever published post – pancreatoduodenectomy non – chylous ascites , conservatively treated .

P 103

IMPROVEMENT IN SURVIVAL FOR PATIENTS WITH METASTATIC PANCREATIC CANCER (Pca)

R.Dobrila-Dintinjana, M.Rubinic, N.Ivanis, M.Uravic, A.Depolo, D.Kovac, M.Dintinjana
Internal and Surgical Clinic, University Hospital Rijeka, CROATIA

Aims: To compare two protocols in therapy for stage IV of metastatic pancreatic cancer.
Methods: The tumors were pathologically confirmed and staged by CT, US and laparotomy as needed. All patients were treated ambulatory. Patients whose age was >75, with prior chemotherapy or more than 15% weight loss were excluded. By one protocol patients received cisplatin(P), 5 florouracil(F) and leukovorin(L) for two days every two weeks as out-patients. Other patients received Gemcitabine(G) every 8 days seven consecutive weeks.
Results: 13 patients presenting with metastatic Pca started chemotherapy, 6 patients underwent protocol PLF and 7 patients protocol G. In both groups in about 50 % tumor markers decreased. Partial regression of disease (PRD) on CT-US scan in G group was in 3 months 57 %, and PRD in PLF group was 33 %. We have no mortality rate in first 90 days. 6 months and 1 year survival was 50 % and 33 % in PLF group and 85,7 % and 57,15 % in G group respectivelly.
Conclusions: No sex or age had implications on PRD or survival time in this study. We have higher 1 year survival time in G group than expected. Altough we have small number of patients and altough 1 year survival time is quite short time for evaluation of quality and validity of chemotherapeutic protocol, we can say that G protocol improves prognosis of Pca.

P 104

THE ROLE CONTROLLED LASER THERAPY IN TREATMENT SICK WITH CHOLANGITIS

V.M.Lisienco, M.D.; E.V.Anikina
Urals State Medical academy. Ekaterinburg, Russia

The Purpose: Improvement of results of treatment sick with obstructive cholangitis, mechanical jaundice, liver insufficiency with using controlled laser therapy.

The Methods: Under observation there were 60 patients with cholangitis, mechanical jaundice, liver insufficiency, got controlled laser therapy from 1997 to 1998. Low energy ray of lazer is used in preoperative and postoperative period in the manner of semiconductor, helium-neon and magnetic laser radiation. Laser therapy was conduct intravenous, transcutaneous and endocholedochial by ways. Duration of session of laser therapy is defined with provision for the individual sensitivity to lazer radiation each sick. As checking to efficiency of treatment alongside with biochemical and immunological factors we use the biophysical methods of study of biological liquids of organism (the wheys shelters and biles) – refraction and polarization microscopy.

The Results: Got data speak that ray of lazer promotes the processes earlier regeneration of gepatocitis, has antiedematous, immunocorrective action. It is proved value of method refraction and polarization microscopy in control for conducted treatment and forecast of disease. So in quip phase of disease in biles is noted the high concentration liquid-cristal structures. In process of treatment a bile changes its structure before fundamental solution. This fact we consider the criterion for removing the drainage from biliary ways. Due to the above-mentioned types of treatment the number of hepatic insufficiencies was reduced and as a result of it the number of lethality was reduced from 7.2 to 5%. The average number of days that the patient spent in the hospital was reduced from 27.2 to 19.8

The Findings: 1. Laser therapy complements and perfects the complex treatment sick with cholangitis. 2. The Methods of refraction and polarization microscopy allow to choose individual selecting the dose of laser therapy for each concrete sick. 3. Biophysical methods of study can be used for checking and forecast of efficiency of treatment beside sick with cholangitis, are a criterion of duration external drainage biliary ways.

P 105

FIRST RESULTS WITH CT-CHOLANGIOGRAPHY IN OUR CLINIC

Puhl M., Weszelits V., Doros A., Németh A., Görög D., Perner F.
Semmelweis Medical University, Transplantation and Surgical Clinic, Budapest, Hungary

Aims: The aim of this study was to assess retrospectively the role of CT cholangiography in the diseases of the bile ducts in our clinic.
Matherials and method:41 CT-cholangiography were performed in 38 patients (17 male, 21 female), including 8 with transplanted liver.40-60ml intravenous hepatotrop contrast agents were given and a helical scan set (GE Prospeed Plus) was obtained after 20-40 min., with 3mm slice thickness and 1-2 pitch. Reconstruction were performed every 1-1,5 mm. With an Advantage Windows workstation (GEMS) MIP and SSD technics were used.
Result:35 (85%) examinations were successful. The high SeBi level and poor liver function have limited the diagnostic value. In four cases intraductal stones, in 15 patients stenosis of the bile ducts, in 2 cases tumor and in 2 case injury of the bile ducts were found. In 12 cases the cholangiogram were negative.
Conclusion: CT-cholangiography is a non-invasive, successful method to evaluate the diseases of the bile ducts, also in patients with transplanted liver.

P 106

THE ROLE OF THREE-DIMENSIONAL CT -ANGIOGRAPHY IN LIVER TRANSPLANTATION CANDIDATES

Weszelits V., Puhl M., Doros A., Dabasi G.,Görög D., Perner F.
Semmelweis Medical University, Transplantation and Surgical Clinic, Budapest, Hungary

Purpose: To assess the hepatic arterial supply in transplantation candidates with 3D-CT-angiography
Material and Method: 3D CT-angiography were performed in 75 patients (7-62 years). Intravenous contrast agent was given, and two helical scan sets (GE-Prospeed Plus) were obtained. Axial images were reconstructed every 1 mm and 3D CT-angiograms were obtained by using an Advantage Windows workstation (GEMS), both MIP and SSD techniques were used. The anatomy was categorised by Michels classification. 29 patients underwent conventional angiography also, and 33 patients underwent liver tarnsplantation.
Results: 69 (92%) examination were diagnostic and successful: the major arteries supplying the liver were delineated on the images. In 6 cases technical failure occured. In the patients who underwent conventional angiography, or liver transplantation, there were no marked disagreement with 3D CT-angiography.
Conclusion: 3D CT-angiography is a reliable and accurate method to assess the hepatic arterial anatomy.

P 107

INEDIT ETIOPATHOGENIC ASPECTS OF THE LIMY BILE SYNDROME - ELEVEN CASES OPERATED IN TIMIŞOARA

F.C. Rada, I. Sporea, M. Mracec, Domniţa Rada, I.O. Rada

University of Medicine and Pharmacy, Timişoara, România, str. Siret no.6

Limy bile represents a radiological syndrome with no speci ic clinical symptoms and ultrasound features.

Over a period of 20 years (1976-1995), 11 patients (10 female, 1 male) with limy bile syndrome - LBS - were observed for clinical, radiological, intraoperative, postoperative and laboratory fndings. The syndrome was diagnosed on plain roentgenograms in 10 cases and confirmed during the surgical procedure in 9 cases and in one case, LBS was demonstrated by postmortem dissection (cause of death: lung cancer). In one case LBS was discovered during surgery. Eight patients showed associated cholesterol cholelithiasis and among them, in 7 cases the gallbladder was flled with white bile of various consistency, ranging from "milky" to pasty consistency. Two patients presented yellow bile and other 2 with brown bile. The cystic duct and the infundibulum were stone-free in all cases and filled with limy bile in 4 cases. Chemical analyses revealed a composition of 36% calcium carbonate in one case with "milky" bile (postoperative diagnosis) and a proportion of ' 72-96% calcium carbonate in other 10 cases.

Calcium carbonate appears in the gallbladder by concomitant synthesis, crystallization and precipitation from two bicarbonate ions and one calcium ion occurring at a pH of 8 and above. Calcium bicarbonate has increased density than other biliary components and deposits in declivous parts of the gallbladder, achieving gradually a sludging in the presence of pathologic wall alterations (fibrosclerosis). When the bile flow to the gallbladder is stopped (by an impacted stone), the bicarbonate and calcium supply and therefore the calcium synthesis is interrupted.

Conclusions: Limy bile is synthesized in the gallbladder from bile constituents at pH above 8 and affected gallbladder contractility (parietal fibrosis), in absence of an inflammatory process (that would determine a drop in pH level). Once gallstones block the infundibulum or the cystic duct, the limy bile synthesis process is interrupted.

P 108

THE MANAGEMENT OF OBSTRUCTIVE CHOLECYSTITIS BY MICROLAPAROTOMY

Rozsos I., Szira P.
Moritz Kaposi Medical Centre, Kaposvár, Hungary

Aims: Whether early or delayed cholecystectomy has more technical difficulties and postoperative complications in the cases of obstructive cholecystitis seems to be controversial. Question often arises when the gallbladder should be removed. The object was to clarify, in the authors' experience, the optimal time for surgical intervention.
Methods: A total of 2400 cholecystectomies have been performed by micro- and minilaparotomies at our department: 811 (34 percent) with obstructive cholecystitis. These patients have been subclassified into 5 groups according to the first onset of symptomes and the time of surgery.
Results: The operation was performed within 3 days in 52 patients (group I), between the 4th and the 7th day in 109 patients (group II), between the 8th and the 10th day in 54 patients (group III), between the 11th day and the 6th week in 292 patients (group IV) and later than 6 weeks in 304 patients (group V) after the onset of symptomes. Different postoperative complications have been found to be more common in the group III, IV and V.
Conclusion: In the cases of obstructive cholecystitis the authors' grouping may be helpful to estimate the potential postoperative complications and intraoperative difficulties as well. In our experience the optimal time for surgery in the cases of obstructive cholecystitis is within 1 week after the onset of symptomes.

P 109

HOW EASY IS CHOLECYSTECTOMY FOR LITHIASIS OF THE GALLBLADDER.

by
V. SKOUNTZOS, G. KYRATZIS, D. XYPOLYTAS and V. GOUGOUTAS.

From the 2nd Surgical Department, General Peripheral Hospital «KAT», 14561 Kifisia, Hellas.

Aim: Simple cholecystectomy, is well known, as an easy operation, carried out usually by the surgical residents. Although in some patients, sceduled for elective cholecystectomy, major operative problems might arised unexpectedly, on exploration in the operating room, requiring a major operative procedure.

Patients - Methods: Elective cholecystectomies were performed on 1345 patients, over the last 14 years period, from 1985 till 1988. The female, made ratio were 2.3:1 and the mean age of the patients was 61 years. Operative difficulties were encountered in 158 patients (11.37%), requiring more difficult procedures than a simple cholecystectomy, prolongation of the operative time and more complex post operative treatment.

Results: The causative factors of these problems were mainly due to inflammation of the gallbladder in 118 patients (74.66%), such as acute cholecystitis, empyema, gangrene of the gall bladder or choledocholithiasis in 23 patients (14,55%), congenital anomalies of the extrahepatic billiary system in 14 patients (8.84%) and malignant processes in 3 patients (1.8%) were additional factors requiring more complicated procedures.

Conclusion : The operative findings, in a patient scheduled for a simple cholecystectomy, may be different then a simple operation, which usually is carried out by a resident, might be a difficult one, requiring a more experienced surgeon, with better knowledge on this filed and more skillful in the biliary surgery.

P 110

COMPARATIVE STUDY OF INFLAMMATORY RESPONSE IN OPEN AND LAPAROSCOPIC CHOLECYSTECTOMY

Crema,E; Oliveira, C.B.; Silva,AA; Alves, J.R.; Gomes, R.A.S.; Rodrigues Jr.,V. Department of Digestive Surgery of Federal School of Medicine of Triângulo Mineiro, Uberaba – MG, Brazil.

Laparoscopic cholecystectomy has proved to be the best choice for the treatment of symptomatic cholelithiasis. Inflammatory and endocrine changes caused by the anesthetic or surgical procedure by measuring cytokines (IL-1, IL-6, IL-10 and TNF-alfa) and stress hormone levels (growth hormone – GH, cortisol, anti-diuretic hormone – ADH, insulin, glucagon and adrenocorticotropic hormone – ACTH).
Forty-two patients underwent cholecystectomy either open (21 – Group 1) or laparoscopic (21 – Group 2). Serial dosages of cytokines (IL-1, IL-6, IL-10 and TNF-alfa) and hormones (GH, ACTH, ADH, insulin, cortisol and glucagon) were obtained preoperatively (T0) and 24h (T24), 48h (T48) and 72h (T72) postoperatively.
General data (age, Sex, weight, body mass index, surgical and anesthetic duration were not significantly different between groups.
Results obtained from ACTH, insulin, GH and glucagon levels were compared between groups and no statistically significant difference was found either pre- or postoperatively. Cortisol levels obtained at T24, T48 and T72 were significantly greater compared to preoperative values for group.
Plasma cortisol concentration was significantly greater in patients undergoing open cholecystectomy at T24, T48 and T72 compared to the respective values obtained for the laparoscopic surgery group.
Mean levels of Il-1, IL-6 and TNF-alfa found preoperatively in group 2 were lower than those observed in group 1. This finding suggests that the laparoscopic technique caused lower inflammatory reaction. The fact that no difference was found in levels of IL-10, the cytokine responsible for anti-inflammatory expression gives support to our conclusion.
Therefore, it was concluded that surgical stress determined measuring cortisol levels throughout 3 days postoperatively was significantly greater and inflammatory cytokine levels were also greater in open compared to laparoscopic cholecystectomy.

P 111

LOW-INVASIVE METHODS IN SURGERY OF CHOLECYSTITIS

B.S.Briskin, A.V.Bryunin, Yektov P.V., A.N.Gudkov
Clinic of Surgical Diseases, MMSI, Hospital No.81 (Moscow, Russia)

Aims: revealing of engineering features of a minicholecystectomia-MC,definition of the indications to it by realization randomized controlled treal of laparoscopic versus minicholecystectomy. The choice of MC is caused by the absence of intense carbon dioxide pneumoperitoneum.
Methods: Laparoscopy and minilaparotomy methods performed for carrying out cholecystectomy. MC was carried out from the 30- 50 MM cut along the transrectal line to the right ,with use ring retractor, offered by Russell RCG in 1987,based on the method of M.I.Prudkov,1993,with the use of the instruments specially developed by the author.Both methods have been accustomed almost simultaneously for the last3years by one group of surgeons.The data of the period of the development are included in the research.MC is a rather simple and reliable gasless method.
Results: 211 MCwere executed (males-19,females-192) at the age from 17 to 85; 37,9%of them being older than 60 years.In 103(48,8%)cases we have applied MC under epidural anaesthesia.We had no problems with the relaxation and the achievement of adequate access for dissection. In 16,6%- the operation was under the acute cholecystitis.LC was 160 (males-10,females-150)at the age from 17to74,older than 60-17,5%.The experience shows that keeping of the technique correctly, MC is possible under partially intrahepatic gall-bladder, at the expressed adhesion in subhepaticus region,after earlier imposed cholecystostomies under the ultrasonic or laparoscopy control.MCis more preferable under an acute cholecystitis.Conversions were 6,9 %at LC, including 1relaparotomy(0,63%)and reoperation-1,88 %;conversion at MC-4,74 %;the complications have made accordingly- 6,25 % (LC) and 3,32 %(MC),mortality-0%.Among the complications: the bleedings have made accordingly- 3,1% (LC) / 2,37 %(MC),bile leakage-1.88 %(LC), including 1,25%intro and 0,63% after operation, 0 %(MC);common hepatic and bile duct injuries-1,3 %(LC)and 0 %(MC),subhepaticus abscessus-0 %(LC)and 0.95% (MC).There were not any wound infection. Only 1pneumonia was registered after the operation MC. Postoperative hospital stay and return to preoperative functional status and to work differed a little.
Conclusions:the advantages and features of the combination of MC with epidural anaesthesia for the patients with cardiovascular diseases, chronic lungs diseases, who have undergone a lot of operations on abdominal cavity before,for the old men,for the patients with an acute cholecystitis were determined.The necessity of application of an optimal combination of MC, LC and standard conventional cholecystectomia is evidently shown. MC is assimilated easier because of the similarity with the standard one.

P 112

BILIARY COMPLICATIONS OF LAPAROSCOPIC CHOLECYSTECTOMY

Rohde L, Osvaldt A, Borges da Costa MS, Viero P, Wendt LR
Department of Surgery, University of Rio Grande do Sul Medical School, *Hospital de Clínicas*, Porto Alegre, Brazil

Aims: The purpose of this study is to present our experience with biliary complications of laparoscopic cholecystectomy (LC) treated at our university hospital in a six-year period.
Methods: The medical records of 27 patients treated at our university hospital from August 1992 to July 1998 were retrospectively reviewed.
Results: Bile peritonitis secondary to cystic duct stump leak occurred in 12 patients: seven were treated with laparotomy, peritoneal cleansing and cystic duct stump ligation; five patients were trated via laparoscopy, 3 of them also required endoscopic sphincterotomy (residual bile duct stones in 2). Extra-hepatic bile duct injuries were treated in 15 patients: 2 bile duct ligations with clips treated in the early postoperative period with laparotomy and clip removal; 1 total stenosis probably following termal injury diagnosed 20 days after LC that required hepaticojejunostomy; 1 partial stenosis diagnosed 18 months after LC treated with endoscopically placed stent; 2 partial sections of the common bile duct treated with T-tube insertion; 9 high biliary lesions (6 type-II and 3 type-III according to the Bismuth's classification) that required hepaticojejunostomy (5 of these 9 patients had arrived to our hospital with anastomotic dehiscence of biliary reconstructions performed prior to referral).
Conclusions: Compared to the author's previous experience, these results suggest an increased incidence of cystic stump leaks and more frequent reoperations after failed initial repairs than observed before the laparoscopic era. A multidisciplinary approach can be advantageous to treat some cases of biliary complications of LC.

P 113

LAPAROSCOPIC CHOLECYSTECTOMY; A RETROSPECTIVE STUDY OF 870 PATIENTS, SINGEL CENTRE EXPERIENCE

A. Moustafa and M El-Wahsh*
Departments of Surgery, Alzhraa University Hospital, Cairo, Egypt & Royal Free Hospital, London, UK*

Introduction: Laparoscopic Cholecystectomy (LC) is currently the standard procedure for the treatment of cholelithiasis. However possible complications must not be underestimated.
Aim: to analyse and evaluate retrospectively the rate of conversion and the post operative complication of LC.
Patients & Methods: 870 patients who underwent LC (July 1993 – May 1998) due to cholelithiasis were included in our study. Preoperative assessment includes, liver function tests, abdominal ultrasound and selective cases had E.R.C.P. The procedure was carried through two 10 mm and two 5mm ports in 783 patients, and two 10 mm and one 5mm ports in 87 patients.
Results: In 31/870 patients had conversion of the procedure, in 3/31 conversion was mandatory and elective in 28. 12 patients had postoperative complications (4 had jaundice, 2 bile leak, 3 haemorrhage, 1 subhepatic collection, 1 bilateral pneumothorax and 1 gastric fistula). There was only one death after non-eventful recovery. Laparotomy was performed in 6/12. All patients who had successful LC (827) were ambulated out of bed and allowed oral fluids on the same day and the maximum hospital stay was 72 hours postoperatively.
Conclusion: LC is a safe and effective technique. The procedure appears to benefit all component of the health care delivery system.

P 114

CALOT'S TRIANGLE WIDE OPENING TECHNIQUE IN LAPAROSCOPIC CHOLOCYSTECTOMY. A SAFE PROCEDURE?

Philippou P, Chiotis A,Varada E, Dimopoulos A ,Georgiou G,Pakataridis A, Kampouris A.
Department of Surgery, General Hospital of Xanthi, Xanthi, Greece.

Aims: Bile duct injury is a well-documented complication of laparoscopic cholocystectomy (LC). Wide opening of the Calot's triangle as a first step of LC, is mandatory in preventing these injuries. This study aimed to determine the safety of this procedure, based in our experience in laparoscopic cholocystectomy.
Methods: Between January 1994 and October 1998, we performed 200 laparoscopic cholocystectomies in patients with gallstone disease. A standard four-port technique was used according to the "French" method. Gallbladder (GB) neck was initially retracted away from the common bile duct (CBD) with grasper. Anterior GB peritoneum was first stripped, beginning in the region of the GB neck medially to expose cystic duct and cystic artery. Posterior peritoneum was divided next,at a distance from the liver.Cellular tissue was subsequently dissected in the space between GB and liver away from cystic duct and artery until Calot's triangle was widely opened. Then retracting GB neck away from the liver, cystic duct and artery meticulously dissected at a distance from CBD. Cystic artery was divided before the division of cystic duct resulting to the further opening of the Calot's triangle. GB was then detached from the liver. With the above technique we could detect anatomic abnormalities and avoid injuries of major extrahepatic ducts. All procedures were undertaken by Senior Surgeons.
Results: During this period no injury of the CBD,common hepatic duct, right hepatic duct and artery or accessory ducts occured. In 16 patients (8%), the laparoscopic procedure converted to open cholocystectomy because of prominent scarry and inflammatory changes in Calot's triangle. During dissection of the tissue interposed between cystic duct and cystic artery, 4 minor injuries (2%) of the cystic duct occured, but cystic duct stump was safety clipped in all cases.
Conclusion: The results of our study suggest that, Calot's triangle wide opening technique as a first step , is a safe and useful manoeuvre in preventing injuries of major extrahepatic bile ducts in laparoscopic cholocystectomy.

P 115

Ultrasonografic and Operative Comparation of Billious Calculosis

S. Sekulic, P. Simic, R. Kosanovic, D. Zlta
Medical Facylti, Surgical Clinic, Pristina, YUGOSLAVIA

Ultrasonography (US) is a method in diagnossis of hepato-billious tractus. Due to the construction of modern ultrasound facilites this method presents one of the most important method in this field due to the fact that it is: uninvasive method, it does not procedure harmful biological effect, it does not demand contrastive means, there are no counter indications known, and it does not provoke uneasiness to patient.

200 patients were treated ultrasonographically at Surgical Clinic Faculty of Medicine in Pristina. In 119 (59,9%) cases calculus in gallbaldder was localised ultrasonographically and in 131 (65,5%) cases operativelly. Calculus was found in Hartmann's place in 60 (30,0%) cases ultrasonographically and in 65 (32,5%) cases operativelly. Calculus in d. cysticus was operativelly found in 4 (2,0%) cases and it was not found ultrasonographically. Solitary calculosis was found ultrasonographically in 52 (26,0%) cases and it was confirmed operativelly 47 (23,5%) cases. Multiple calculosis was diagnosed ultrasonographically in 148 (74,0%) cases, and operativelly in 153 (76,5%) cases. Anteroposterious radious of gallbladder was found ultrasonographically to be 3 or more than 5 cm long in 109 (54,5%) cases, and operativelly in 111 (55,5%) cases. Gallbladder wall size higher than 3 cm was foun US in 149 (74,5%) cases, and operativelly in 137 (68,5%) cases. Choledolithiasis was US diagnosed in 29 (53,7%) cases and operativelly in 54 cases. Gallbladder carcinom was US diagnosed in 5 (71,4%), and operativelly found in 7 cases 6 gallbladder path carcinomes were not US diagnosed.

Those results show that ultrasonography is a method of choice in gallbladder disseases treatment Accuracy of the method equalls 89,5% on our clinical material.

P 116

COMPLICATIONS OF INTRAPERITONEAL GALLSTONES AFTER LAPAROSCOPIC CHOLECYSTECTOMY"

P. VOULGARIS, D TSANTZALOS, V. PRIMIKIRIS, G. PAPADOPOULOS, S. TSOUPANOS, N. VASILADIOTIS.
1 sr HOSPITAL IKA - ATHENS- 2N° DEPT OF SURGERY

Between the years 1993 and 1998 one thousand eight hundred seventy six (1 876) laparoscopic cholecystectomies have taken place in our clinic. During the laparoscopic procedure gallstones fell into peritonian cavity in 132 of them (7%). Four patients from the 132 appeared post operation complications due to the gallstones in the peritonium cavity. One developed abscess in the front abdominal wall eight months post operatively, respectively to the site of the trocar insertion. Another developed intestinal obstruction two years later, and the other two subfrenic abscess three and four months later. The first patient submitted drainage under local anaesthesia, the second open laparotomy, which followed by symphysiolysis and the last two drainage under CT-Scan surveillance.
During the LC procedure the incidence of falling gallstones in the peritoneal cavity is 7-40%. In our series the percentage fluctuated up to 7%. The appearance of the related complications was 3% and 0.2% over all. We suggest the fallings stones must be selected as many as possible in order to prevent our patients from post operative complications. According to our opinion there is no any reason to convert the procedure to an open laparotomy for such a thing.

P 117

OPEN (MINI) VERSUS LAPAROSCOPIC CHOLECYSTECTOMY

M. Jeremic. M. Stojanovic, M. Stojiljkovic, Lj. Jeremic
Surgical Clinic, Clinical
Center Nis, Yugoslavia

Aims: Mini laparotomy cholecystectomy (ML) has similar characteristics like laparoscopic cholecystectomy (LC), but the advantages of this method are direct visualization and palpation of this region. The aim of this study is to compare the values of mini laparotomy and laparoscopic cholecystectomy.

Methods: The authors analyzed two groups (200 patients each): group ML - mini laparotomy; group LC- laparoscopic cholecystectomy. They looked out durability of operation, hospitalization alimentation reappearance, intraoperative and postoperative complication, pain intensity (Mc Gill score), metabolic perioperative response (CPK, LDH, AST), esthetic results, reappearance of working activity and economic aspects.

Results: Durability of operation ratio MULC has been 43 / 61 min. Alimentation reappearance has been established 24 hours after OP similarly in both groups. Intraoperative complications were more frequent in LC group (2/0): main bile duct section in one case, and biliary peritonitis in one case following cystic duct clip's falling-down. Conversion rate is 3% in LC group, but increasing incision in ML group in 2.5% (choledocholithiasis in 3, cholecystoduodenal fistula in 2 cases). There was no mortality. Wound infection occurred more frequently in ML (4% versus 2% in LC group). Postoperative hospitalization has been shorter in LC (1 ,6 days versus 2.9 in ML). Postoperative pain, according Mc Gill score, didn't showed significant difference. Metabolic response (necrosis enzymes) has increased in ML group (statistical significance). Reappearance of working activity is better in LC (10.5 versus 16.2 days in ML). Esthetic results are better in LC. In our health insurance system, LC is more expensive than ML. Because of the shorter operative time and lower intraoperative complication rate, mini laparotomy cholecystectomy is valid alternative to laparoscopic cholecystectomy, especially indicated from social, personal or technical reasons.

P 118

LOW INTRAABDOMINAL PRESSURE DURING LAPAROSCOPIC CHOLECYSTECTOMY

Capsambelis P., Palli E., Vithoulkas K., Tsagaropoulos K., Panagopoulos G., Lagodimos D., Tsoucalas M., Kounadi Th.

Department of Surgery-General Hospital of Zante-Greece

The Authors report their experience in performing low intra-abdominal pressure (7mmHg) during laparoscopic cholecystectomy (LC).

There were 80 patients (group A, 40 pts. and group B, 40 pts.) treated by means of LC in our department during the year 1998. The mean intra-abdominal pressure in group A and in group B were 14mmHg and 7mmHg respectively. The groups were similar as regards age, sex, BMI, ASA grade, postoperative abdominal scars and severity of the gallbladder disease.

The median operative time was 60 min and 75 min in groups A and B respectively. Insertion of an additional port was required in group B (8 pts. 20%). Patients from group A had more frequently pain on their shoulders (6 in group A and 2 in group B, 15% and 5% respectively). The analysis of our data showed no differences between group A and group B in terms of: post-operative pain, use painkillers and postoperative hospital stay (24h-36h).
Cardiopulmonary complications during the operation were related to the group A especially the high-risk patients.

The low intra-abdominal pressure during LC is more safe method because it is minimize the haemodynamics problems. It is indicated for old patients and those with cardiopulmonary problems.

P 119

ADVANTAGES OF HARMONIC SCALPEL (ULTRACISION) IN LAPAROSCOPIC SURGERY

S. Skaltsas, E. Gonia, E. Tsaniklides, A. Pachydakis, G. Stamatopoulos, S. Ôriantafyllides
Patission General Hospital, 1st Surgical Clinic, Athens, Greece

Aims
To prove the superiority of the use of the Harmonic Scalpel in the Laparoscopic Surgery

Methods
130 cases were examined in terms of operative time, perioperative and postoperative bleeding and length of hospital stay.

Results
The Harmonic Scalpel is creating a much smaller in depth burned surface making the healing of the damaged tissue quicker and is at the same time very efficient in closing firmly the small biliaries making the postoperative complications rare and the recovery time shorter.
When in use, it produces a small cloud of vapor wich vanishes quickly, so use of suction wich affects the pneumoperitoneum is limited and very close camera takes are possible. That is the reason for reduced operative time.

Conclusions
The Harmonic Scalpel is more effective and less destructive than the electrosurgery. There is no postoperative bile leakage, postoperative hemorhage is less probable, healing is accomplished faster and the patient rehabilitates sooner.

P 120

ADVANTAGES OF THE LAPAROSCOPIC OVER OPEN CHOLECYSTECTOMY

Cvijanovic R., Zoricic D., Farkas E., Milosevic K.

Clinical Center Novi Sad, Institute for Surgery, Clinic for Abdominal and Endocrine Surgery, Novi Sad, Yugoslavia

Aims: Attempts to the establish minilaparotomy in order to minimize postoperative complaints didn't achieve desired results, but introducing laparoscooic cholecystectomy gave substantial changes.
Methods: The prospective study in the last one-year period was done. The study consists of two groups patients, first group with the 100 patients operated on by laparoscopic cholecystectomy, and the second group with the 100 patients operated on by classic cholecystectomy. All available data were analyzed, especially duration and intensity of the postoperative pain, patient's postoperative mobilization, complications and costs.
Results: During classic, open cholecystectomy there is section of the muscles with nerves, which cause postoperative pain. This leads to delay in patient's mobilization postoperatively. Possibility of seroma, hemathoma, wound infection formation, as well as herniation is up to 12%. After laparoscopic cholecystectomy postoperative pain is less intensive and lasts one, or two days. Mobilization of the patients is more rapid, so the postoperative complications are very rare. Convalescence is incomparably shorter after laparoscopic operation, which decrease hospital and overall expenses.
Conclusions: Advantages are at the laparoscopic side; therefore it is unjustified to start with classic cholecystectomy.

P 121

IS LAPAROSCOPIC CHOLOLANGIOGRAFY FEASIBLE AND USEFUL AS A ROUTINE PRACTICE ?

N.Apostolopoulos . F.Karvelas . P.Dimopoulos . S.Adamopoulos . A.Papatsoris .

General Surgical Clinic . "Saint Andrews" General Hospital of Patras Hellas (Greece)

AIM : Evaluation of the usefulness and the risks of the routine laparoscopic cholangiography in our hospital .

PATIENTS AND METHODS : We studied 185 patients , where elective laparoscopic cholecystectomy with intraoperative cholangiography took place . There was a preoperative suspicion of chololithiasis for 34 of the patients .

RESULTS : Intraoperative cholangiography was succeeded in 162 patients (rate 90%) . In 2 patients (rate 1%) the billiary duct was injured during cholangiography . From the patients without preoperative indication of chololithiasis 1 patient had chololithiasis which was shown during the operation . From the group with preoperative indications of chololithiasis , 8 had lithiasis of the billiary duct . which was shown intraoperative and in 3 patients the intraoperative cholangiography was not possible . In 4 patients (rate 2,47%) the cholangiography showed possible injury of the billiary duct during the dissection .

CONCLUSION : The intraoperative cholangiography as a routine practice is feasible and useful during the laparoscopic cholecystectomy , but the risk of injuring the billiary duct is high .

P 122

SPECTRUM AND MANAGEMENT OF COMPLICATIONS AFTER CHOLECYSTECTOMY

Samy Osman, Mohamed K. El-Ammary
From the General Surgery Department, Sohag Faculty of Medicine, South Valley University, Egypt

Background: Death is an uncommon complication of open or laparoscopic cholecystectomy. The rapid introduc tion of laparoscopic cholecystectomy has been associated with apparently increased incidence of bile ducts injury which has provoked worldwide concern.

Patient and Method: The true incidence and mechanism of post-cholecystectomy complications wheather open or laparoscopic during the last 6 years in our hospital were studied.

Results: Open cholecystectomy was associated with biliary complications as retained stones, leakage of bile, bile duct injury Unusual lte biliary complications were retained gall bladder remnant containing stones and ampullary stenosis consequent to passatge of calculi or operative manipulation. A long cystic duct remnant has been implicated as a cause of postoperativd symptoms. Laparoscopic specifically complications were bile leakage, major bile duct injuries which was the most heralded complication and management are discussed.
Conclusion: Both open and laparoscopic cholecystectomy are highly safe and effective procedures for the treatment of patients with symptomatic gallbladder disease. Toay, adverse outcomes after open cholecystectomy are largely limited to elderly patients with co-morbid conditions and complicated biliary tract disease. Although infequent major biliary complicationsstill occur and have been slightly more common in the initial experience with laparoscopic cholecystectomy.

P 123

LAPAROSCOPIC TREATMENT OF ACUTE CHOLOCYSTITIS (EMPYEMA , HYDROPS).

P. Dimopoulos, N. Apostolopoulos, F. Karvelas, S. Adamopoulos and A.Papatsoris.
General Surgical Clinic, "Saint Andrews" General Hospital of Patras, GREECE.

Aim: Acute lithiasic cholocystitis with empyema or hydrors is thought to be an absolute contraindication for laparoscopic surgical treatment. We try to oppose this point of view.

Patients and Methods: We studied 17 patients (9 men and 8 female) with acute cholocystitis and empyema or hydrops. The average age was 63,2 years (29-78). The preoperative diagnosis was simple cholocystitis. During the laparoscopic operation we discovered that it was cholocystitis complicated with empyema or hydrops. We used veress needle to remove the content of the gallbladder. After we conceived the gallbladder with alligator forceps. The tissue dissection at the Calot triangle was always difficult, mainly because of the stone, which was wedged at the Hartman bursa. After the legation of the elements, the detachment of the gallbladder took place. We placed drainage for 48 hours and we gave double antibiosis for 3 days.

Results: Cholocystectomy was succeeded in all 17 patients (rate 100%). In 5 patients (29,4%) we had to leave a part of the parries of the gallbladder at the side of the liver. In 6 patients (35,2%) the gallbladder opened and the stones were removed by mechanic capture or by lavage through drainage tubes from the trocar (10mm). The average operation time was 90min (60-150). Postoperative analgesia was still less than analgesia in open cholocystectomy. There was no local collection. There was 1 purulence from the exit trocar of the gallbladder. The average nursing time was 4,1 days. Also there was no death.

Conclusion: Cholocystitis with empyema or hydrops should be treated with laparoscopic operation. The only difficulty is during the tissue dissection at the Calot triangle, which however is more difficult at the open operation.

P 124

THE MANAGEMENT OF ACUTE CHOLECYSTITIS AND THE LAPAROSCOPIC SURGERY"

V. PRIMIKIRIS, D. TSANTZALOS, P. VOULGARIS, S. TSOUPANOS, P. PAVLOPOULOS.
21° SURGICAL DEPARTMENT - 1 sT NOSPITAL IKA, ATHENS

The application of laparoscopic procedure in cases with acute cholecystitis creates rational hesitations. From January 19□'7 to May 19□8 four hundred fourteen L.C. took place. Thirtyeight of them were cases with acute cholecystitis. Four of them were gangrenous. All patients underwent laparoscopic operation by the surveillance of experienced surgeons. Eleven cases converted to open laparotomy (2,8 %). The mean hospitalization for L.C was 2,6 days while for the converted ones was 5,6 days. There was no mortality or any other major complication. Laparoscopic cholecystectomy seems to be a safe procedure even in cases with acute infection. The experience and the well custom to the technique allows us to be optimist for the results.

P 125

LAPAROSCOPIC CHOLELYSTECTOMY IN ACUTE LITHIASIC CHOLECYSTITIS

Dr. A. COTÎRLEŢ, Dr. E. TINCU, Dr. M. BUJOR
HOSPITAL MOINEŞTI – SURGICAL DEPARTAMENT – ROMANIA

DIM: Results evaluation of laparoscopic cholecystectomy in acute cholecystitis.
MATERIAL AND METHOD: Between 1 I 1996 – 31 XII 1998. We performed 80 laparoscopic cholecystectomies for histopathologically proved acute lithiasic cholecystitis. We studied clinic and echographic diagnosis, operative moment, conversion rate, operative time, postoperative morbidity and hospitalization. The cholecystectomy was performed within 72 hours in 20 patients (trial I), 4 to 7 days in 36 patients (trial II) and over 7 days in 24 patients (trial III).
RESULTS: Diagnosis of acute lithiasic cholecystitis was always possible by clinical examinations and ultrasonography. We performed 7 conversions in patients of trial II and 9 of trial III. The mean operative time was 70 minutes postoperative morbidity consisted in 2 bile leakages in the liver bed, 1 subhepatic abscess, 2 right pleural effusion. The mean hospitalization was 4,5 days.
CONCLUSIONS: 1. Urgent laparoscopic cholecystectomy is a benefic act for acute lithiasic cholecystitis.
2. The operative moment is the most important factor of influence on conversion rate, operative time and postoperative morbidity.

P 126

PARTIAL AUXILIARY LIVER TRANSPLANTATION IN DOGS

Ahmed A. Maharan, Gamal A. Ahmed, Bahjat A. Thabit, Mohamed M. El Shafie, Hassan B. El-Badawy, Mustafa A. Hassanien and Golnar M. Fathy*
Department of Surgery and Anaesthesia
*Faculty of Medicine Assiut University

This work included 30 healthy mongrel dogs weighting between 10-25 kgs (mean 17.5 kgs). The dogs were divided into 2 main groups.
I. The first group was subjected to partial auxiliary autotransplantation. The immunological factors were behind this choice. The left lobe of liver in 5 dogs was dissected and transplanted in the right flank or pelvic regions of the same animals. The outcome of these animals was not encourging. This enforced us tho change the procedure to be homotransplantation in the second group.
II. In the second group heterotopic transplantation was studied in 25 cases as follows:
1 - Subgroup II-A: was subjected to partial auxiliary transplantation without porto-caval shunt in 10 cases.
2 - Subgroup II-B: was subjected to partial auxiliary transplantation and porto-caval shunt in the same sitting (10 cases) in order to minimize the effect of functional competition which is usually developed between the host liveer and the graft.
3 - In subgroup II-C: we started firstly by porto-caval shunt and after 3 weeks we transplanted the graft.
We can concluded that:
1. Auxiliary transplantation will be simple, safer and may be more convenient in all diseases which do not require hepatectomy.
2. Portal blood represents an absolute factor for functioning of the graft.
3. Auxiliary transplantation is more suitable as we leave the host liver in its place.
4. The auxiliary grafts from a living related donor will be more convenient after further confirmatory and complementary studies on animals.

P 127

Liver resections for intrahepatic stones

R. Čolović, D. Bilanović, M. Jovanović, S. Zogović

First Surgical University Hospital, Institute of Digestive Diseases, Clinical Center of Serbia, Belgrade, Yugoslavia

Intrahepatic stones had been regarded as a disease of far east countries, but it turned out not to be rare in the western world as well. We registered it in 1,21 % of all biliary stone disease patients. Surgical treatment is necessary in majority of these patients. In some cases liver resections may be necessary.
Over a 13 year period we did segment II nad III liver resections in 15 pts and segment V resection in one pt. 11 men and 5 women. Recurrent attacks of cholangitis were registered in 75 % of patients. Twelve patients (75 %) had been operated before elsewhere from 1 to 3 times and 26 different procedures have been carried out (11 cholecystectomies, 6 choledocholitotomies and "T" tube drainage, 5 choledochoduodenostomies, 2 choledochojejunostomies, 1 distal gastrectomy and 1 hydatide cyst operation). Besides liver resection we performed 20 additional procedures either to correct previous improper procedures or to improve biliary drainage. There was one postoperative death (6,25 %). A number of minor complications were registered in 7 patients (50 %). The average hospital stay was 37 days. All 15 patients have been followed up from 8 to 153 months (average 55 months). A favorable result is registered in all patients.
We conclude that if properly indicated liver resection may be extremly useful in the treatment of some patients with intrahepatic stones.

P 128

INDICATIONS OF THE CHOLEDOCHODUODENOSTOMY BY BENIGN AND MALIGNANT DISEASE OF THE CHOLEDOCHUS DUCT AND HEAD OF PANGREAS

A.Koussidis, G.Koussidis, A.Apsokardou, I.GeorgiadisSurgical Department, General Hospital of Chios - Greece

Aims: The aim of this communication is to point out the value of choledochoduodenostomy of benign and malignant disease of the choledochus duct and the head of the pancreas.

Methods: During the last decade 76 choledochoduodenostomies were performed in our clinic for benign and malignant disease of the common bile duct and head of the pancreas. In 51 patients multiple choledocholithiasis was the reason for the surgical intervention. The age of the patients was in the range of 40 to 85. 29 patients were females and 22 were males. 25 patients were operated for cancer of the head of the pancreas. The age of the patients was in the range of 50 to 88. 11 of them were females and 14 were males. Majority of the patients in both groups was above the age of 70.

Results: The 51 patients operated for multiple choledocholithiasis were completely healed. No cases of post operative cholangiitis were presented neither in the short nor in the long term. The 25 patients submitted to choledochoduodenostomy for cancer of the head of the pancreas exhibited significant improvement of their health state. The postoperative period of survival was in the range of 6 to 42 months. Of this group only one patient aged 84,died on the 14th postoperative day.

Conclusions: Choledochoduodenostomy constitutes a surgical method that contributes to the complete healing of patient with benign disease of the common bile duct. In malignancies of the head of the pancreas the method contributes to the prolongation and improvement of the quality of life post operatively.

P 129

Reconstruction and restore operations on offliver bile ducts

A.A. Ashrafov
Azerbaijan Medical University, Baku, Azerbaijan

At the period of last 10 years in our clinic 285 patients underwent surgery because of different non-tum or diseases of offliver bile ducts. The patients age varied from 16 to 84 years old. There were 191 female and 94 male patients. All the necessary clinical laboratory tests and also special methods were used. Almost all the patients were performed on ultrasonographic investigation, which helped in 86 percent of cases. In 13 cases fibroscopic retrograde cholan giopan creatography was used. (FRCPG) In 11 cases computer tomography was used. 244 patients were diagnosed choledocholithiasis, fibrosis of the opening of bile duct into the duodenum was diagnosed at 23 patients, combination of choledocholithiasis and fibiasis of the opening of bile duct into the duodenum was found in 18 cases, 17 of 285 patients were operated on the fist day of entering to the clinic with acute cholecystitis and choledocholithiasis, complicated by peritonitis. 220 patients were operated on their 2 –5 day of entering to the clinic. 48 patients in satisfactory condition were operated on later the fifth day.

In 98 of 285 operated patient was a necessity of performing reconstruction and restore operations, because of abnormality at bile flow into the duodenum. The operations named the creation of various types of biliodigestive anastom osises choledochoduodenoanastom osises were created at 55 patients. In 21 cases was used a double drainage of common bile duct. Papillotomy with plastic surgery performed in 15 cases. At the rest patients, because of duodenostasis, was used hepaticojejunoanastomosis in combination with Braun anastomosis or with Rue method separated small intestine. 3 patients died out from 98. (3.1% mortality). Cause of death in 2 cases was bile peritonitis and in 1 case was the tromboemboly of pulmonary artery.

P 130

CICATRICIAL STENOSIS OF THE PROXIMAL COMMON HEPATIC DUCT. A REPORT OF 11 CASES

Speranzini, M.B., Mittelstaedt, W., Deutsch, C., Aunha, J.C., Waisberg, J., Bromberg S.H.
Faculdade de Medicina do ABC - Santo André

Aims: Eleven patients with cica tricial stenosis in the junction area of hepatic ducts were evaluated.
Methods: In all patients the injury occured during choolescystectomy and no operative cholangiography was performed. In 3 patients the injury was recognized during the initial cholecistectomy. Ten patients had been operated on at least one time to correct the injury in other Service. Four cases had duct or peritoneal drainage. There was an attempt of reanastomosis in two cases. Five patients had a bilio-digestive anatomosis performed in variable occasions. Two patients were reoperated 5 times, one patient 3 times. The others were submitted to one or 2 reoperations. There were a period of 1 to 72 months between the unjury and last reoperation, Jaundice was the most common presenting manifestation since it appeared in all patient except one. Five patients had biliary cirrhosis.
Results: Roux-en-Y hepaticojejunostomy was carried out in all cases after enlarging the biliar stoma by longitudinal section on the left hepatic duct and performing a termino-terminal anastomosis. The 10 or 12 cliber Kehr drain used was taken out after the control cholangiography, carried around the second postoperative week. Concerning the long term results, one patient died of recurrent cholangitis six months after the 6th reoperation and one patient 14 months after the 4th reoperation of liver failure. Both had biliary cirrhosis. Two patients, remained assymptomatic for 60 months and 3 patients for 24,37 and 56 months.
Conclusions: The importance of preventing this severe complication is stressed by the authors. Patients with such lesions need be referred to specialized centers where well trained suergeons are available. The technique herein presented seems us to be a good options.

P 131

Scintograhic Confirmation of Obstruktive Icterus and It's Surgical Treatment

S. Sekulic, R. Kosanovic, B. Lazic, P. Simic, D. Zlta

Medical Facylti, Surgical Clinic Pristina, YUGOSLAVIA

Hephatobillious Scintigraphy (HBS) is nuclear-medical method for functional-morphological research of hepathobillious fractus. HBS is used for diagnossis and differential diagnossis of sholestasis, icterius, functional dissorders of hepathobillios fractus, condenital anomalies of billious fractus etc. Specific derivates of DA marked with tehnicium (99m Tc) are used in HBS method.

In 1997. 3508 patients with GIT disseases were treated at Surgical Clinic, Faculty of Medicine in Pristina. 368 billious tractus operations were performed during the period. 74,5% of patient were female and 25,5% male. Average age of patients was 55,3 years. 99 (26,9%) patients were operated due to obstructive icterious during the period. In 54,4% of cases cause of the obstruction was choledolituiasis, in 7,3. The cause was gallbladder carcinom, in 6,1%. The cause was gallbladder paths carcinom, in 22,2%. The cause was Irancreas head tumors, in 5,1% of cases the cause was liver carcinom, in 3,0%. The cause was liver echinococus and done on 31 (31,3%) patients with obstructive icterus for confirmation, using 3 mCi 99m TC i DA. Mantaining of the pharmac occured: on liver level in 6 (19,4%) cases (liver carcinom, gallbladder carcinom-explorative aparatomy and biopsy); on choledohus level in 15 (48,4%) cases (gallbladder paths carcinom, gallbladder carcinom-sholedohotomy, resection with Roux curve); on dvodenum level 10 (32,3%) cases (pancreas head tumor, Stenossis papile Water inclaviated calculosis-explorative laparatomy with biopsy, pancreatectomy, papilectomy, choledohotomy, choledoduodenostomy).

We have omly confirmed or annuled disseases that we could not diagnosse by means of other method, HBS. Accuracy in diagnossis helps the surgeon to chose and prepare method and aproach to procedure.

P 132

"MUCASAL-GRAFT" METHOD IN BILE DUCT INJURY TREATMENT.

Raczyanska S., Dybicki J., Draczkowski T., Kostro J., Witczak-Malinowska K.

I Department of Surgery Medical University of Gdansk, Poland
Ul. Debinki 7, 80-211 Gdansk, Poland

Aim: Mucosal-graft is a very rare method of treatment of biliary tract injuries. The aim of our study was to present the result of such treatment.
Methods: In the years 1970-1998, 56 reconstruction procedures were performed. 43 patients were admited with existing bile duct injuries, 37 of them underwent at least one atempt of reconstruction. In 14 cases type III, and in 9 type IV stenosis ac. to
Bismuth's classiffication was found. In 17 patients "mucosal-graft" technique was used: in 15 - the ductal hepaticus was anastomosed to the jejunum, and in 2 to the duodenum. In type III
stenosis single drainage was performed, in type IV - double drainage on two separate stents was done.
Results: Two patients died out of 17 operated using the mucosal-graft technique (first - on the 6th postopertive day due to hepato-renal insufficiency, the second - 3 month after the operation due to
cerebral insufficiency). The remaining 15 patients have a patent anastomosis.
Conclusion: The mucosal-graft is an effective method of treatment
of high biliary injuries, associated with a good long term effect.

P 133

PERIOPERATIVE CHOLANGIOGRAPHY. EXPERIENCE IN 2930 CASES

S. Skaltsas[1], A. Pachydakis[1], E. Tsaniklides[1], E. Gonia[1], M. Chaniotakis[1], A. Giannakakis[1], B. Kekis[2]
1. Patission General Hospital, 1st Surgical Clinic, Athens, Greece
2. Athens Medical Center, Athens, Greece

Aims
Although Intraoperative Cholangiography (IC) has been a routine procedure in several centers in the past is nowadays been accused of misleading the surgeon. This tendency is due to other diagnostic and therapeutic procedures that prove IC to give false positive and false negative results in numerous cases.

Methods
For the last 25 years information was accumulated about patients who underwent IC with or without findings. The data was compared to the findings of the surgical exploration of the biliary tree as well as with the ERCP findings.

Results
Intraoperative Cholangiography was proved to be useful only in: 1) cases were the anatomy and the morphology of the biliary tree should be examined preoperatively according to the surgeon 2) During laparoscopic surgery altered in open surgery due to probable injury or unusual anatomy of the biliary tract. 3) During surgery in patients where there was failure to perform ERCP

Conclusions
IC should be performed only in strictly selected patients because it can mislead the surgeon to unnecessary surgical manipulations.

P 134

STRATEGY OF SPHINCTEROTOMY IN THE EXTRAHEPATIC BILIARY DISEASE

S. Skaltsas, E. Tsaniklides, A. Pachydakis, S. Triantafyllides, A. Giannakakis
Patission General Hospital, 1st Surgical Clinic, Athens, Greece

Aims
Since the introduction of Laparoscopic Surgery the number of ERCPs performed has enormously augmented.Our aim was to determine the proper timing for performing ERCP in patients with extrahepatic biliary disease to be surgically managed.

Methods
We selected our patients in terms of combined history, liver function tests and ultrasonography. None of these criteria alone was efficient in the patients selection. Patients with only asymptomatic gallblader stones were excluded.

Results
ERCP proved to be useful in patients were there was suspicion of unusual morphology of the biliary tree as well as in patients with a high suspicion of common bile duct stones. Even in cases were there was anatomic or other problems and the patient finally underwent surgery, ERCP proved to be most useful to the surgeon showing the exact coordinates of the problem.

Conclusions
Selective preoperative ERCP can prevent a Cholocystectomy from being a complex operation including management of a possible lithiasis of the bile duct. The operation becomes of a lower mortality and morbidity and in case of failure accomplishing ERCP there is always the reserved solution of a subsequent operation.

P 135

N.ECONOMOU-V.ARGITIS-A.KARKALETSIS-A.KYRIAKIDIS-A.ALIFRAGIS-J.ADAMAKIS-M.KANARA-J.CHRONIS-G.ANTSAKLIS.
"Acute peritonitis caused by diseases from the biliary tract.The 5-year experiance of our surgical department."
Surgical department of Sismanoglion G.H.Athens,Greece.
Acute peritonitis as a complication of a disease from the biliary tract,occurs in 0,16% of urgent surgical operations.This study includes 19 patients which were hospitalized between Sept.' 92 and Sept.' 98.
The commonest cause was cholelithiasis and the patients aged 70,5 years m.o.
The surgical treatment of choice was cholecystectomy and common bile duct exploration
Morbidity and mortality rates were 22,6% and 50% respectively.
In conclusion,these patients are ofter extremly ill,urgently operated and diagnosed with a delay.These are the main reasons for the high morbidity and mortality rates they present.
For any problems please contact with E-mail:lakonia@otenet.gr
Thank you.

P 136

MANAGEMENT OF BILIARY TRACT STENOSIS IN LIVER TRANSPLANT RECIPIENTS: ROLE OF RADIOLOGY AND INTERVENTION

Doros A .,Weszelits V., Puhl M., Dabasi G.,Görög D., Perner F.
Semmelweis Medical University, Transplantation and Surgical Clinic, Budapest, Hungary

Aims: to show the variety of biliary complications after orthotopic liver transplantation, and the endoscopical and radiological diagnostic and therapeutic possibilities. Methods: In our institute from jan.1996 to jan.1999 64 orthoto liver transplantation were performed.. The incidence of intra- or extrahepatical bile duct stenosis was 11% (in the literature 9-30%). The main causes were ischemic or inflammatory injury of the bile ducts, and the surgical technical problem in the choldocho-choledochal anastomosis site. The diagnosis of biliary complications is based on laboratory datas, sonography, cysticus drain cholangiography scintigraphy, MRCP, CT and CT-cholangiography, ERCP and PTC. The therapy can be surgical reanastomosis, endoscopical (temporary or permanent stent placement), or using the percutan transhepatic approach
(drainage, bilioplasty, self-expandable stent placement).For follow up US, CT and CT-cholangiography , scintigraphy and MRCP can be used.
Results: We performed 15 PTC/PTD in 8 patients. 6 patients had katheter bilioplasty. All the patients with previous bilioplasty developed restenosis. 5 self expandable stents were placed in 4 patients. One patient has two stents. The patient with 2 stents and 2 patient with 1-1 stent are doing well for 30, 12 and 5 months. One patient had surgical
reanastomosis, three patients had retransplantation. One patient with stent died in the first week due to acute hepatic failure not related to the stent.
Conclusions: In cases of biliary tract complications in liver transplant patients radiology plays a major role in the diagnosis and interventional therapy. The modern imaging modalities (
CT/cholangiography, MRCP with 3D reconstruction) help to plan surgical or inteventional therapy. Concerning the patients general status endoscopic temporary stent placement, or percutaneous external, or external-internal drainage are the method of choice, but in selected cases bilioplasty (especially in the intrahepatic ducts) and (even primary) self-expandable stent placement are good alternatives with acceptable long term results.

P 137

Endoscopic treatment of benign biliary strictures after laparoscopic and open cholecystectomy

L. Topa, Á. Pap*
2nd Dept. of Int. Medicine, St. Imre Hospital, and *Central Hospital of the Hungarian Railways, Budapest, Hungary

The damage of the biliary tree is a rare, but severe complication of open and laparoscopic cholecystectomy. The rate of biliary injury is 0.1-3% and 1% after laparoscopic (LC) and open (OP) cholecystectomy, respectively. The most important factor is the routine of surgeons. The cause of the common bile duct stricture used to be the damage of the biliary tree by the inappropriate insertion of the clip after LC, and the prolonged Kehr-drainage following choledochotomy after OP.

We analysed data on 2863 endoscopic retrograde cholangio-pancreatographies made in our department between 1995 and 1997. **Patients:** 36 cases with benign postoperative biliary strictures (1,2%): 21 cases after OP, and 15 cases after LC. **Diagnosis of biliary stricture:** *in LC cases*, bile leakage through the abdominal drain remained after surgery; *in OP cases*, the extraction of Kehr-drain (average duration 6 weeks) was followed by obstructive jaundice: dilated intra- and extrahepatic biliary ducts were shown by ultrasound, and elevated alkaline phosphatase, GGT and bilirubine levels occurred in the serum. **Endoscopic treatment:** complete endoscopic sphincterotomy was followed by stent implantation into the common bile duct in every case. In two cases a Wall-stent placement was necessary. Simple drainage was made in 17 patients, double drainage in 15 cases. In addition, one case got three, and one four drains. Naso-biliary drainage was needed in 16 cases for the management of suppurative cholangitis. The follow-up of patients was continuos. **Results:** *1. In the LC group:* endoscopic stent removal has been performed in 11 patients, while two patients lost their drains spontaneously. The mean time of stent removal was 5,5 months. In the present, the drains in the common bile duct still remained in four patients. *2. In the OP group:* the removal of stent was possible only in 7 cases (these patients had multiple stents). In this group, 14 cases still have the drains at this moment. The mean time of stent-removal was 8,4 months.

Conclusions: The postoperative benign strictures of the common bile duct can be treated successfully with endoscopic stent-placement, a procedure which seems to be effective and safe. The duration of stent-placement was shorter in the LC group. Finally, after multiple stent placements the success-rate was higher compared to the simple stent-holder group.

P 138

LAPAROSCOPIC CHOLECYSTECTOMY AND CANCER OF THE GALLBLADDER

L.Tóth, K.Takáts, Z.Balika, J.Felker, Anna Szilágyi

Surgical Dept. of City Hospital MÓR

Pathological Dept., County Hospital Székesfehérvár, Hungary

According to literature data the histological examination of the exstirpated gallbladder reveals carcinoma in 2-7% of the cases. Cancer of the gallbladder is diagnosed preoperatively only in one fifth of the patients. Histological examination following 1420 laparoscopic cholecystectomies reveled an early stage carcinoma in 4 cases and an infiltrative carcinoma in one cases. For a 3-48 months follow-up period 4 patients have been tumor- and symptom-free. 1 patient is alive with tumor.
Authors review the results of surgery of gallbladder carcinomas. In the case of a preoperatively suspect malignant process an open surgery is indicated. If histology confirms carcinoma an individual decision on reoperation should be made, depending upon the site and extent of the tumor.

P 139

PROGNOSTIC FACTORS FOLLOWING AGGRESSIVE RESECTION AND TRANSPLANTATION FOR HILAR CHOLANGIOCARCINOMA

B J Ammori, T Mahmood, K R Prasad, S G Pollard, J P A Lodge
Departments of Hepatobiliary Surgery, St. James's University Hospital, Beckett Street, Leeds LS9 7TF, UK

AIMS To define the prognostic factors after surgical resection of hilar cholangiocarcinoma.
METHODS: Between January 1991 and July 1998, 36 patients underwent laparotomy for radiologically operable hilar cholangiocarcinoma. Twenty nine patients underwent resection (local resection 2, major liver resection 19, orthotopic liver transplantation 8). Survival analyses were performed by the Kaplan-Meier method. Univariate survival analysis was assessed by the log-rank test. Multivariate results were confirmed using the Cox regression model. The end point in the analysis was death due to any cause. Eighteen variables were studied including age, sex, extent and type of resection, pathological variables (TNM stage, differentiation, resection margin involvement, caudate lobe involvement, perineural or vascular invasion) and adjuvant therapy.
RESULTS: Hospital mortality was 9.5% for resection alone and 13.8% when liver transplantation was considered. The Kaplan-Meier 3-year actuarial survival for resection alone, transplantation and 'no resection' was 37.4%, 31.3% and 0% respectively. Univariate analysis identified male sex and poor tumour differentiation in patients who underwent resection and age <45 years in all resected and transplanted patients as factors with a statistically significant value. Cox analysis, however, identified poor tumour differentiation to be the only independent prognostic factor in patients who underwent resection alone.
CONCLUSIONS: Satisfactory medium-term survival can be achieved with aggressive resection and transplantation for hilar cholangiocarcinoma. Prognosis after resection is mainly determined by tumour differentiation.

P 140

HOW TO IMPROVE THE RESULTS OF TREATMENT OF PROXIMAL BILE DUCT CANCER

V. Vishnevski , V. Koubishkin, A. Chzhao , R. Ikramov

Institute of surgery , Moscow , Russia .

Aims: To evaluate the possibility of radical and palliative resection in pts. with advanced Klatskin tumors in view of long term results and quality of life.
Methods: II and III stages operations (radical and palliative excision of the tumor) were done in 61 pts with Klatskin tumors
Results: In heavy jaundiced pts. with III-IYA stages of the tumors (68,9% of all pts) two and three stages operations were done. Postoperative mortality was 3 / 4,9% /. 4 pts were treated by intraductal radiotherapy. Actuarial survival in 1, 2, 3, 4 and 5 years were 100%, 87.5%, 87.5%, 75% and 53%. All pts lived more than 1 year with good life quality. 4 pts were operated in the late period for local recurrency (reconstruction of the anastomoses on PTD).
Conclusion : radical and palliative resections are justified in pts with III and IYA stages of Klatskin tumors.

P 141

CANCER OF THE COMMON BILE DUCT: COMBINED PERCUTAN TREATMENT

Vigváry Z, Tarján Z, Makó E Dept. of Radiology, Semmelweis Medical University, Budapest, Hungary

Aim: Our purpose is to demonstrate the feasibility of combined interventional radiological and intraluminal radiation treatment in patients with obstructive jaundice caused by malignant masses.
Methods: In a patient with obstructive jaundice caused by nonoperable cholangiocarcinoma originating from the common bile duct the following palliative treatment was applied: after percutaneous biliary drainage intraluminal Cs 137 irradiation with LDR after loading was applied (32 Gy, 24 h). The irradiated lumen was stented by percutaneous transhepatic intervention applying double endoprothesis.
Results: The intervention was well tolerated well and ensured free bile flow. The patient died due to the progression of the disease 19 months later free of jaundice.
Conclusions: We conclude that intraluminal irradiation in combination with biliary percutaneous intervention is a feasible and promising treatment to increase the efficacy of palliative percutaneous drainages in patients with obstructive jaundice caused by malignant masses.

P 142

PORT SITE METASTASIS OF OCCULT PRIMARY TUMOUR

[x]Rahóty P., [x]Besznyák I., [x]Sulyok Z., [xx]Péter I, [x]Farkas E.
[x]Department of Surgery, National Institute of Oncology
[xx]Diagnostic and Experimental Tumour Pathology Centre
1122 Budapest, Ráth Gy. u. 7-9.

In line with spreading of the minimally invasive surgical technique appearance of new complications like the so-called port site metastases can be reckoned with.
Analysis of endoscopic cholecystectomy data in Hungary shows an incidence of port site metastases in 0.03‰. The authors observed a tumour metastasis of unknown primary at the site of epigastric port of laparoscopic cholecystectomy performed 14 months before. Twenty four months after reintervention their patient is free of symptoms and complaints. Referring to this case literature dealing with the incidence of port site metastases is reviewed. Attention is drawn to the necessity of in-depth investigation and entire intraoperative endoscopic exploration to be performed prior to endoscopic surgical interventions.

P 143

SURGICAL TREATMENT OF MALIGNANT TUMORS AT THE BIFURCATION OF THE CHOLEDOCHAL DUCT

V. Paizis, G. Panetsos, A. Polydorou, M. Theodorakopoulou, E. Tzirakis, D. Kalatzopoulos, K. Megalokonomos, K. Sykiotis
Surgical Department, Hippokration Hospital, Athens, Greece

During the last seven years we have treated in our Department 28 patients with malignant tumors at the bifurcation of the choledochal duct. This group of patients was composed by 10 males and 18 females with mean age 61 and 68 years respectively. Their diagnostic work up included: abdominal ultrasound, computerized tomography with IV contrast and/or MRI and endoscopic retrograde cholangiopancreatography (ERCP).
They were stage (according to Bismuth classification) to stage I (6 patients), stage II (11 patients) and stage III (11 patients). We considered a tumor resectable if there were no hepatic or regional lymph node metastases. Three of the patients, (Bismuth stage I, 10%) underwent resection of the tumor and regional lymph node resection with Roux en y reconstruction after intraoperative stent placement. In five patients a paliative bypass of the tumor was performed. In three patients a transhepatic - transdermal catheter was placed (Terblance) while the remaining seventeen patients were treated non surgically. Thirteen had a stent placed with an ERCP and four through a PTC. We only had problems with catheter oclusion in five patients, that had an ERCP guided stent placement that required a PTC to had a better biliary decompression. The mean survival of the surgically treated group was 18 months computed to 10 months of the non surgically treated patients.

P 144

CASE OF CARCINOMA OF CYSTIC DUCT ET ADENOMA OF GALLBLADDER

Vukmirovic B; Varicak N; Saric P; Djurovic D; *Trifunov S; *Gligoric D.
Department of General Surgery et*Department of Patohistology
Health Centre"dr.R.Simonovic",Vojvodjanska 75,25000 Sombor,Yugoslavia
Key Words:Cystic-Duct surgery,Bile-Duct neoplasms,opstructive jaundice

Aim was to report a case of carcinoma of cystic duct(CCD) together with adenoma cholecystae.

We compared only 36 cases(including this)CCD published in literature(1,2).We admited 56 year old man with symptoms of biliary colic.Obstuctive jaundice tended to progres then to regres.Ultrasonography indicates polypus in fundus of gallbladder.Operation was performed on December 2.1996.Intraoperative-cholangiography(CHIO)was attempted through the cystic duct but was given up as duct was impassable.Gallbladder was then surgicaly removed together with entire cystic duct.Choledochotomy followed and then,through choledochal duct,CHIO which did not show any signs of obstructive or external compresion of the choledochal duct.Following cholangioscopy T tube was placed and subsequently removed following normal cholangiographic finding.Patohistological examination led us to real diagnosis;Adenocarcinoma ducti cystici(pT1,Nx,Mx).Adenoma vesicae felleae.Cholecystitis chronica.

Patient is still being observed(25 months) and there are no signs of either local recurrencesor metastatic changes.Ten of 21 cases vere lived less than 18 months,and 11 vere lived longer than 18 months.

Symptoms of CCD were unspecific,topographic area occupied by cystic duct was small, so that preoperative diagnosis usually is seldom possible.Postoperative, patohistological examination of cystic duct led us to true diagnosis,brings us to question as to wheather the surgery perfomed was radical.After each cholecystectomy, in addition to patohistological examination of gallbladder it is necessary also to examine cystic duct especially in patients with acalculous cholecystitis and obstructive jaundice of an unknown case.

P 145

PRIMARY CARCINOMA OF THE GALLBLADDER EXPERIENCE OF 18 CASES IN ASSIUT UNIVERSITY HOSPITALS

Mohammed M. El Shafie
Department of General Surgery, Faculty of Medicine, Assiut University

Carcinoma of gallbladder is not a rare entity. This study presents 18 cases (15 remales and 3 males) of histologically proven primary carcinoma of the gallbladder among 866 patients operated in the General Surgery Department of Assiut University Hospital for different biliary troubles during the last 4 years. In only five cases the diagnosis of gallbladder tumour was suggested preoperatively by the help of CT scan and abdominal sonography. In 83.3% of cases (15 out of 18) galistones were associated. Diagnosis wqas confirmed only by laparotomy and histopathological examination. Adenocarcinoma (77%), undifferentiated carcinoma (16%) and squamous cell carcinoma (5%) were the pathological types of the tumours. Areas of spred included liveer bed, portahepatis and caeliac lymph nodes. Distant metastasis included mesenteric lymph nodes, bones and umblicus.

Clinical presentations included pain, fever, vomiting, jaundice, dyspepsia and upper right quadrant mass. Surgical manoeuvers included laparotomy and external billiary drainage, gastrojejunostomy and wedge hepatic resection. 1The mean survival time postoperatively wa 7 months with 2 cases living for 18 and 22 months.

The best hope to improve this dismal lies in earlier cholecystectomy in patients with calcular or benign gallbladder disease.

P 146

DONOR AND RECIPIENT PENTOXIFYLLINE PRETREATMENT IMPROVES VIABILITY OF LIVERS PROCURED FROM NON-HEART-BEATING DONORS

Astarcioglu H., Karademir S. Ünek T., Özer E., Atila K., Coker A., Astarcioglu I.
Dokuy Eylül University Hospital, Izmir, Turkey

Pentoxifylline pretreatment of graft recipients was shown to protect against liver graft failure from ischemia-reperfusion injury after orthotopic rat liver transplantation. It has also been shown that pentoxifylline protects against normothermic ischemi-reperfusion injury to liver in lobar ischemia model in the rat. Whether pentoxifylline can benefit the liver procured from non-heart-beating donors (NHBDs) with up 9 hours of cold ischemia is unknown. Donor and recipient rats were pretreated with pentoxifylline (50 mg/kg) 1 hour before the cardiac arrest and transplantation respectively. Transplantation was performed in the rats with donor cardiac arrest from 0 to 30 and 60 minutes with additional 1 hour or 9 hours cold ishemia times as pentoxifylline pretreated groups (n=10/group). The same number of liver transplantations was done in each paired control group without donor and recipient pentoxifylline pretreatment. Pentoxifylline treatment was continued for 5 days postoperatively (25 mg/kg) in surviving recipients. Recipient survival rates, serum enzymes and histopathological examination of post-reperfusion (6 th hour) liver biopsies were analysed. The survival rates were significantly improved in the groups treated with pentoxifylline (in both 1/2 hr. and 1 hr. warm ischemia + 9 hr of colt ischemia) vs controls (p=0.03 and p=0.005 respectively). On conclusion, donor and recipient pentoxifylline pretreatment improves viability of livers procured from NHBDs.

P 147

NEW ASPECTS IN TREATMENT OF ECHINOCOCCOSIS CYSTS.

S.A.Dadvani, A.N.Lotov, G.H.Musaev, F.P.Kovalenko
Moscow Medical Academy, Surgical clinic № 1, Moscow, Russia

Purpose: study of the parasite's biology and improvement results of surgical treatment of echinococcosis cysts.
Materials and methods: between 1986 and 1999 in Surgical clinic N 1 Moscow medical Academy were treated 148 patients with echinococcosis cysts. Up to middle of the 1990-th year the treatment of echinococcosis cysts was carried out on the standard techniques, from a beginning 90-th more actively have begun to be applied minimally invasive technologies. Together with Institute of parasitology and tropical medicine on experimental models on rats studied biology of the parasite, interaction of the parasite and the owner organism, reaction of the parasite on surgical intervention. On the basis of experimental researches and biological tests we was carried out search more effective protozoicides, studied a liquid and brood capsule of the man's echinococcosis cysts by means the microscopy.
Results of research: there revealed, what even at long term of an echinococcosis cyst's destruction in detrite and brood capsule can be kept a live protoscolexs or acephalocysts of the parasite. For the first time in the world the new aspect in duplication of the parasite is revealed. Established, that as against the earlier known fact development acephalocysts from brood capsule of an environment of the echinococcosis laters can develop as well from protoscolex at any stage of the parasite's life. Established, that widely distributed protozoicides at the standard exposition during operation not always cause destruction all elements of the parasite, in particular acephalocysts, who contribute for a relapse of disease.
Conclusions: the received results testify to necessity of some correction of intraoperative processing of cysts and dictate necessity of application with this purpose new, more effective antiparasitic agents.

P 148

GALLSTONE ILEUS OF THE SIGMOID COLON
Case report
Koželj M., Kavalar R., Horvat M.
Teaching Hospital Maribor, Slovenia

In the last 20 years we experienced 27 patients with the gallstone ileus of the small bowel antecedent by the cholecystoduodenal fistulas. According to the literature the most frequent are cholecystoduodenal (70 %), cholecystocolonic (13,5 %), cholecystogastric (11 %) fistulas. The etiology of the fistulas is chronic and acute inflammation of the gallbladder together with gallstones. We report a case of 80 years old female patient with chronic lymphatic leukaemia (CLL), myocardiopathia and with the gallstone ileus of the sigmoid colon.
The patient was admitted to the department of internal medicine with ill-defined symptoms of abdominal pain and suspected worsening of the CLL. US examination of the upper abdomen showed empty gallbladder with thickened wall. Plain X-ray examination of the abdomen revealed aero-liquid levels and distention of large and small intestine. Because of the worsening of the clinical picture she was urgently operated without any further investigations.
After total medial laparotomy we found an enormous dilatation of large bowel caused by a large, hard »tumour mass« in the sigmoid colon. Because of the impression that we are dealing with malignancy, our first intention was to perform Hartman procedure. After dissection of the resected colonic segment, we found a huge gallstone, which led us to cholecystocolonic fistula. We performed cholecystectomy and subtotal colectomy with ileo-sigmo anastomosis.
For histopathologycal examination we received 87 cm long part of the large bowel and the gallbladder. The wall of the bowel was dilated , mucosa was oedematous and in the distal part of the resected specimen ulcerated. The lumen of the bowel was filled up with faeces and 4 cm off the distal resection margin the lumen was obliterated with 8,5x5x5 cm big and 85 g heavy gallstone. 27 cm from the proximal resection margin a mural defect of 3 cm in diameter was discovered. Microscopically non-specific ulcers of mucosa, partial haemorrhagic infarction of the intestinal wall and fistula of the bowel wall were found. Microscopic examination of the gallbladder showed signs of chronic cholecystitis and focally elements of the adenocarcinoma with minimal invasion.
The postoperative course was prolonged with signs of myocardial decompensation, transitory renal failure and wound inflammation. CLL remained stabile.

P 149

MINIINVASIVE SURGICAL TECHNIQUE FOR HYDATIDE LIVER CYSTS

Saenko V., Lopoushanskii Y., Chornyy V., Boulanov K.
Department of Biliary Surgery
Institute of Clinical & Experimental Surgery, Kiev, Ukraine

Aims: to evaluate results of miniinvasive surgical approach in patients with hydatide liver cysts (HLC).

Methods: 46 patients (27 women and 19 men, aged 18-72) with HLC were subjected to surgical treatment during 1992-1998. Solitary cysts were found in 40 (87%), multiple - in 6 (13%) cases. Cysts were localized in the right liver lobe in 36 (78%), in left lobe - in 10 (22%). The size of cysts varied from 3,5 to 30 cm. Miniinvasive surgical approach included precise visualization of vascular and biliary structures under intraoperative ultrasound guidance and using of ultrasound aspirator for enucleation of cysts (30) or liver resection (16). Patient's follow-up ranged 12-60 months.

Results: no intraoperative complications occurred. Mean blood loss was 110 ml, mean operative time was 125 min. No patients required blood transfusion. Early postoperative complications were transient and of minor importance. There were no postoperative episodes of bile leakage. The mortality was nil. During the follow-up no recurrence of HLC was observed.

Conclusions: using of the miniinvasive approach improves considerably either early or remote results of surgical treatment in patients with HLC.

P 151

WHIPPLE'S PROCEDURE (PANCREATICODUODENECTOMY), MANSOURA EXPERIENCE
El-Ebidy G., Fathy O., Soltan A., Abd el-Wahab M., El-Hak N., Abu Zid M., Abu El-Enin A.
Gastroenterology Center, Mansoura University, Mansoura, Egypt

Aims: To review the experience of Gastroenterology Surgical Center in Mansoura University as regards outcomes of Whipple procedure of pancreaticodudenectomy.
Methods: Between January 1990 and August 1998, 95 consecutive patients of pancreatic head and periampullary carcinoma underwent pancreaticodudenectomy. Main presention was obstructive jaundice in 85 patients (89%)). Mean serum bilirubin was 5.5±2 mg%. Preoperative ERCP was done in 69 patients (72.6%) as a diagnostic toal and for decompression of the obstructed biliary system as well. Preoperative abdominal CT scan revealed a resectable mass in 60 patients (63%) with vascular encasement in 9 cases. Pancreatico-duodenectomy was done using Whipple procedure with preserving in 5 cases. Pancreaticofejunostomy was done in 49 cases (51.5%) and pancreaticogastrostomy in 46 cases (48.5%).
Results: From total of 95 patients we had 61 males and 43 females with mean age of 58±11 years. The number of resections per year increased from 5 cases in 1990 to 40 resections in 1998. Histopathology revealed pancreatic head carcinoma in 62 cases (65%), ampullary carcinoma in 17 cases (18%), cholangio carcinoma of the distal third of conunon bile duct in 12 patients (13%) and duodenal tumor in 4 patients (4%). The median intraoperative blood loss was 1000cc, median units of blood transfusion was 2 and the median operativer time was 5 hours. Hospital mortality occured in 6 patients (6.3%) mostly due to pancreatic fistula. Hospital staw was 20 ± 8 days. Postoperative complication involved pancreatic fitula in 15 patients (15.8%) being mostly after pancreaticojejunostomy in early years of performance. Pancreatic fistula complicats only one case after pancreatico gastrostomy out of 46 cases (2%). All cases managed consevatively except 2 cases where total pancreatectomy was needed to control the fistula. Reoperation for bleeding pancreaticogastostomy or gastojejunostomy was done in 5 cases. Intraperiotoneal collection in the lesser sac occure in 3 cases treated with ultrasonography-guided tube drainage.
Conclusion: Pancreatico-duodenectomy could be performed safely for the malignant disorders of the pancreas and perianpullary region. The rate of complications decreases with pancreaticogastrostomy and with high volume experience.

P 152

MYOELECTRICAL ACTIVITIES OF THE STOMACH BEFORE AND AFTER LAPAROSCOPIC CHOLECYSTECTOMY

Nabil Gad El-Hak, M.D.
Gastroenterology Surgical Center, Mansoura, University Mansoura, Egypt

The effects of chronic calcular cholecystitis and of laparoscopic cholecystectomy (LC) on gastric myoelectrical activities have not been well documented.
Aim: Was to investigate the pattern of gastric myoelectrical activities in patients having chronic calcular gall bladder disease and to evalute the effect of LC on EEG.
Methods: 46 patients (20 male, 25 female, mean age 41 years) with chronic calcular cholecystitis were included in the study. Gastric myoelectrical activities was measured using surfacce electrogastrography (EGG). The study was performed to all patients before and one year after LC. The EGG recording was made for 0.5 hour in the fasting state and 1.5 hour in the postprandial state. Power spected analysis was applied (1). The peercentage of abnormal waves (outside the range of 2.4-3.7 cycles/min) (2). The amplitudeof the gastric slow waves.
Results: EGG abnormal frequency was detected in 16 patients (34.8%) before LC (preprandial abnormatities in 12 and postprandial in 9 patients). One year following LC the EGG abnormal frequency was detected in 6 patients (13%) (4 had preprandial and 2 postprandial abnormalitics). The EGG peak power decreased after meal in 2 patients (4.4%) before LC compared to 13 patients one year after surgery.
Conclusion: This study suggested that gastric dysrhythmias decrease one year after LC but there is an increas in the percentage of patients with decreased poer peak after meal.

P 153

PRIMARY CARCINOMA OF THE GALLBLADDER: A WESTERN SURGICAL EXPERIENCE.

Frena A, Martin F, La Guardia G, Catalano PL
Regional Hospital of Bolzano, 2nd Surgical Dept., Bolzano, Italy

Aims: primary carcinoma of the gallbladder (GC) is a progressive lethal disease with an incidence of 2 %. The survival of the patients with GC depends strictly on depth of tumor invasion. We evaluated the results of our surgical series according to the pTNM classification and the stage groupings designated by the American Joint Committee on Cancer in 1992.

Methods: a retrospective analysis of a fifteen-years experience was performed. Of the 69 patients with GC observed at our institution between November 1993 and December 1998, a "curative" operation was carried out in 25 patients (36,2%). The most common presenting symptom was pain (78,6%) in the 13 patients with Stage I-II and jaundice (41,7%) in the 12 patients with Stage III-IV. Of 25 patients, 15 underwent cholecistectomy and 10 had an extended operation (6 cases of cholecistectomy and liver segmentectomy IV or IV-V; 2 cases of Whipple procedure; 1 case of Whipple procedure and liver segmentectomy IV; 1 case of cholecistectomy and bile duct resection).

Results: survival time according to Kaplan-Meyer is 81,8% after 1 year, 63,6% after 2 years, and 18,1% after 5 years for the Stage I-II patients; 27,2%, 0, and 0 for the Stage III-IV patients respectively. Moreover, one-, two-, and five-years survival rates were 69,2%, 53,8%, and 15,2% in the patients treated by cholecistectomy; 30,0%, 0, and 0 in the patients who underwent an extended surgical approach.

Conclusions: the Stage I-II patients represent a minority of cases of GC: they have a localized disease and surgical treatment provides the opportunity of a good survival. The Stage III-IV patients are not curable: the survival rates demonstrated that surgery is only a good palliation. Extended operations for advanced stages are associated with a poor prognosis.

Digestive Surgery

Author Index Vol. 16, (suppl 1): 1999

The Abstracts of the European Congress of the International Hepato-Pancreato-Biliary Association (IHPBA)

KARGER
Fax +41 61 306 12 34
E-Mail karger@karger.ch
www.karger.com

Digestive Surgery

Contents Vol. 16, (suppl 1): 1999

KARGER

Fax +41 61 306 12 34
E-Mail karger@karger.ch
www.karger.com

70 **First report of cavoportal hemitransposition in pediatric reduced size liver transplantation**
U. Hanack, Th. Lorf, R. Talaulicar, R. Canelo, J.-H. Schiffmann, B. Ringe (Germany)

Safe usage for hepatic transplant of graft livers procured from old donors (from 70 to 87 years old)
M. Cescon, A. Mazziotti, G.L. Grazi, G. Ercolani, C. Quintini, R. Montalti, A. Cavallari (Italy)

Anatomic variations of the hepatic artery: Classification and their significante in liver transplantation
E.S. Felekours, A.C. Tsamandas, G. Blesios, S. Pierrakakis, D. Karavias, D. Álexiou, N. Setakis, S. Salakou, K. Tepetes, E. Papalapmros, E. Bastounis (Greece)

Liver tumor IV.

71 **Extensive surgery for hilar cholangiocagcinoma: Early results**
J.P.A. Lodge, B.J. Ammori, G.V. Miller, K.R. Prasad, S.G. Pollard (U.K.)

Surgical treatment of hepatocellular carcinoma
F. Geissler, H. Witzigmann, A. Tannapfel, D. Uhlmann, I. Hanss (Germany)

Hepatocellular carcinoma in cirrhotic patients. Our experience with echo-guided radiofrequency percutaneous ablation
S. Puleo, G. Azzarello, M. Astuto, R. Lombardo, I. Di Carlo (Italy)

72 **Increased survival after liver resection for HCC in cirrhosis gives the procedure additional efficacy**
G.L. Grazi, A. Mazziotti, G. Ercolani, F. Pierangeli, R. Montalti, M. Del Gaudio, A. Cavallari (Italy)

Results of operations for primary malignant hepatic tumurs
P. Tóth, I. Takács, Cs. András, M. Szappanos, G. Varga, P. Sápy (Hungary)

Early surgical results of liver resections
I. Takács, P. Tóth, Cs. András, A. Vágvölgyi, L. Halász, P. Sápy (Hungary)

Hepatic resection for cancer in the elderly
A. Chiappa (Italy), A.P. Zbar (U.K.), F. Biella (Italy), E. Bertani (Italy), C. Crotti (Italy), C. Staudacher (Italy)

73 **Liver tuberculosis (Selective damage)**
A. Severtsev, N. Mironov, E. Nikolaenko, V. Laptev, Yu. Gribunov, E. Merzljakova, E. Ivanova, V. Nazarenko, Z. Zemskova, L. Sedova, E. Tupikova (Russia)

Quality of life in patients with observed and resected focal nodular hyperplasia
M. Mössinger, K. Fronhoff, S. Nadalin, G. Tusch, R. Raab, A. Weimann (Germany)

Liver tumor V.

74 **Risk factors in liver surgery — A new score**
P. Lamesch, I. Tanev, I. Geißler, J. Hauss (Germany)

Does small HCC correspond to early tumor stage?
A. Weimann, S. Hoeberg, H. Lang, H.J. Schlitt, G. Tusch, R. Raab J. Klempnauer (Germany)

Preoperative segmental liver mass evaluation
O. Tsiroulnikova, A. Filin, A. Semenkov, S. Gautier (Russia)

75 **Surgical classification of liver tumours**
S. Gautier, O. Tsiroulnikova (Russia)

General anaesthesia for patients with liver diseases: Intravenous or inhalated anaesthesia?
K. Darvas, M. Tarjányi, K. Pinkola, Zs. Molnár, P. Kupcsulik, L. Flautner (Hungary)

p53 mutation in cholangiocarcinoma is associated with worse prognosis after surgical resection
R. Havlik (U.K.), L.R. Jiao (U.K.), E. Sbisa (Italy), A. Tullo (Italy), C. Saccone (Italy), K. Honda (U.K. , R.R. Ragai (U.K.), N.A. Habib (U.K.)

Large hepatic hemangiomas: To treat or not to treat?
P. Bercolo, D. Borzomati, M. Caricato, A. Granai, A Esposito, A. Arallani (Italy)

76 **Hepatic cavernous haemangiomas — Diagnostic tools and choice of surgical procedures**
J. Raposo, H.V. Dias, J.L. Correia, M.J. Queiros, Medeiros (Portugal)

HPB Egypt

77 **Partial auxiliary liver transplantation in dogs**
A.A. Mahuran, G. A. Ahmed, B. A. Thabit, M.M. El Shaije, H.B. El-Badawy. M.A. Hassanien, G.M. Fathy (Egypt)

Primary carcinoma of the gallbladder experience of 18 cases in Assuit University Hospital
M.M. El Shafie (Egypt)

Spectrum and management of complications after cholecystectomy
S. Osman, M.K. El-Ammary (Egypt)

78 **Whipple's procedure (pancreaticoduodenectomy). Mansoura experience**
G. El-Ebidy, O. Fathy, A. Soltan, M. Abd El-Wahab, N. El-Hak, M. Abu Zid, Abu El-Enin (Egypt)

Myoelectrical activaties of the stomach before and after laparoscopic cholecystectomy
N. G. El-Hak (Egypt)

Video Session

79 **Hepato-jejunal anastomosis in loop excluded by laparoscopy in the treatment of iatrogenic ligature of the bile duct**
E. Crema, A.A. Silva, D.A. Ferreira, C.B. Oliveira , Jr. A. Martins, Jr. Alves (Brazil)

Laparoscopic management of common bile duct calculi by choledochotomy in selective patients
C. Karaliotas, N. Kouris, A. Liosis, S. Lanitis, S. Doukas, E. Papaevangelou (Greece)

Operative technique of laparoscopic pancreatectomy
B.J. Ammori, A. Vezakis, D. Davides, M. Larvin, M.J. McMahon (U.K.)

80 **Fibrin sealing in the prevention of pancreaticojejunostomy leakage — Experimental study**
M. Stoianović, M.Jeremić, M. Stojiljković, Z. Cvetković, P. Stojanović D. Gmijović, V. Savić, V. Djordjević, V. Katić, M. Kostov (Yugoslavia)

The difficult cholecystectomy
G. Svanis, G. Velimezis, J. Antoniades, V. Patrikakos, A. Banter, G. Mitropapas, E. Perrakis (Greece)

Possibilities of new surgical unit — plasma flows — in liver surgery
A. Severtsev, E. Brekhov, N. Mironov, E. Ivanova, V. Laptev, N. Suslov, V. Bashilov, E. Tupikova (Russia)

Video assisted modality for safe decompression of large hepatic hydatid cysts
C. Karaliotas, N. Kouris, A. N-Papaevangelou, G. Tsiripidis, S. Lanitis, H. Chatziagelli, E. Papaevangelou (Greece)

81 **Extended right hepatectomy for hepatocellular carcinoma**
G. Ercolani, A. Mazziotti, G.L. Grazi, F. Pierangeli, M. Cescon, A. Cavallari (Italy)

Hemangiectomy: The surgical treatment of choice in the hepatic cavernous hemangioma
J. Grondona, R. Bracco, A. Michetti, M. Duhalde (Argentina)

Iatrogenic lesion of the main bile duct: Cholangio-jejunostomy as definitive treatment
G.B. Doglietto, S. Alfieri, C. Carriero, F. Pacelli (Italy)

Hemihepatic vascular exclusion for right segmentectomies in cirrhotic patients using an extraglissonian anterior approach to the portal pedicle
G. Batignani, S. Passini, F. Tonelli (Italy)

82 **Liver surgery and "basket ball" metastasectomy by means of high pressure waterjet method**
F. Jakab (Hungary)

83 **In vivo assessment of hepatic tissue oxygenation with graded hypoxia**
El-Desoky A.A., Seifalian A.M., Davidson B.R. (U.K.)

Tissue engineering using hepatocytes under flow bioreactor conditions on 3-dimensional biodegradable polymer prior to implantation
Pollok J.M. (Germany), Török É. (Germany), Ma P.X. (USA), Kaufmann P.M. (Germany), Topp S. (Germany), Kluth D. (Germany), Rogiers X.(Germany)

The effect of liver blood flow and function on hepatic indocyanide green clearance in cirrhosis measured directly in a cirrhitic animal model
Jiao L.R., El-Desoky A.A., Seifalian A.M., Habib N., Davidson B.R. (U.K.)

84 **A large cirrhotic animal model**
Jiao L.R., Havlik E., Seifalian A.M., Li Y., Davidson B.R.,Habib N. (U.K.)

Quantitative detection of hepatic tyssue hypoxia with near infrared spectroscopy
Seifalian A.M., El-Desoky A.A., Cope M., Delpy D.T., Davidson B.R. (U.K.)

Soluble tumor necrosis factor α-receptor II (sTNFα-RII) and acute phase plasma proteins have similar kinetics during the experimental liver regeneration in rats
Fülöp A.K., Pócsik É., Karabélyos Cs., Kiss Á., Dobozy O., Falus A. (Hungary)

Angiogenesis in hepatocarcinoma on cirrhosis evaluated by CD 34 immunohistochemistry
Lupo L., Marzullo G., Gentile A., Martines G., Caputi L., Aquilino F., Pollice L., Memeo V. (Italy)

85 **Hepatectomy and colonic mucosa: An experimental study**
Çoker A., Aydýn., Atilla K., Çoker I., Huseyinov A., Özer E., Karademir S., Astarczoðlu H., Astarczoðlu (Turkey)

Expression of the E-cadherin cell adehesion complex in hepatocellular carcinoma
Syrigos K.N:, Karayiannakis A.J., Tsioulos D., Papanikolaou Sp., Simatos G., Papanikolaou D., Riza F., Karatzas G. (Greece)

Protective effects of exogenous coenzyme Q in rat liver exőposed to ischemia-reperfusion
Nardo B., Catena F., Turi P., Cavallari G., Genova M.L., Bonacorsi E., D'Aurelio M., Formiggini G., Merlo Pinch M., Lenaz G., Principe A., Mazziotti A., Cavallari A. (Italy)

Role of nutritional status on mithocondrial injury in a rat model of fatty liver
Nardo B., Caraceni P., Grattaglliano I., Catena F. Turi P., Cavallari G., Domenicali M., Dall'Agata M., Vendemiale G.L., Altomare E., Bernardi M., Principe A., Mazziotti A., Cavallari A. (Italy)

86 **River regeneration and cancer: What is the role of angiostatin?**
Drixler T.A., Gebbink M.F., Ritchie E.D., Aarsman C.J., Reyerkerk A., Voest E.E., Borel Rinkes I.H. (The Netherlands)

Expression of heat shock protein 70 (HSP70) after laser thermotherapy of an adenocarcinoma transplanted into rat liver
Tranberg K.-G., Ivarsson K., Bruun A., Stenram U. (Sweden)

Physical and pharmacological intraoperative methods for the final haemostasis on the raw liver surface
Severtsev A., Mironov N., Brekhov E., Ivanova E., Repin I., Merzljakova E., Gaidukova N., Barinov V., Bashilov V., Gribonov Zu., Tupikova E. (Russia)

Expression of metallothionein in the liver after 70% partial hepatectomy in rats
Theocharis S.E., Skaltsas S., Spiliopoulou C., Margeli A.P., Koutselinis A. (Greece)

87 **The usage of criopreserved biological medicines in the treatment of obturation jaundice**
Mamchich V.I., Subbota N.P., Kebkalo A.B., Palamarchuck V.I. (Ukraine)

Risk factors of variceal bleeding in patient with advanced liver cirrhosis
Boulanov K.I. (Ukraine)

Percutaneous sclerotherapy (PS) of simple liver cysts (SLC)
Polysalov V.N., Granov D.A., Prozorovskij K.V., Oelshchuk N.V. (Russia)

Neuroendocrine tumors metastatic to the liver (NTML): Role of transcatheter treatment
Polykarpov A.A., Tarazov P.G., Granov D.A., Zeadeh A.A. (Russia)

88 **"Ukrain" in treatment of the fatty liver in chronic active alcoholic patients**
Zemskova M.V., Zemskov S.V. (Ukraine)

Abnormalities of carbohydrate metabolism and immune parameters in patients with hepatitis C and alcohol-related chronic liver disease
Pusztay M., Nemesánszky E., Csepregi A., Horányi M. (Hungary)

Etiological factors and treatment of hepatic abscess
Yettimis E., Kalokerinos E., Barsamidakis N., Kourcounakis N., Karagiannis A., Polyzoes C., Dahambre S., Melayes Z., Polymeropoulos Th. (Greece)

Cholecysto-jejunostomy as a substitute for cholecystectomy in portal venous thrombosis
Penteado S., Machado M.C.C., Jukemura J., Cunha J.E.M., Montagnini A.L. (Brazil)

89 **Endoscopic ligation of esophageal bleeding varices previously treated by endoscopic sclerotherapy**
Caputi Iambrenghi O., Pannarale O., Scardigno A., Simone M., Verzillo F., Memeo V. (Italy)

Hepatic veno-occlusive disease caused by oral contraceptives
Borka K., Illyés G., Fischer M. (Hungary)

Pathology of liver involvement in non-Hodgkin's lymphomas
Marković M., Basić H., Nikolić D., Lazarević V. (Yugosléavia)

The surgical treatment of the hepatic hydatid cyst in surgical clinic No. III Ţirgu-Mures
Bara T., Bancu S., Esianu M., Zamfir D., Butilca F., Marian D., Borz C., Jimboreanu O., Butiurca A., Frandes D. (Romania)

90 **Was it a simple cyst or a lethal lesion? An unusual presentation of peliosis hepatis**
Karademir S., Astarcioğlu H., Sağol H., Ak D., Çoker A., Astarcioğlu I. (Turkey)

Successful revascularization of the late hepatic arterial thrombosis by interpositional saphenous vein graft in living related liver transplantation
Astarcioğlu H., Karademir S., Koçdor M.A., Akgür F., Olguner M., Çoker A., Astarcioğlu I. (Turkey)

The kidneys and alcohol — What is the relationship in liver cirrhosis?
Apetrechioaie C., Diculescu M., Pitigoi D., Tudor C., Jinga M., Oproiu A.A.A. (Romania)

Diagnosis of portal hypertension — Endoscopy or ultrasound? What is the best?
Diculescu M., Apetrechioaie C., Tudor C., Pitigoi D., Oproui A. (Romania)

91 **The management of intrabiliary ruptured hydatid disease of liver**
Koksal N., Muftuoglu T., Uzun M.A., Gunerhan Y., Kurt R. (Turkey)

Evaluation of ultrasound guided aspiration biopsy of focal liver lesions
Tarján Z., Winternitz T., Járay B., Haj H., Forgács B., Tóth G., Galgóczy H. (Hungary)

Factors associated with hepatic cirrhosis development in chronic hepatitis C
Constantino A., Ramalha F., Serejo F., Fatela N., Glória H., Lopes J., Marinho R., Raimundo M., Velosa J., Moura M.C. (Portugal)

Little-invasive surgery in the treatment of echinococcosis of liver and lungs
Aliev M., Seysembaev M., Adylkhanov C., Narzhanov B., Kenzhebaev A. (Kazahstan)

92 **Surgery of portal hypertension**
Arynov N., Shirtaev B., Nashanov Dh. (Kazahstan)